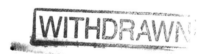

SAUNDERS SOLUTIONS IN
VETERINARY PRACTICE

SMALL ANIMAL
ONCOLOGY

Biographies

Rob Foale qualified from the Royal Veterinary College, University of London in 1996 having previously completed a BSc in Physiology and Pharmacology at King's College, University of London in 1992. After a four-year period in mixed general practice he joined the medicine service at the University of Cambridge Veterinary School as a resident and completed this programme in 2003. He obtained his RCVS Diploma in Small Animal Medicine in 2003, his ECVIM diploma in 2005 and is a recognized European Specialist in Internal Medicine. At present Rob is head of Internal Medicine and a director at Dick White Referrals in Suffolk, UK with active research in developing gene therapy for canine diabetes mellitus and the identification of genetic susceptibility loci in canine lymphoma. He is married to Jackie and they have three children.

Jackie Demetriou also qualified from the Royal Veterinary College, University of London in 1996. She spent 1 year in mixed general practice before moving to the Royal (Dick) School of Veterinary Studies, University of Edinburgh where she completed a 1-year internship in small animal studies in 1998 and a 3-year residency in small animal surgery in 2001. She then took up the post of temporary lecturer at Edinburgh University before moving to the University of Cambridge in 2002 where she currently holds a lectureship in Small Animal Surgery. She obtained her RCVS certificate in Small Animal Surgery in 1999, her European College of Veterinary Surgery Diploma in 2002 and she is a recognized European Specialist in Small Animal Surgery. She has published papers on airway surgery and thoracic disease and her main clinical interests are oncological and upper airway surgery.

For Elsevier:

Commissioning Editor: Robert Edwards
Development Editor: Ewan Halley
Project Manager: Kerrie-Anne McKinlay
Designer: Charles Gray
Illustrator: Merlyn Harvey

SAUNDERS SOLUTIONS IN
VETERINARY PRACTICE

SMALL ANIMAL
ONCOLOGY

Series Editor: **Fred Nind** BVM&S MRCVS

Rob Foale

BSc BVetMed DSAM DipECVIM-CA MRCVS
Consultant in Small Animal Medicine, Dick White Referrals, Suffolk, UK
Special Lecturer in Small Animal Medicine, School of Veterinary Medicine and Science,
University of Nottingham, UK

Jackie Demetriou

BVetMed CertSAS DipECVS MRCVS
Lecturer in Small Animal Surgery, The Queen's Veterinary School Hospital, University of
Cambridge, Cambridge, UK

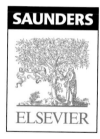

SAUNDERS

ELSEVIER

Edinburgh   London   New York   Oxford   Philadelphia   St Louis   Sydney   Toronto   2010

SAUNDERS
ELSEVIER

First published 2010

ISBN: 978-0-7020-2869-4

British Library Cataloguing in Publication Data
A catalogue record for this book is available from the British Library

Library of Congress Cataloging in Publication Data
A catalog record for this book is available from the Library of Congress

Notice

Knowledge and best practice in this field are constantly changing. As new research and experience broaden our knowledge, changes in practice, treatment and drug therapy may become necessary or appropriate. Readers are advised to check the most current information provided (i) on procedures featured or (ii) by the manufacturer of each product to be administered, to verify the recommended dose or formula, the method and duration of administration, and contraindications. It is the responsibility of the practitioner, relying on their own experience and knowledge of the patient, to make diagnoses, to determine dosages and the best treatment for each individual patient, and to take all appropriate safety precautions. To the fullest extent of the law, neither the Publisher nor the Authors assume any liability for any injury and/or damage to persons or property arising out of or related to any use of the material contained in this book.

The Publisher

your source for books,
journals and multimedia
in the health sciences
www.elsevierhealth.com

Working together to grow
libraries in developing countries

www.elsevier.com | www.bookaid.org | www.sabre.org

ELSEVIER   BOOK AID International   Sabre Foundation

The
publisher's
policy is to use
**paper manufactured
from sustainable forests**

Printed in China

Contents

Introduction

Saunders Solutions in Veterinary Practice series is a new range of veterinary textbooks that will grow into a mini library over the next few years, covering all the main disciplines of companion animal practice.

Readers should realize that it is not the authors' intention to cover all that is known about each topic. As such the books in the *Saunders Solutions* series are not standard reference works. Instead they are intended to provide practical information on the more frequently encountered conditions in an easily accessible form based on real-life case studies. They cover that range of cases that fall between the boringly routine and the referral. The books will help practitioners with a particular interest in a topic or those preparing for a specialist qualification. The cases are arranged by presenting sign rather than by the underlying pathology, as this is how veterinary surgeons will see them in practice.

It is hoped that the books will also be of interest to veterinary students in the later parts of their course and to veterinary nurses.

Continuing professional development (CPD) is mandatory for many veterinarians and a recommended practice for others. The *Saunders Solutions* series will provide a CPD resource which can be accessed economically, shared with colleagues and used anywhere. They will also provide busy veterinary practitioners with quick access to authoritative information on the diagnosis and treatment of interesting and challenging cases. The robust cover has been made resistant to some of the more gruesome contaminants found in a veterinary clinic because this is where we hope these books will be used.

Joyce Rodenhuis and Mary Seager were the inspiration for the series. Robert Edwards has overseen their writing and production. The series editor and the individual authors are grateful for their foresight in commissioning the series and their unfailing support and guidance during their production.

ONCOLOGY

As the advances in preventive health care, nutrition and general husbandry that were developed in the 20th century begin to have their effect on the general pet population, companion animals are, on average, living longer lives. Cancers are not limited to older animals, but it is certainly the case that they become more common as pets age.

In parallel with these changes in the incidence of neoplastic conditions, there have been advances in the drugs, surgical techniques and radiotherapy facilities available for treatment. Where a diagnosis of a malignancy was once an automatic indication for euthanasia, many of these cases can now be offered treatment which will give a significant extension to life and that extended life will be lived with relatively little compromise from the disease or the treatment.

The authors and editor hope that this book will help to open your eyes to what is now possible for the treatment of these cases and inspire you to offer such treatments to your clients.

Fred Nind
Series Editor
2010

1 How to obtain the perfect biopsy

Obtaining a diagnosis is one of the most important steps in the management of the cancer patient. Obtaining a biopsy *before* the surgical procedure is performed is best clinical practice in the majority of cases as it provides a pre-treatment diagnosis, helps the clinician plan the surgery and can provide the owner with a more accurate prognosis. There are a number of methods of obtaining samples from the tumour and the choice is based on a number of factors including:

- Tumour location
- Suspected tumour type
- Safety of the procedure
- The patient's clinical status
- Cost
- Equipment availability
- The surgeon's preference.

With the exception of diagnostic cytology, all other techniques listed in Table 1.1 involve tissue sampling and histological interpretation.

CLINICAL CASE EXAMPLE 1.1 – CYTOLOGY

Signalment

5-year-old male neutered boxer dog.

Presenting signs

A 5-cm diameter subcutaneous mass located over the left hip.

Clinical history

Four months previously, the dog had presented with a 2-cm mass located in the region of the left hip. The veterinary surgeon had excised the mass; however, the owners declined histopathology so the diagnosis was not determined. The mass gradually recurred and the dog was referred for further evaluation and treatment (Fig. 1.1).

> **CLINICAL TIP**
>
> Bear in mind when explaining a management plan that many pet owners may not realize the importance or relevance of obtaining a final diagnosis when excising a mass. Consider including histopathology costs as an integral part of the surgical 'package'.

Differential diagnosis

- Mast cell tumour
- Soft tissue sarcoma
- Sebaceous adenoma
- Cutaneous haemangiosarcoma.

Diagnostic options

As the mass had been previously undiagnosed and had recurred, any future treatment would be dependent on an accurate diagnosis. If surgical excision was indicated, definitive surgery can then be planned. An excisional biopsy in this case would not be indicated. Options for obtaining a diagnosis, therefore, include cytological sampling, needle-core or incisional biopsy. Using a punch biopsy may not be an appropriate choice in this case due to the location of the mass in the deeper subcutaneous tissues. Therefore, in this case a fine needle aspirate was opted for initially as the procedure was the least invasive of all the biopsy options, inexpensive, easy to perform and results were made available rapidly.

To perform a fine needle aspirate the only tools required are:

- 21–23 gauge needles
- 3–10 ml syringes
- Glass microscope slides
- Cytological stains
- A good microscope with oil immersion (Figs 1.2–1.7).

Table 1.1 Biopsy techniques

Biopsy technique	Advantages	Disadvantages	Indications/examples
Cytology	Inexpensive Simple, rapid procedure Minimal equipment Immediate results Minimal restraint	Non-diagnostic specimens Tissue architecture not evaluated	Bone marrow Lymph nodes Cutaneous/subcutaneous masses Body cavity fluids Impression smears

Needle core	Minimally invasive
	Rapid procedure
	Well-preserved tissue sample
	High diagnostic yield
	Can be done under sedation/local
	  anaesthetic
	Inexpensive
	Easy procedure
		Needle core instruments
		  required
		Smaller tissue sample
		  compared with incisional
			Any externally located mass
			Any internal lesions (kidney, liver,
			  prostate) with the aid of
			  ultrasound guidance or during
			  open surgery

Punch	Larger tissue sample
	Easy procedure
		Sample obtained limited by
		  depth of punch
		Superficial lesions only
		Invasive procedure
		General anaesthetic often
		  required
			Superficial cutaneous lesions
			Parenchymatous organ (liver,
			  spleen) biopsy during open
			  surgery

Incisional	Larger tissue mass
	Useful when needle core or punch
	  methods prove non-diagnostic
		Invasive procedure
		General anaesthetic mostly
		  required
		More expensive
		Biospy tract may compromise
		  future surgery
			When other biopsy methods have
			  been non-diagnostic
			Ulcerated and necrotic lesions
			  (e.g. oral masses)

Excisional	Can be both diagnostic and therapeutic
	May be cost effective
	Diagnosis always obtained
	Can evaluate completeness of excision
		In most cases may
		  compromise future
		  treatment options and
		  prognosis
			Reserve for 'benign' skin lesions
			  and tumour excision where
			  treatment is not dependent on
			  tumour type (mammary masses,
			  single splenic mass, single
			  pulmonary mass)

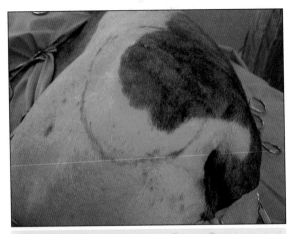

Figure 1.1 *Case 1.1* The appearance of the mass before treatment

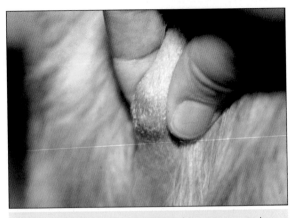

Figure 1.2 *Case 1.1* Step 1. Clip and prepare area to be aspirated. Stabilize mass with one hand

Figures 1.2–1.7 The steps involved in performing a fine needle aspirate or capillary method aspirate on a cutaneous or subcutaneous mass

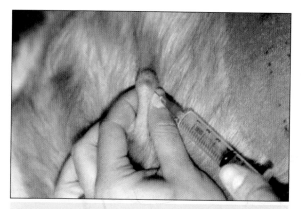

Figure 1.3 *Case 1.1* Step 2. Insert needle into mass with syringe attached and apply negative pressure to the syringe. The needle can be redirected within the mass but aspiration should be ceased if fluid is observed within the hub of the needle

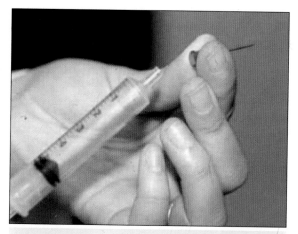

Figure 1.5 *Case 1.1* Step 3. Release negative pressure whilst the needle is within the mass and remove the syringe with the needle attached. Aspirate air into the syringe and reattach needle (or for the capillary sampling method attach a sterile, air-filled syringe)

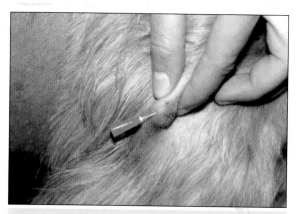

Figure 1.4 *Case 1.1* Step 2 can be carried out alternatively using the capillary method. Here a needle is used without a syringe to obtain a needle core sample of cells by swiftly moving the hub of the needle backwards and forwards within the mass

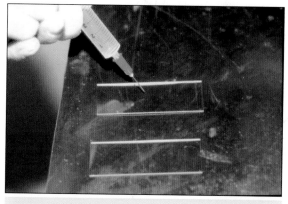

Figure 1.6 *Case 1.1* Step 4. Expel air and contents of needle onto a clean glass slide

---

CLINICAL TIP

For masses that are very vascular or that contain fluid cavities the capillary method may improve diagnostic yield by reducing blood or fluid contamination and increasing the relative cellularity of the sample. Similarly, the syringe method may be more suitable for solid tumours, such as a soft tissue sarcoma.

The smears should be air dried and the sample should be thin enough to dry within 1 minute. The best cytology stains to use in clinical practice are the Romanowsky stains (such as Wright's stain, Giemsa stain and May-Grünwald-Giemsa stain) as these provide clear detail of both the nuclear and cytoplasmic structures. They are relatively quick to prepare and these stains will also stain bacteria if they are present. The 'rapid' stain kits such as 'Diff-Quik' are highly useful and obviously extremely convenient but it is important to realize that these may not always stain the granules within mast cells clearly, thereby leading to potential confusion in the diagnosis. In such a situation, Toludine blue stain will identify mast

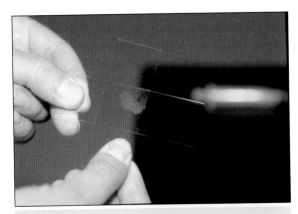

Figure 1.7 *Case 1.1* Step 5. Prepare the slide by placing another slide on top of the aspirated material and gently slide the two slides away in opposite directions. The slide is then air dried and stained

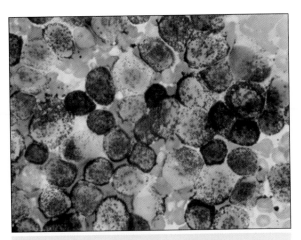

Figure 1.8 *Case 1.1* Mast cell tumour aspirate, revealing the classical 'granular' appearance of the cytoplasm

cell granules. The use of Toludine blue may be especially useful in poorly differentiated mast cell tumours in which the granularity can be low.

> **NURSING TIP**
>
> With regular use, all stains will become exhausted and so it is important to regularly replace the stains as directed by the manufacturer. Exhausted stains will lead to poor cytological interpretation and frustration within your clinic, so this is an important job!

Diagnosis

The specimen obtained in this case was of diagnostic quality and a diagnosis of a mast cell tumour (Fig. 1.8) was made.

Mast cells tumours are classified as being a round cell tumour, which means they exfoliate as discrete round cells with clear margins and a rounded nucleus. Other tumours in the round cell category include lymphoma, histiocytoma, plasmacytoma and transmissible venereal tumour (which does not occur naturally in the UK but may theoretically be seen in imported dogs). Mast cells contain azurophilic granules in their cytoplasm which stain a crimson-purple colour with Romanowsky stains, therefore usually making their identification relatively straightforward but the number of granules present in different tumours can vary considerably depending on the tumour grade. In the hands of an experienced cytologist, aspirates can be helpful to indicate the tumour

grade, as low-grade mast cell tumours usually have well-defined and uniform nuclei with a high number of granules in each cell. The more poorly differentiated the tumour is, then the fewer the number of cytoloplasmic granules there are, the more prominent the nucleoli are and the degree of variation in cell size (anisocytosis) and nuclear size (ansiokaryosis) increases. The use of silver staining of the nucleolar organizing regions ('AgNOR staining') can also be used to help predict the grade of a tumour on aspirate samples, thereby adding further detail and diagnostic use from a simple aspirate. However, histopathological analysis will still be required to obtain accurate grading information.

For this case a fine needle aspirate provided an accurate diagnosis although providing a definitive grade for this tumour type is not possible by cytology alone as explained above. However, by submitting the entire tumour after excision, a tumour grade can be assigned and the completeness of surgical excision evaluated. In this and similar cases, knowledge of the tumour type preoperatively allows careful surgical planning. Additionally, appropriate staging of the disease can be performed by means of thoracic radiographs, local lymph node assessment and hepatic and splenic ultrasound examination. The mass was excised with 2-cm lateral margins and one fascial plane deep and the wound deficit was repaired using a local transposition flap (Figs 1.9 and 1.10).

Outcome

The dog made an uneventful recovery from surgery and healed well. The histopathology confirmed the mass to be a grade II (intermediately differentiated) mast cell

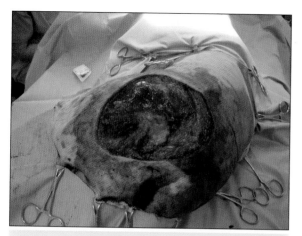

Figure 1.9 *Case 1.1* The wound deficit after the mass was excised with 2-cm margins

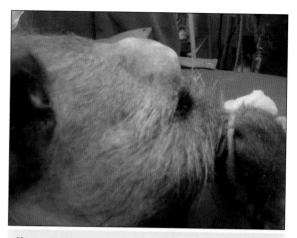

Figure 1.11 *Case 1.2* The appearance of the mass in the area of the right frontal sinus following aseptic preparation for the needle core biopsy

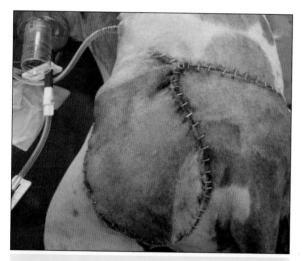

Figure 1.10 *Case 1.1* A local transposition flap has been used for reconstruction of the skin deficit

tumour with complete margins and there was no evidence of recurrence 2 years post-operatively.

CLINICAL CASE EXAMPLE 1.2 – NEEDLE CORE BIOPSY

Signalment

9-year-old male neutered cross breed dog.

Presenting signs

A 4 × 4 cm raised mass in the area of the right frontal sinus.

Clinical history

The mass had appeared 3 months previously and gradually increased in size over this period of time (Fig. 1.11). Initial treatment with anti-inflammatory drugs did not result in any improvement. Radiographs revealed increased soft tissue opacity of the right frontal sinus with evidence of bone lysis surrounding it. No evidence of metastasis was observed on thoracic radiographs. Cytological examination of fine needle aspirates of the mass indicated a possible diagnosis of a squamous cell carcinoma (SCC).

Differential diagnosis

- Frontal sinus tumour
  - Carcinoma
  - Osteosarcoma
  - Lymphoma
- Primary bone tumour
  - Osteosarcoma
  - Chondrosarcoma
- Soft tissue sarcoma.

Diagnostic options

Cytology had been performed with a suspected diagnosis of SCC. However, histological confirmation of this diagnosis was necessary *before* aggressive surgery in this area was contemplated so that a complete treatment plan could be formulated which might involve adjunctive treatment with radiotherapy or chemotherapy. The least invasive method of obtaining a pretreatment biopsy in this case that would also allow the obtaining of tissue from within the frontal sinus was by a needle core biopsy. The sampling in this case was performed under general anaesthesia after an MRI was performed on the skull.

Needle core biopsy provides a quick and easy way of obtaining a tissue sample. It can be used on externally or internally (usually in combination with ultrasound guidance) located masses and can be performed using local anaesthetic and sedation, providing a cost-effective and less-invasive option to clients, compared with incisional biopsy. As the initial incision and tract made by the instrument is small, there is little risk of disruption of the tumour and subsequent tumour seeding, although removal of the biopsy tract is recommended at the definitive surgery. It is therefore important to consider what surgical approach will be required before the biopsy is obtained to ensure that any needle tract will be able to be easily excised at surgery. Although designed as disposable instruments needles can be reused after sterilization with ethylene oxide and performing the skin incision with a scalpel blade before insertion of the needle will delay blunting of the tip and extend the life span of the instrument. In core biopsy the typical needle size is 18 Gauge–14 Gauge and comprises an inner notched stylet with an outer cannula (Figs 1.12–1.14).

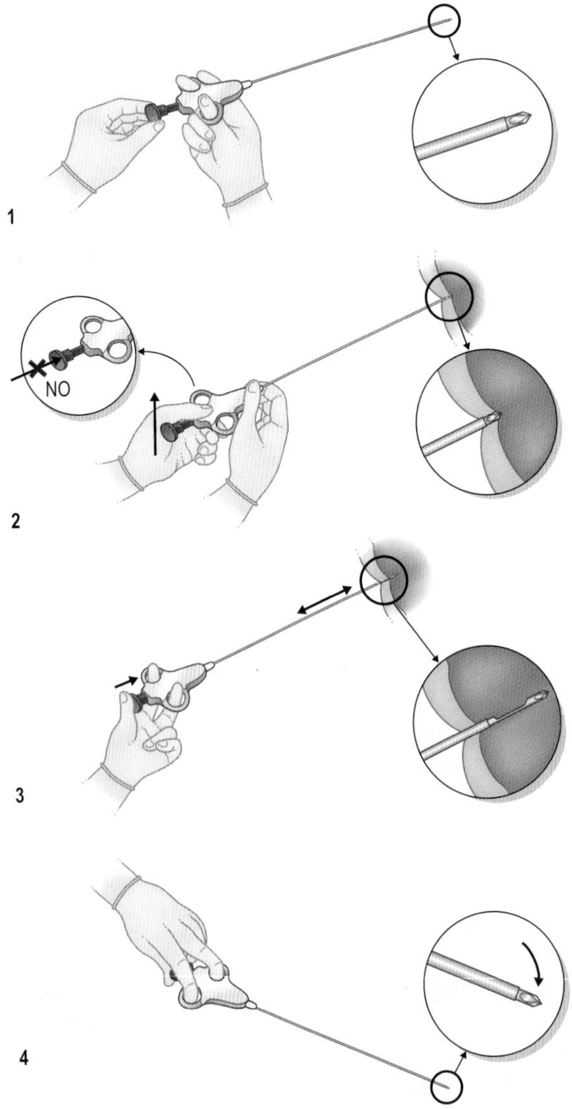

CLINICAL TIP

If this technique is unfamiliar it may be useful to practice using a needle core biopsy instrument on a piece of fruit such as an apple or kiwi before applying it to a mass.

If possible, perform several biopsies at varying levels using the same initial incision to increase the probability of obtaining a diagnostic specimen.

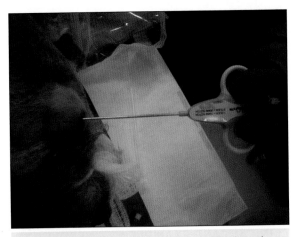

Figure 1.13 *Case 1.2* Step 1. An initial incision is made with a number 11 blade. The needle of the biopsy instrument is manually inserted and the sample is taken by activating the spring-loaded instrument. When discharged, the inner stylet of the needle advances rapidly to a distance usually of 1–2 cm. The outer cannula follows immediately behind the inner cannula to capture the acquired sample and the entire instrument is withdrawn

Figure 1.12 Needle core biopsy technique

Figures 1.13, 1.14 Needle core biopsy

1

2

NO

3

4

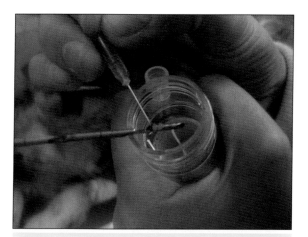

Figure 1.14 *Case 1.2* Step 2. After withdrawing the outer cannula the tissue specimen is gently removed from the notch within the inner stylet with a fine gauge needle and placed into a formalin pot. A sample can also be rolled onto a microscope slide to create an impression smear which can be sent for cytological evaluation

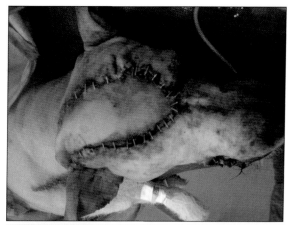

Figure 1.16 *Case 1.2* A postoperative photograph after the surgery was completed

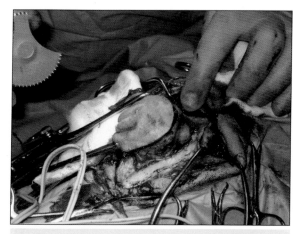

Figure 1.15 *Case 1.2* An intraoperative photograph of the mass within the frontal sinus and overlying skin

Diagnosis

Histopathology on the specimens submitted in this case confirmed a diagnosis of squamous cell carcinoma. MRI revealed the mass to be localized within the frontal sinus without penetration into the brain and thoracic radiographs did not reveal any evidence of metastasis. In this case, both cytology and histopathology were utilized to obtain an accurate initial diagnosis, which was essential in this situation before surgery was contemplated. The imaging indicated that macroscopic disease was amenable to surgical resection with radiotherapy a potential

postoperative adjunctive therapy. The tumour was excised en bloc with surrounding tissues (including the right eye) and the skin closed using a caudal auricular flap (Figs 1.15, 1.16).

CLINCIAL CASE EXAMPLE 1.3 – PUNCH BIOPSY AND EXCISIONAL BIOPSY

Signalment

7-year-old male entire German shepherd dog.

Presenting signs

Acute haemoabdomen.

Clinical history

The dog presented acutely with pale mucous membranes, tachypnoea and ascites. A peritoneal tap revealed a haemoabdomen. Abdominal radiographs and ultrasonography revealed a single assymetric splenic mass measuring approximately 10 cm × 8 cm. No further abnormalities could be detected and thoracic radiographs were within normal limits.

Diagnostic options

In this case a presurgical biopsy was not obtained for three reasons. Firstly this is one example when the type of treatment would not be altered by prior knowledge of the tumour type, i.e. a splenectomy or partial splenectomy is indicated whether the mass is a benign or malignant lesion. Secondly the diagnostic value of a fine needle aspirate from a spleen is low due to the effects of haemodilution. Thirdly with any suspected case of haemangiosarcoma there is a risk of tumour seeding with aspirates or needle core biopsy as the needle is withdrawn. Furthermore with single splenic masses that are solitary and have not ruptured, aspiration may cause rupture of the tumour and a haemoabdomen. For this reason an exploratory laparotomy was performed with the view to excisional biopsy of the spleen. On exploration the liver had small (5 mm) nodules over the surface that were biopsied using a skin punch biopsy instrument (Figs 1.17, 1.18).

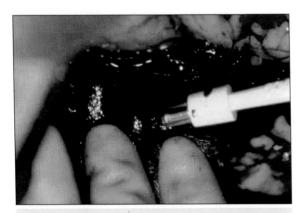

Figure 1.17 *Case 1.3* The punch biopsy is directed over the lesion and rotated until it has penetrated to an adequate depth. The sample can be grasped carefully with atraumatic forceps and the base of the sample excised using small iris scissors

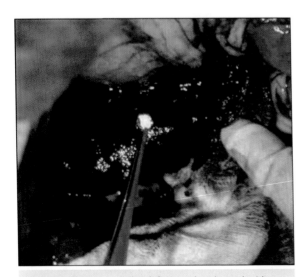

Figure 1.18 *Case 1.3* The deficit can be plugged with a haemostatic agent to effectively control haemorrhage

CLINICAL TIP

Using a punch biopsy instrument is an ideal method of obtaining biopsies from the surface of the liver and spleen intraoperatively. The sample is shorter and wider than a needle core, and haemorrhage from the remaining deficit can be controlled using a haemostatic agent such as commercially available collagen or gelatine.

Diagnosis

The spleen was submitted for histopathology and a diagnosis of haemangiosarcoma made. The histopathology from the liver also confirmed metastatic spread. This case therefore illustrates how more than one biopsy technique can be used for an individual case in both the diagnosis and staging of disease.

Outcome

The dog underwent an echocardiogram to see if there was right auricular involvement in the disease but this was normal. The dog was then given doxorubicin by slow intravenous infusion once every 2 weeks with the treatment aim being to give five cycles in total. However, sadly the dog re-presented collapsed just before the fourth treatment was due to be administered (i.e. 10 weeks postoperatively) and was found to have developed haemoabdomen again, presumably due to haemorrhage from the hepatic metastases. The dog was therefore euthanized.

CLINICAL CASE EXAMPLE 1.4 – INCISIONAL BIOPSY

Signalment

4-year-old female entire Labrador dog.

Presenting signs

Left rostral mandibular mass. The mass was proliferative and friable.

Clinical history

The oral mass had been noted after the dog had presented with signs of halitosis and oral bleeding (Fig. 1.19). Radiographs of the mandible demonstrated some bone destruction of the mandible surrounding the left canine tooth. The left submandibular lymph node was palpably enlarged. There was no evidence of metastasis on thoracic radiographs.

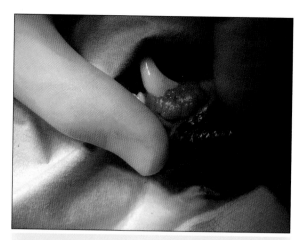

Figure 1.19 *Case 1.4* The appearance of the intraoral mass before incisional biopsy

Figures 1.19–1.21 Incisional biopsy

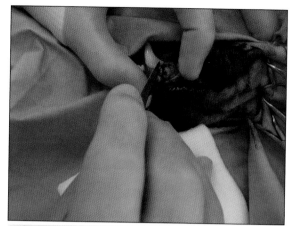

Figure 1.20 *Case 1.4* The incisional biopsy obtained using a Number 10 blade. Haemorrhage was controlled by direct pressure

Differential diagnosis

- Epulis
  - Fibrous
  - Ossifying
  - Acanthomatous
- Squamous cell carcinoma
- Malignant amelanotic melanoma
- Fibrosarcoma.

Diagnostic options

Both the local lymph node and the oral mass require investigation before surgical options are considered. Knowing the tumour type before surgery will provide owners with a prognosis but also aid adjunctive treatment decisions if complete surgical resection is not feasible. The local lymph node can be easily assessed by fine needle aspiration. To obtain a diagnosis from the mass a large sample is required, as often, oral tumours are associated with a high proportion of ulceration, necrosis and inflammation which can penetrate deep beyond the surface. Cytology, needle core biopsies and punch biopsies may therefore not be adequate so, in these cases, an incisional biopsy is recommended. Due to the denervation associated with some of these proliferative masses a general anaesthetic for the incisional biopsy procedure is often not necessary.

The procedure is simply carried out with a scalpel blade under aseptic conditions. If performed in the skin it is preferable to include a portion of normal tissue in addition to the mass that is being sampled. The subse-

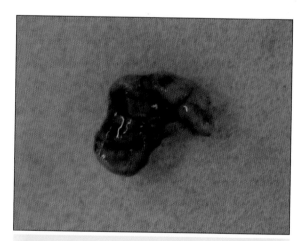

Figure 1.21 *Case 1.4* The incisional biopsy sample obtained from the mandibular mass

quent deficit can be sutured or, as with this case left to heal by secondary intention, after haemorrhage is controlled (Figs 1.20 and 1.21).

> ### CLINICAL TIP
>
> When performing an incisional biopsy it is important to obtain a deep wedge sample that extends beyond any surface inflammation.
>
> Always bear in mind when planning the biopsy incision that the tract will have to be removed in the final surgical procedure.

Diagnosis

The left submandibular lymph node aspirates were consistent with reactive inflammation. The incisional biopsy of the oral mass revealed a diagnosis of an acanthomatous epulis. The dog was treated with a unilateral rostral mandibulectomy and complete surgical margins were obtained.

Outcome

Immediately after the operation, the dog was managed with opioid and non-steroidal anti-inflammatory medication, using the opioids for 48 hours and the NSAIDs for 5 days. The dog ate soft food without difficulty the night of the procedure and was discharged with instructions to feed soft food for the next 10–14 days. The dog remained tumour free at 2 years after the operation.

2 Principles of cancer surgery

In most cancer patients, obtaining a preoperative diagnosis before contemplating surgery is desirable. Knowledge of the type and possible grade of the tumour will allow the surgeon to answer the following questions:

1. Is surgery indicated?
2. Is a potential cure possible?
3. What margins of resection are required?
4. Are further diagnostics recommended, i.e. additional staging?
5. Is adjunctive treatment either pre- or postoperatively an option?
6. Is additional surgical planning for adequate reconstruction indicated?
7. Is this type of surgery within the surgeon's capabilities?

SURGICAL MARGINS

The key to successful surgical cancer management is very much dependent, in the majority of cases, on obtaining margins of normal tissue in addition to the main tumour mass. Even using this approach will not guarantee the complete removal of the tumour as there are often tumour cells that infiltrate the surrounding normal tissue in the form of 'satellite' or 'skip' metastasis (Fig. 2.1). Therefore in most circumstances there is a greater likelihood of complete local excision when wider margins are taken. The exact distance recommended depends on the tumour type, biological behaviour and anatomical location. For example with low- or intermediate-grade mast cell tumours a margin of 2 cm laterally is recommended and results in the complete excision of the majority of tumours. Deep margins must not be disregarded. However, often tumours lie over naturally resistant anatomical barriers such as fascia, ligaments and tendons which are resistant to tumour spread and therefore if a fascial plane is included in the deep margin this would normally be sufficient as an adequate surgical margin.

There are four basic types of tumour resection depending upon the location of the surgical margin:

1. **Intracapsular**. The mass/tumour is removed from within the capsule in pieces. This method is only suitable for benign conditions.
2. **Marginal**. The tumour is removed through the reactive zone, including all or most of the pseudocapsule. This method will not be adequate for malignant tumours as satellite and skip metastases would remain. However, for benign masses, such as lipomas, this type of resection would be adequate.
3. **Wide**. The tumour is removed with its pseudocapsule, the reactive zone and a margin of normal tissue. The tumour and capsule are not entered and the width of the excision is determined preoperatively after obtaining a suitable biopsy which would indicate the tumour type and biological behaviour. With aggressive malignant tumours, there would still be a risk of recurrence due to skip metastasis. This type of resection would be suitable for the majority of intermediate-grade mast cell tumours and low- to intermediate-grade sarcomas.
4. **Radical**. The tumour is removed en bloc with the tissue compartment within which it lies. This surgery is indicated for high-grade malignant tumours, particularly those which have traversed across or through multiple fascial planes. This type of surgery would be indicated for appendicular osteosarcomas (amputation), phalangeal carcinomas (amputation), thoracic wall sarcomas (rib resection).

SURGICAL TECHNIQUES

The first attempt at complete excision will always give the best results with locally aggressive and/or malignant tumours. If an excisional biopsy has been previously performed with tumours such as soft tissue sarcomas then the chances of complete excision and therefore a

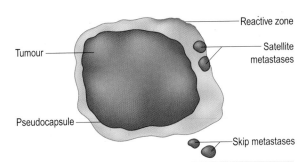

Tumour

Pseudocapsule

Reactive zone

Satellite metastases

Skip metastases

Figure 2.1 This diagram illustrates typical tumour anatomy of a soft-tissue sarcoma and demonstrates the presence of metastases outside the main tumour mass

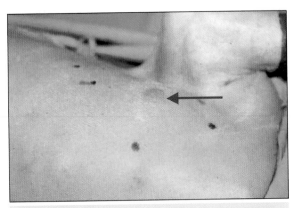

Figure 2.3 A mast cell tumour (location shown by the red arrow) previously diagnosed on aspirate with 2-cm margins marked out with a sterile marker pen

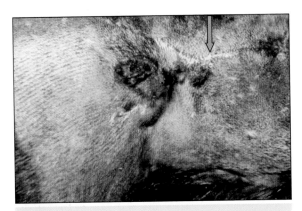

Figure 2.2 This dog has had recurrence of a mast cell tumour following excisional biopsy of the original tumour with incomplete margins (arrow indicates previous scar) on the lateral thoracic wall. The second surgery will be made difficult as now both the gross recurrence and previous scar will have to be included in the second excision

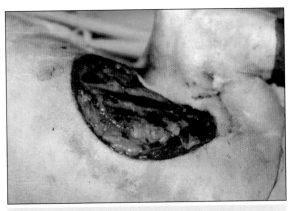

Figure 2.4 After excision with 2-cm minimum lateral margins and including the underlying fascial plane. Histopathology confirmed an intermediate-grade mast cell tumour with complete margins of excision

potential cure are reduced. This is because disruption to the tumour from the first surgery can result in tumour seeding to surrounding tissues. Furthermore, disturbance of normal tumour margins can make identification of 'normal' versus 'abnormal' tissue difficult and also there will be less available local skin for adequate closure. For these reasons a second surgery normally requires even greater margins of excision compared with the first (Fig. 2.2). The exception to this rule is when the tumour type will not affect future treatment options (e.g. mammary tumours, single pulmonary and splenic masses) and in these situations, excisional biopsy is acceptable.

Known malignant tumours should be removed with an adequate margin of normal tissue. Recommendations are that locally aggressive tumours be removed with a minimum of 2 cm margins in the lateral planes and one fascial plane in the deep margin. It is not enough to just 'shell' out the tumour and then go back and remove further tissue as this may cause seeding and lead to recurrence. Attempts must be made to avoid disruption to the tumour and perform the excision by cutting through normal, disease-free tissue only (Figs 2.3, 2.4).

Tumours should always be handled carefully and if possible other means of tumour retraction other than using the hand should be used. This can be in the form of stay sutures, Allis tissue forceps or laparotomy sponges (Fig. 2.5). This will help to avoid tumour cell seeding into local, surrounding tissues. Lavage of the excision site

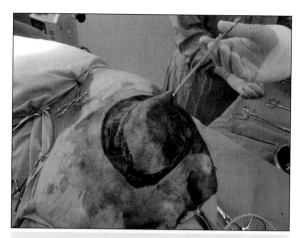

Figure 2.5 This is a case of a mast cell tumour excision demonstrating the use of Allis tissue forceps for tumour handling during dissection

with sterile physiological saline before closure may also be utilized to reduce the number of tumour cells remaining in the wound.

Tumour surgery can be considered as 'contaminated' so recommended surgical procedures to avoid the risk of tumour seeding or spread include:

- Changing surgical gloves before closing normal tissues (e.g. abdominal wall closure)
- Performing 'clean' surgeries before cancer surgery if two or more procedures are planned under the same anaesthesia.

Some tumours exfoliate more readily than others, e.g. epithelial tumours compared with mesenchymal cell tumours, so the risk of transferring cells from the tumour to normal tissue will vary according to tumour type.

SURGERY AS PART OF MULTIMODAL THERAPY

Even if complete excision is not possible, surgery can be effectively utilized as part of a multidisciplinary approach in combination with radiotherapy and/or chemotherapy. Therefore treatment of a cancer patient should not be declined on the basis that the tumour is not completely resectable, or indeed considered ineffective until after a combined management protocol has been explored and offered to the owner. It is becoming more commonplace,

in fact, to *preferentially* select multimodal therapy over a single treatment option, as often, this approach maximizes benefits and minimizes side effects. This is why it is often worth discussing a case with a specialist oncologist before any surgical procedures are undertaken so that all cases can have appropriate treatment plans developed.

CLINICAL CASE EXAMPLE 2.1 – SURGERY AND RADIOTHERAPY

Signalment

7-year-old male neutered Hungarian viszla.

Presenting signs

A 4-cm diameter mass on the lateral aspect of the right elbow.

Clinical history

The mass had appeared 2 months previously and had rapidly grown to 4 cm by the time of presentation. Tru-cut (needle core) biopsies had been taken which revealed a diagnosis of an intermediate-grade soft-tissue sarcoma (Fig. 2.6). Thoracic radiographs were negative for the presence of metastatic disease and local lymph nodes were not palpable.

Management options

At the time of presentation and after staging, it appeared that the main management aim was local disease control. As soft-tissue sarcomas are locally aggressive, and typically, tumour cells extend beyond the pseudo-capsule, they should be removed with 2–3-cm margins of normal tissue laterally and include one fascial plane deep. To achieve this in this area, surgical reconstruction using a local flap, such as a thoracodorsal axial pattern flap, would have to be used to ensure a tension-free wound closure. Using surgery alone in this way is one management option and a reasonable choice if radiotherapy was not available. A disadvantage of this approach is that morbidity associated with this extensive surgery (flap failure) is increased so an alternative option would be to carry out a 'debulk' or more conservative operation, whereby the majority of the tumour burden is removed (cytoreductive therapy) and the remaining microscopic disease is treated with postoperative radiotherapy. This treatment protocol was selected in this case.

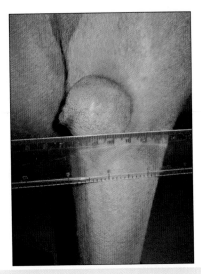

Figure 2.6 *Case 2.1* The appearance of the soft-tissue sarcoma preoperatively

Figures 2.6–2.8 Cytoreductive surgery for a self-tissue sarcoma

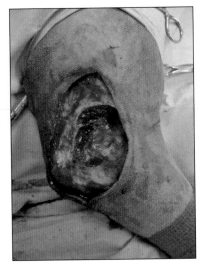

Figure 2.7

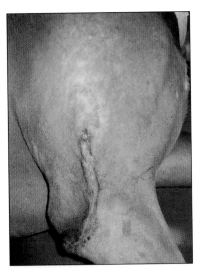

Figure 2.8

Figures 2.7, Figure 2.8 *Case 2.1* Cytoreductive surgery for the soft-tissue sarcoma resulted in a tension-free primary closure that healed without complication prior to radiotherapy

CLINICAL TIP

If cytoreductive surgery is performed with a view to postoperative radiotherapy then careful discussion with a specialist oncologist is strongly advised before the surgery is performed. It is also extremely helpful for the radiotherapy planning to take detailed photographs pre- and postoperatively (Figs 2.6, 2.7, 2.8).

Outcome

Radiotherapy was performed using 4 fractions of 900 cGy once a week and was commenced 10 days after suture removal and confirmation of wound healing. The patient was re-examined every 6 months for recurrence and remained free of detectable disease 2 years after treatment.

CLINICAL CASE EXAMPLE 2.2 – SURGERY AND CHEMOTHERAPY

Signalment

6-year-old neutered male doberman.

Case history

A 2-week history of progressively worsening right fore-limb lameness.

Clinical signs

The dog had started to limp after returning from a walk 10 days prior to presentation and had been prescribed a short course of nonsteroidal anti-inflammatory (NSAID) medication by the referring veterinary surgeon. However, despite this treatment the lameness did not improve and when the course of NSAIDs was completed, the lameness progressed rapidly such that the dog was hardly weight-bearing at presentation and examination revealed the presence of a bony swelling on the distal aspect of his radius. Radiographs revealed the presence of an osteolytic lesion within the radius with an accompanying periosteal reaction, as shown in Figure 2.9.

Differential diagnosis

- Primary bone tumour
  - Osteosarcoma
  - Chondrosarcoma
- Metastatic bone tumour.

Management options

In light of the radiographic findings, the diagnosis was a bone tumour, likely to be a primary bone neoplasm. Because of the degree of pain he was obviously in for him to be non-weight-bearingly lame, the decision was made not to biopsy the mass because it was felt that knowledge of the tumour type would not affect the initial treatment (i.e. the limb required amputation if any treatment was to be considered), but knowledge of the tumour type would influence whether or not postoperative chemotherapy should be recommended. Therefore, the prescapular lymph node was carefully searched for, but was found not to be palpable. Left and right lateral inflated thoracic radiographs were obtained which revealed no gross metastatic disease, so the dog underwent a full fore-quarter amputation. Histopathology confirmed the tumour to be an osteosarcoma.

Outcome

The dog received chemotherapy in the form of alternating carboplatin and doxorubicin given once every 3 weeks for a total of six treatments in combination with bisphosphonate treatment. The dog was alive and well with no evidence of pulmonary metastasis at 12 months postsurgery.

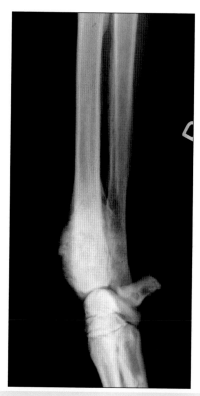

Figure 2.9 *Case 2.2* The lateral radiograph of the radius revealing the presence of a bone tumour in the radius. Image courtesy of Dr Martin Owen, Dick White Referrals

CLINICAL TIP

The life expectancy of a dog in which an appendicular limb osteosarcoma is diagnosed is significantly increased by the administration of postoperative chemotherapy as described above and therefore such treatment should always be discussed with owners if at all possible and the treatment started approximately 2 weeks after the surgery.

OTHER PREOPERATIVE AND POSTOPERATIVE CONSIDERATIONS FOR THE CANCER PATIENT

Although surgical techniques, including margin evaluation and preoperative planning according to tumour type and behaviour, are important elements of oncological surgery, there are several other additional factors that also need to be considered.

Antimicrobial prophylaxis

The use of perioperative antibiotics is beneficial in those surgeries classified as clean-contaminated or contaminated. However, the decision to administer perioperative antibiotics is also based on a number of other criteria including patient factors and local wound factors. Patient factors such as old age, poor nutritional status and other concurrent disease are often features of cancer patients, which result in an increased risk of infection. Additionally, local factors such as local wound immunity and blood supply also have a potential impact on infection rates. For these reasons the infection rates in veterinary cancer patients are significantly higher than other types of surgeries and this may influence the decision to use antibiotics perioperatively. What is more important, however, is *how* to use antibiotics during surgery to afford maximum efficacy. There is definitive evidence that antibiotics are most useful when given before surgery rather than after surgery. Indeed there is also evidence to suggest that giving antibiotics only after surgery not only has no effect on the prevention of infection but actually may *increase* infection rates. The goals of antimicrobial treatment of the cancer patient in preparation for surgery are:

- Never use antibiotics as a substitute for good surgical practice and technique, good hospital infection control policies and patient care.
- The timing of antibiotic administration is critical. Minimum inhibitory concentrations of the drug must be present at the incision site for the entire duration of the surgery. Therefore it is recommended that only intravenous drugs are used and administered at least 30 minutes, but no greater than 60 minutes, prior to the first incision. This is to ensure that adequate tissue concentrations of the drug are present at the site of the surgical wound at the point of possible wound contamination.
- The frequency of administration of antibiotics depends on the pharmacokinetics of the individual drug. For example, for some drugs such as the beta-lactams, repeating administration every 2–3 hours is recommended to ensure tissue concentrations of the drug do not fall below the minimum inhibitory concentration (MIC).
- There is no evidence to suggest that continuing the use of antibiotics beyond the surgical period is beneficial in those patients where the antibiotic is being used prophylactically.

Nutrition and fluid therapy

Cancer has an enormous impact on the nutritional status of affected patients for multiple reasons which are beyond the scope of this chapter to discuss in detail. It is also well known that if left untreated, protein–energy malnutrition is associated with a number of complications including:

- Delayed wound healing
- Anaemia and hypoproteinaemia
- Decreased immune function
- Poor function and eventual failure of the gastrointestinal, cardiovascular and pulmonary systems.

Due to these adverse effects it is vital that feeding the cancer patient pre- and postoperatively is considered a veterinary and nursing priority. Consideration should be given to calculation of the nutritional need of the patient, consideration of the type of food to be given and how it will be given (enterally versus parenterally). The placement of various tubes (nasoesophageal, oesophagostomy, gastrostomy and jejenostomy) to assisted enteral feeding is becoming more commonplace as an adjunctive surgical procedure and many of these can now be placed noninvasively either by percutaneous endoscopic insertion or by laparoscopic means. In addition to nutrition, the administration of effective fluid therapy preoperatively, intraoperatively and postoperatively is also important, particularly in those patients that are compromised and have fluid deficits that require correction.

> **NURSING TIP**
>
> All hospitalized patients, but especially cancer patients, should have their daily calorie requirements calculated and their dietary management planned in the light of this. All cancer patients must receive high quality nutrition whenever possible.

ANALGESIA

Many cancer patients presenting for surgery will have discomfort and/or frank pain as a result of their disease and this has an impact on the provision of analgesia, both before and after surgery. If there is any question of whether or not a patient has discomfort as a result of their tumour they should receive analgesia. Initially, a combination therapy approach of a nonsteroidal anti-inflammatory drug (NSAID) and an opioid such as buprenorphine, is the best recommendation. The main concern for patients who obviously have a painful focus, such as an osteolytic bone tumour, is that the pre-existing pain will cause the phenomenon known as 'wind-up', by which the perception of pain actually increases over time due to mechanisms within the central nervous system (CNS). This, therefore, means that ensuring they are as pain-free as possible during the diagnostic procedure is essential, as good analgesia in this period will reduce the wind-up effect. For surgery, analgesia needs to be planned beforehand, with good-quality analgesia being administered in the premedication and then being maintained in the postoperative period. In the authors' hospitals it would be routine to provide NSAID medication along with methadone in the pre-med and for fentanyl to be administered intraoperatively if there is indication of pain (by increased heart rate, respiratory rate, elevated blood pressure, etc). Post-operatively, patients who have undergone procedures that are known to be potentially painful should be hospitalized for 24–48 hours, receiving both opioid and NSAID medication before being discharged, usually with a further 5 days of NSAID medication. The question of which NSAID to use is difficult, as different patients show differing responses to different drugs. However, in the light of the possible antineoplastic effects of meloxicam, the use of this drug should always be considered, especially if the tumour being treated is epithelial in origin.

A slightly different approach to administering 'blanket analgesia' post-operatively is to use a 'pain scoring' system, such as the Composite Measure Pain Score (CMPS) system. This assesses many descriptor options within six behavioural catagories, thereby generating a pain score based on the sum of the rank scores. This is now used routinely within the author's hospital with assessments being made every 2–4 hours for all surgical patients, enabling much better and more accurate analgesia administration. This approach also allows accurate assessment when multiple analgesic agents (such as opioids plus constant-rate infusion lignocaine or ketamine) are used, thereby ensuring treatment toxicity is minimized whilst analgesia is maximized and patient recovery times are optimized.

3 Principles of cancer chemotherapy

A basic understanding of the mechanisms of action and particular uses of chemotherapy is vital if we are to give the best-quality, compassionate and safe care to our cancer patients. It is important to remember that people can suffer markedly during chemotherapy, so from the outset we have to explain that in veterinary medicine it is generally considered ethically unjustifiable to allow our patients to experience such side effects, so we will attempt to make our chemotherapy side-effect-free where possible (which should be the majority of cases). However, in order to achieve this aim we have to use lower dosages than those used in human medicine with the inevitable consequence that veterinary chemotherapy usually has a lower success rate in terms of remission rates and durations when compared to such treatment in humans.

Although cancer development is an extremely complex series of events at a genomic level, cancer cells only vary from normal cells in six main ways. They:

- Have self-sufficient growth ability
- Are insensitive to natural antigrowth signals
- Are able to evade preprogrammed cell death (apoptosis)
- Have limitless replicative potential
- Are able to promote sustained angiogenesis
- Are able to invade tissue and develop metastasis.

Tumours develop, therefore, because of an imbalance between normal cell growth/division and natural cell death. As a result, understanding the cell cycle is fundamental to understanding cancer biology. The cell cycle has four phases, as shown in Figure 3.1.

Most normal cells are in the G_0 stage, obviously depending upon their location and function, but it is important to remember that cells in G_0 may still act as a reservoir from which further tumour cells may develop. In addition, the cell cycle is important clinically because many therapeutic modalities used in oncology only affect dividing cells, so the cell cycle specificity of various treatments may affect the choice and efficacy of treatment used. As a general rule, chemotherapeutics are either cell cycle specific or cell cycle nonspecific.

Chemotherapy drugs can act by damaging DNA and thus preventing cellular replication, inducing apoptosis, or they may interfere with a specific phase of the cell cycle. Actively dividing cells are obviously more sensitive to DNA damage.

BASIC CONCEPTS OF TUMOUR GROWTH

Most tumours are detected late in the course of the disease, at which stage there are many millions of cells making up the tumour (e.g. a mass of approximately 1-cm diameter contains 10^9 cells whilst an average 20-cm mass contains 10^{12} cells). Tumour cell growth pattern generally follows 'Gompertzian' growth kinetics; that is, initially exponential cell division resulting in a rapid growth phase but as cell numbers increase the rate of cell division starts to tail off. This means that because large tumours contain a very high number of cells, only a small proportion of them will be dividing when compared to when the tumour was very small, and therefore there will be fewer cells that are susceptible to chemotherapy. Conversely, smaller tumours with a higher growth fraction theoretically have a greater potential response to chemotherapy because they contain a greater number of proliferating cells. This principle is illustrated graphically in Figure 3.2.

This graph also illustrates why surgical debaulking and follow-up chemotherapy or radiotherapy can theoretically be useful in tumours which display sensitivity to the follow-up treatment. By reducing the number of cancer cells in the mass, the growth curve can be shifted to the left, thereby generating a possible window of opportunity for the adjunctive treatments to be more effective than they would otherwise be without the surgery. Obviously, inherent tumour resistance, vascular supply and the type and grade of the tumour all impact

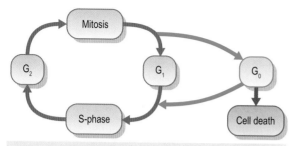

Figure 3.1 The four phases of the cell cycle S = period of DNA synthesis; G_1 = RNA and protein synthesis; G_2 = second period of RNA and protein synthesis and G_0 = resting cells

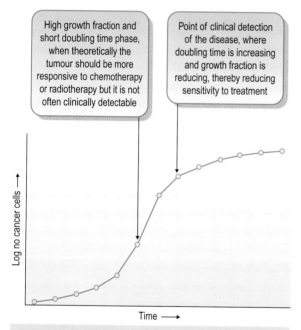

High growth fraction and short doubling time phase, when theoretically the tumour should be more responsive to chemotherapy or radiotherapy but it is not often clinically detectable

Point of clinical detection of the disease, where doubling time is increasing and growth fraction is reducing, thereby reducing sensitivity to treatment

Figure 3.2 Rate of tumour cell growth relating to clinical detection and response to medical management

proliferative diseases such as lymphoma. There are therefore four main indications to use chemotherapy:

1. In patients with a tumour with known (or strongly presumed) sensitivity to chemotherapy, e.g. lymphoma, multiple myeloma, transmissible venereal tumour
2. As an adjunctive treatment to surgery aiming to eradicate or reduce occult micrometastases (e.g. in canine osteosarcoma and haemangiosarcoma)
3. In patients for whom palliative treatment for systemic or metastatic cancer is required and for whom surgical management is not considered viable
4. To sensitize tissues to the effects of radiation therapy.

OUR GOALS: to control the cancer and prolong survival while still maintaining a good, acceptable quality of life.

DRUG DOSAGE AND TIMING

The aim of chemotherapy is to administer the maximum possible doses at the shortest possible dosing interval (dose intensity). Any decrease in the administered dose can result in a significant reduction in drug efficacy, so giving optimal doses is vital. The efficacy of chemotherapy can be further enhanced in many situations by administering chemotherapy using several different drugs that have different mechanisms of action, known as 'combination chemotherapy'. To make this as effective as possible without causing toxicity, several rules need to be followed:

- Administer therapies as close together as the maximal tolerable dose allows (therefore the most effective dose in most cases is very near to the toxic dose)
- Do not use drugs with overlapping drug toxicities simultaneously
- Use drugs with known activity against the tumour of interest.

In a clinically detectable tumour (i.e. approx 10^9 cells or more) the tumour will not contain a homogeneous population of cells. It has been hypothesized that tumours develop intrinsically resistant cell lines because of their inherent genetic instability, leading to the observation that in any tumour containing > 10^6 cells, drug resistance will often already have developed. This led to the development of multidrug protocols based on the activity of individual drugs against a specific tumour type, drug toxicity and mechanism of actions. The aims of combination chemotherapy therefore are to:

on this principle so it is not possible to apply it to all conditions. However, the basic theory that chemotherapy and radiotherapy work most effectively on microscopic disease does generally apply, hence multimodal treatment should always be undertaken if possible.

INDICATIONS FOR CHEMOTHERAPY

Chemotherapy is rarely effective in veterinary medicine if used as the sole treatment modality, except in lympho-

- Maximize cell kill but maintain an acceptable toxicity range
- Broaden the range of therapy against a heterogeneous tumour population
- Prevent/slow the development of new resistant lines.

TOXICITY

The most clinically important toxicoses include **b**one marrow suppression, **a**lopecia and **g**astrointestinal toxicity (i.e. a 'BAG' of adverse effects).

Bone marrow toxicity

This is caused by damage to the rapidly dividing bone marrow stem cells and it occurs because chemotherapeutics are nonselective; they have the potential to kill any rapidly dividing cells and this includes normal bone marrow cells. Bone marrow toxicity can be assessed by taking blood for a complete blood count (CBC) and blood smear examination. Chemotherapy should be delayed in any patient with a neutrophil count of < 2.5 × 10^9/L or a platelet count < 50.0 × 10^9/L. Possible clinical signs associated with myelotoxicity include those related to sepsis, petechial or eccymotic haemorrhage and pallor and weakness. However, anecdotally in the authors' experience, inappetance and marked lethargy are the complaints most commonly cited by the owners of animals with leucopaenia, whilst pyrexia is the most common clinical finding. Usually only patients with clinical signs should be treated, with treatments including:

- Following careful aseptic techniques
- Minimizing trauma and controlling any bleeding if thrombocytopaenic
- Culture of urine, blood and any other exudates which may be significant
- The administration of broad-spectrum antimicrobials, intravenous fluids and/or blood-product transfusions etc., as required.

Recombinant human granulocyte–monocyte colony-stimulating factor (GM-CSF) boosts endogenous production of neutrophils but its use is not routine in veterinary medicine, firstly because the bone marrow usually recovers naturally within approximately 5 days following administration of a chemotherapeutic, and secondly because antibodies can develop to GM-CSF within a few weeks of administration.

It is obviously important to discontinue the drugs that induce bone marrow suppression until blood counts have recovered, but then it would be usual to re-institute the therapy, albeit at a reduced dose. Most animals with chemotherapy-induced leucopaenia respond well to treatment as long as the problem is identified and treated rapidly, and will often only have a hospitalization period of approximately 3–5 days.

Alopecia

This is an uncommon complication but can be seen in dogs with constantly growing hair coats, such as Afghan hounds and old English sheepdogs. The author has also seen periorbital and facial alopecia in West Highland white terriers and Scottish terriers given doxorubicin (Figs 3.3, 3.4). Cats can lose their whiskers, especially with long-term vincristine therapy but more generalized alopecia is less common in cats than in dogs. If affected, the hair coat normally regrows on completion of the chemotherapy.

Gastrointestinal toxicity

The obvious clinical signs of gastrointestinal (GIT) toxicity are vomiting, anorexia and diarrhoea. The development of such signs is either secondary to direct damage to GIT epithelial cells or via efferent nervous stimulation of the chemoreceptor trigger zone or the higher vomiting centres. Anorexia is certainly a relatively common side effect after the administration of many chemotherapeutics, but this usually only lasts 24–36 hours. If there is a major concern regarding GIT toxicity

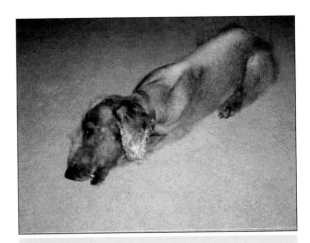

Figure 3.3 A Bedlington terrier which developed generalized alopecia following doxorubicin therapy as part of a modified Madison-Wisconsin protocol to treat mesenteric lymphoma. He went into permanent complete remission and his hair regrew on cessation of his treatment

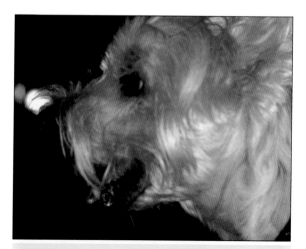

Figure 3.4 A West Highland white terrier which developed periorbital alopecia after receiving doxorubicin, also as part of a Madison-Wisconsin protocol, used to treat his multicentric lymphoma

then post-chemotherapy administration of antiemetics may be justified, and certainly, the author frequently recommends 5-day courses of an antiemetic (maropitant or metoclopramide) after a patient has received doxorubicin or carboplatin.

Chemotherapy-induced diarrhoea usually responds to conservative treatment (no food for 12–24 hours, oral rehydration fluids and a bland, easily digested diet for the following 3–5 days). Some cases may require the use of treatments such as metronidazole for 5–7 days. If the diarrhoea is accompanied by significant signs of systemic illness then a blood sample for CBC analysis should be obtained to ensure that the animal has not become neutropaenic. The faeces should also be cultured for pathogenic bacteria with follow-up antibiosis based on the bacteriology results where appropriate. However, in general, as with bone marrow toxicity, GIT toxicity is rarely a major problem if the chemotherapy has been administered at the correct dose and frequency and if owners have been correctly counselled and supported by the clinical team.

Other than the 'BAG' of side effects, there are several other major possible problems associated with chemotherapy treatment:

1. Cardiac toxicity. This is a well-recognized possible complication of doxorubicin therapy. Doxorubicin is known to induce dilated cardiomyopathy (DCM) with high cumulative doses and is also associated with transient arrhythmias during administration. In human medicine the incidence of doxorubicin-associated cardiomyopathy is quoted as being up to 1% with a total dose of 500 mg/m^2, rising to over 10% with total doses of 600 mg/m^2. However, in veterinary medicine, dogs appear to be more sensitive to the cardiac toxicity of doxorubicin compared to people and this effect is possibly exacerbated by the fact that doxorubicin is most commonly used in cases of canine lymphoma and there is a predilection for this condition in some breeds of dog that are also more prone to developing DCM. The current recommendation therefore is to not exceed a total dose of 180 mg/m^2. Some authors have recommended using total doses of up to 240 mg/m^2 in small-breed dogs in whom concurrent cardiac monitoring is performed but the safety of this has not been clearly proven. It is therefore advisable to use doxorubicin with caution in breeds of dog predisposed to DCM, and routine ECG and echocardiographic assessment are also recommended in appropriate cases. It may also be advisable to auscultate or perform continuous ECG monitoring whilst administering doxorubicin in patients for whom there is any concern regarding cardiac function and the administration should not be over a period of less than 20 minutes.

2. Haemorrhagic cystitis. This can develop following cyclophosphamide administration, due to the production of a metabolite of cyclophosphamide called acrolein that is directly toxic to the bladder epithelium. Cyclophosphamide-induced haemorrhagic cystitis can be difficult to treat when it develops so it is worth asking owners to undertake regular dipstick assessment of the animal's urine whilst it is receiving cyclophosphamide and if there is any indication of the presence of blood in the urine, cyclophosphamide therapy should be stopped immediately and substituted with an alternative alkylating agent (e.g. chlorambucil or melphalan). Treatment of the cystitis is usually symptomatic, with antibiotics, anti-inflammatory analgesics and urinary glycosoaminoglycan supplements having all anecdotally been reported to be beneficial. Intravesicular administration of dimethyl sulphoxide (DMSO) has been reported to be successful in some cases and this has been used successfully in the authors' hospital. The concurrent administration of frusemide at the same time as cyclophosphamide also appears to reduce the incidence of this problem.

3. Neurotoxicity. This has been reported following administration of vincristine (peripheral neuropathy), 5-fluorouracil (seizures and disorientation) and cis-

platin (deafness). The neurological signs following the administration of 5-fluorouracil are significant in cats so the use of this drug is contraindicated in this species.

4. Severe cellulitis. Doxorubicin, actinomycin D, vincristine, vinblastine and mechlorethamine are known to cause a severe localised cellulitis if extravasated during administration. Briefly the treatment for this is:

- Stop injection if there is any suspicion at all that there has been, or may have been extravasation
- Carefully examine the catheter and surrounding tissue, looking for perivascular swelling/'blown vein' appearance
- If extravasation is confirmed, attempt to aspirate drug and 5 ml of blood if possible back into the administration syringe
- Apply an ice pack and topical steroid cream to the affected area. The intravenous administration of Dexrazoxane has also been recommended if doxorubicin extravasation occurs
- Refer to a surgical specialist for possible surgical lavage and wound management. The level of treatment required will depend on the amount of soft-tissue damage that develops but may include the use of wet-to-dry dressings to remove necrotic tissue, careful daily bandage changes, reconstructive surgery and in a worst-case scenario, possibly even amputation of the limb.

For this reason it is mandatory that all intravenous chemotherapeutic agents are administered through a well-placed intravenous catheter and never directly via a needle or butterfly catheter. Placement of the catheter must follow standard aseptic techniques and ensure that the catheter is securely fixed in place (Figs 3.5–3.12).

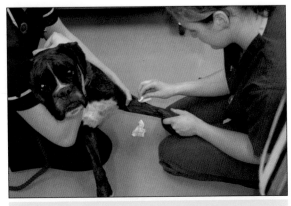

Figure 3.6 After clipping the hair from over the vein to be used, the skin should be cleaned with an antibacterial solution such as Hibiscrub and then surgical spirit which is allowed to dry

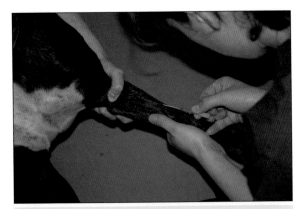

Figure 3.7 With the animal appropriately restrained, the catheter is placed into the vein. If the catheter appears to pass through the vein and not stay within the lumen, use of this vein should be abandoned and an alternative vein used

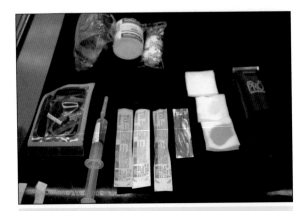

Figure 3.5 Preparation of the equipment required to place an intravenous chemotherapy catheter

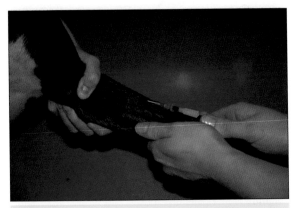

Figure 3.8 Once blood has been seen in the hub of the stylette, the catheter is then carefully advanced off the stylette

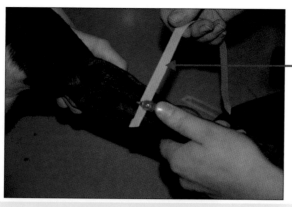

Sticky side of tape facing up, placed underneath and wrapped over the catheter hub before being wrapped around the leg, thereby ensuring that the tape is well attached to the catheter as well as to the leg

Figure 3.9 With the catheter fully advanced, the stylette is removed and the catheter taped in place. Fixing the catheter in place by firstly ensuring that the tape used is adhered to the catheter as shown above is recommended

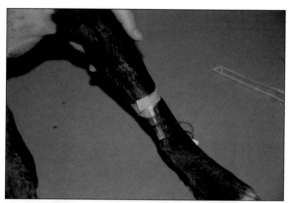

Figure 3.10

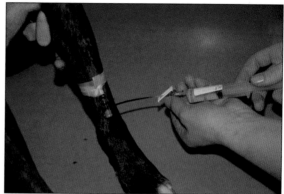

Figure 3.11

Figures 3.10 and 3.11 Once the catheter has been secured with one or two further pieces of tape, a T-port is attached and the catheter patency assessed by withdrawing blood. Once satisfied that the catheter is well placed and patent, it is then thoroughly flushed using 10-ml sterile saline

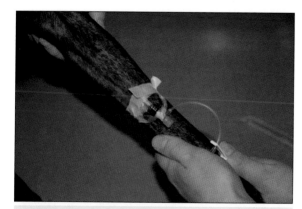

Figure 3.12 The T-port itself is then taped in place in the same manner as the catheter before a bandage is placed over the whole catheter to keep it clean and prevent the patient from trying to remove it!

COMMONLY USED DRUGS IN VETERINARY CHEMOTHERAPY

The following case examples illustrate the mechanism of action and possible toxicities of the more commonly utilized veterinary chemotherapeutics.

Case 3.1

A 7-year-old neutered female boxer dog presented with generalized lymphadenopathy identified on a routine prevaccination health check. Fine needle aspirates were obtained from her prescapular and popliteal lymph nodes which confirmed the diagnosis to be lymphoma. Flow cytometry confirmed the lymphoma to be B-cell in origin whilst abdominal ultrasound revealed no abnormalities to be visible in the liver or spleen and the thoracic radiographs were unremarkable. She was therefore diagnosed with grade IIIa multicentric lymphoma (see Appendix 1). The owner elected to treat with high-dose COP protocol, which is a combination of cyclophosphamide, vincristine (tradename 'Oncovin') and prednisolone.

1. Cyclophosphamide is classed as an alkylating agent (as are chlorambucil, melphalan, lomustine and hydroxyurea). It works by binding to DNA strands by inserting an alkyl group, thereby inhibiting protein synthesis. This class of drugs is cell cycle non-specific. Cyclophosphamide can be given by oral or intravenous administration and once absorbed it is rapidly converted by the liver to active metabolites which are then excreted in an inactive form via the urine. It can be used in lymphomas, leukaemias, soft-tissue sarcomas and feline mammary neoplasia, almost always in combination with other agents. The main potential toxicities seen with cyclophosphamide are bone marrow suppression (with the nadir 7–14 days after treatment and recovery seen 5–10 days after the nadir) and sterile haemorrhagic cystitis (which can result either from a single dose or following long-term administration but usually develops early in the administration period). The formation of the causal cyclophosphamide metabolite acrolein can be prevented by the simultaneous administration of mesna, which is a uroprotective agent and the concurrent administration of frusemide with cyclophosphamide has also been reported to reduce the incidence of the problem. However, as the incidence of haemorrhagic cystitis is low in veterinary medicine, the use of mesna or frusemide is not routine. As described previously, cyclophosphamide-induced haemorrhagic cystitis can be difficult to treat and although the clinical signs usually do resolve once the cyclophosphamide treatment is stopped, this may take several months, during which time the patient can be difficult to manage. The main differential diagnosis is bacterial cystitis, so a full urinalysis and culture on a cystocentesis sample should be performed in patients suspected of having haemorrhagic cystitis. If any patient develops, or is suspected to have developed, haemorrhagic cystitis following the administration of cyclophosphamide, it must not be given cyclophosphamide again and a substitute alkylating agent used instead (Fig 3.13).

2. Vincristine (Oncovin). This is classified as a plant alkaloid and like vinblastine, is derived from the periwinkle plant. Its mechanism of action is to bind to the microtubules present at mitosis to prevent the

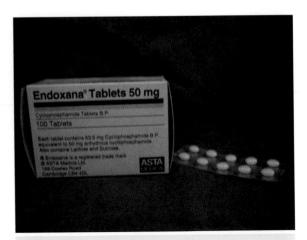

Figure 3.13 Cyclophosphamide can be given by oral or intravenous administration

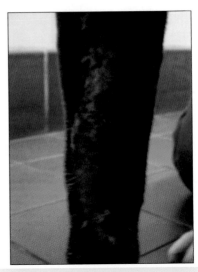

Figure 3.14 A Staffordshire bull terrier with marked skin and subcutaneous tissue damage following the administration of vincristine using a needle rather than an intravenous catheter. The veterinary surgeon did not think any of the vincristine was administered perivascularly but the dog started to display signs of discomfort within 12 hours of the injection

normal formation and function of the mitotic spindle, thus arresting the cell division in metaphase. It can only be administered by intravenous injection and following administration it is excreted via hepatic metabolism into faeces. It is used in lymphomas, transmissible venereal tumour (where it can be used as a sole agent with high success rates) and possibly mast cell tumours. It has also been described as useful in metastatic haemangiosarcomas when combined with doxorubicin and cyclophosphamide in the VAC protocol. The toxicities described with vincristine include a severe perivascular reaction following accidental extravasation (Fig. 3.14), constipation (unusual but possibly more likely to occur in cats) and peripheral neuropathy. It generally causes only moderate myelosuppression, although the risk of myelosuppression may be increased if it is administered concurrently with L-asparaginase.

3. Prednisolone. This is a steroid hormone that acts by binding to cytoplasmic receptor sites which then interact with DNA and prevent cell division. Prednisolone is also directly toxic to lymphocytes. It is metabolized in the liver with the non-toxic metabolites excreted predominately via urine. The toxicities described for prednisolone relate to its glucocorticoid action, i.e. polyuria, polydipsia and polyphagia, iatrogenic Cushing's disease, lethargy and, more rarely, behavioural changes. It is a useful treatment for lymphoproliferative neoplasia and mast cell tumours.

Case 3.2

A 12-year-old neutered female lurcher presented with a 10-day history of progressively worsening lethargy and inappetance. She was drinking more than normal but not vomiting. The owner had also noticed that she was intermittently lame but had put this change down to arthritic disease. Her complete blood count revealed a marked elevation in her total white cell count with a significant thrombocytopaenia and a mild non-regenerative anaemia. Abdominal ultrasound and thoracic radiographs were unremarkable so a bone marrow aspirate was obtained and this showed that the dog had chronic lymphocytic leukaemia (CLL). The dog was therefore treated with a combination of chlorambucil and prednisolone.

- Chlorambucil ('Leukeran'), like cyclophosphamide, is an alkylating agent that is metabolized by the liver to the active form and eliminated via urine and faeces. It is only available as a tablet and it is used in the maintenance phase of treatment of some lymphomas, as a substitute for cyclophosphamide and in the treatment of chronic lymphoid leukaemia. It is a less efficacious drug than cyclophosphamide but its toxicities are also described as mild compared to other agents. In the authors' experience it is usually very well tolerated by both cats and dogs and can be extremely useful in some cases of lymphoma when

used with prednisolone or as a substitute drug instead of cyclophosphamide.

Case 3.3

An 8-year-old neutered male Jack Russell terrier presented with clinical signs of lethargy, suspected urinary incontinence and increased thirst. Clinical examination revealed a mild lymphadenopathy and congested scleral blood vessels. The serum biochemistry revealed a marked hyperglobulinaemia, which when assessed further with serum protein electrophoresis revealed a monoclonal γ-globulinaemia. A bone marrow aspirate was obtained which confirmed the presence of large numbers of neoplastic plasma cells, thereby diagnosing him with multiple myeloma. The dog was successfully treated by a combination of melphalan and prednisolone.

- Melphalan ('Alkeran' tablets, melphalan injection) is a phenylalanine derivative of nitrogen mustard that acts as an alkylating agent and is used in veterinary medicine mainly to treat multiple myeloma, although like chlorambucil it can be used as an alternative to cyclophosphamide in conditions such as lymphoma. Myelosuppression (particularly after prolonged administration) manifesting as thrombocytopenia is reported but is usually mild.

Case 3.4

A 5-year-old male golden retriever presented due to the owner finding 'a lump' on his right hind leg on the palmar aspect of his stifle. Clinical examination, however, revealed that the dog had generalized lymphadenopathy and hepatosplenomegaly. Fine needle aspirates of the enlarged lymph nodes revealed that more than 50% of the cells present were lymphoblasts, thereby diagnosing with grade IVa multicentric lymphoma. The dog was treated with a modified Madison-Wisconsin protocol, which is a combination of L-asparginase, vincristine, cyclophosphamide, doxorubicin and prednisolone.

- Doxorubicin ('Adriamycin') is classified as an antitumour antibiotic and its main mechanism of action is to form stable complexes with DNA, thereby inhibiting further DNA synthesis. It is administered as a slow intravenous infusion over 20 minutes diluted with 0.9% sterile saline. The author generally injects the doxorubicin into the injection port of a fast-running 0.9% saline drip (100 ml bag) but the doxorubicin solution can also simply be added directly to the drip bag and allowed to run in over the same 20-minute timeframe. If it is placed in the drip bag, it is essential to remember to have at least 20 ml of sterile saline ready to flush the bag through to make certain the optimum dose is given, but also to ensure that the intravenous catheter is totally flushed clean before being removed. Following administration it is metabolised predominantly by the liver, resulting in 50% of the metabolites being excreted in the bile, but they are also excreted via the kidneys and can very occasionally cause a red discolouration of the urine for up to 2 days. Doxorubicin is a potent chemotherapeutic agent with a broad spectrum of activity against many tumour types such as lymphomas, sarcomas, carcinomas and mammary neoplasia. It can, however, cause significant toxicity reactions. Immediate side effects that are histamine-mediated and manifest as allergic reaction and shock can occasionally be seen within 5 minutes of commencing administration, so it is advisable to premedicate all patients receiving doxorubicin with intravenous chlorpheniramine ('Piriton'). Following administration, some patients may exhibit gastrointestinal, alopecic and bone marrow toxicity, in particular, neutropaenia. Gastrointestinal toxicity can be manifested as anorexia (24–48 hours post treatment), vomiting (2–5 days post treatment) and diarrhoea (3–7 days post treatment) and is probably the most common toxicity seen following the use of doxorubicin. If leukopenia or thrombocytopaenia develops, patients usually have a nadir at 7-10 days post treatment and will have recovered by day 14. As outlined earlier, cardiotoxicity is also a significant total dose-limiting effect, hence the current recommendations to stop doxorubicin after a total dose of 180 mg/m^2 in most patients (Fig. 3.15).

- L-asparaginase is a bacterially derived enzyme that degrades L-asparagine, thereby depriving growing cells of this amino acid, and as a result, causing inhibition of protein synthesis. However, many tumour cells are able to increase the activity of their endogenous asparagine synthetase and thus become resistant to the antitumour effects of L-asparaginase quite rapidly. Also, antibodies to the foreign bacterial protein frequently develop after drug exposure leading to resistance and a significant risk of allergic reactions after the second or third usage. If an anaphylactic reaction occurs it will usually develop within 1 hour following administration. L-asparaginase has also been associated with the development of acute pancreatitis in a small number of dogs. It is given as either a subcutaneous or intramuscular injection and the resulting metabolites are excreted via both urine and faeces. L-asparaginase is used to treat lymphoma and lymphoblastic leukaemias, usually in combination with other agents, as it does not induce a substantial remission when used alone to treat lymphoma. Furthermore, a recent study has suggested that the omission of L-asparaginase from CHOP-based lymphoma protocols does not significantly alter the remission rates or remission duration, so its use as a primary agent in lymphoma is now in question. It can, however, be useful as a rescue agent or as the first drug in a protocol in situations when immunosuppression that may be caused by other cytotoxics would be better avoided (e.g. concurrent lymphoma and *Ehrlichia* infection).

The golden retriever in question went into complete remission and treatment was stopped after 6 months. The dog stayed in remission for a further 13 months before relapsing, at which point rescue treatment was given in the form of oral lomustine ('CCNU').

- Lomustine is given orally, usually once every 3 weeks in the dog and every 3–6 weeks in the cat. It acts as an alkylating agent and has been shown to have action against lymphoma, mast cell tumours, some brain tumours and fibrosarcomas. It is metabolized by oxidation in the liver and the metabolites are excreted via the urine. The main toxicity associated with the use of lomustine is neutropaenia, which can be severe and usually manifests at 7–14 days following treatment if it develops. A small number of animals have been reported to develop severe, potentially fatal hepatotoxicity after having been given lomustine. The risk of this developing increases with increasing numbers of treatments. It is therefore recommended that serum markers of hepatocellular damage (ALT in particular) are regularly assessed in patients receiving

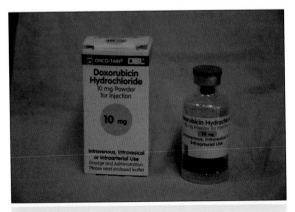

Figure 3.15 Doxorubicin is classified as an antitumour antibiotic

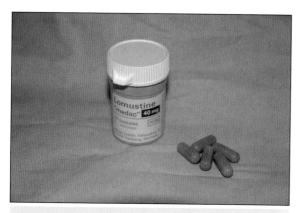

Figure 3.16 Lomustine acts as an alkylating agent

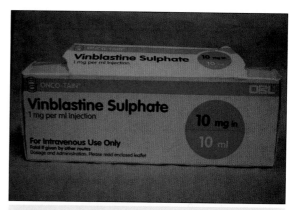

Figure 3.17 Vinblastine is the salt of an alkaloid from the periwinkle plant

lomustine and that treatment should be stopped if the hepatocellular markers rise (Fig. 3.16).

Case 3.5

A 4-year-old neutered male Labrador developed multiple raised, erythematous cutaneous masses in the region of his left shoulder. Fine needle aspiration revealed the masses to be mast cell tumours and histopathology confirmed them to be grade III. The owner opted for adjunctive chemotherapy in the light of the aggressive nature of the tumour grading and treatment was given using vinblastine and prednisolone.

- Vinblastine is the salt of an alkaloid from the periwinkle plant that is only given by intravenous injection, usually once every 14 days. Its mechanism of action is to interfere with microtubular assembly in a similar manner to that of vincristine. It is also known to interfere with glutamic acid utilization, thereby preventing purine synthesis, the citric acid cycle and urea formation. Following administration it is metabolized by the liver and is primarily excreted in the bile. Like vincristine, vinblastine is generally well tolerated but some dogs do develop mild neutropaenia or anorexia and vomiting (Fig. 3.17).

The dog in question initially responded well to the treatment, with the tumours becoming non-palpable within 20 days of starting his treatment. He developed no side effects as a result of treatment except for polydipsia and polyphagia. Sadly, however, he re-presented at vinblastine injection number 6 (i.e. 12 weeks into his treatment) with acute-onset extensive pitting oedema and ecchymotic bruising affecting his head and neck

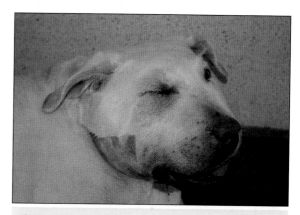

Figure 3.18 *Case 3.5* The appearance of the dog with the grade III mast cell tumour at relapse, with marked facial oedema, oral haemorrhage and cutaneous ecchymoses. The dog was also extremely weak and had vomited

(Fig. 3.18). He was also dyspnoeic and vomiting. In the light of his rapid deterioration, considered most likely to be due to massive histamine release as a result of mast cell degranulation, the owners requested that he be euthanized.

Case 3.6

A 6-year-old neutered female German shepherd dog presented due to progressively worsening lethargy and polydipsia. On examination it was noticed that her mucous membranes appeared very reddened. Her complete blood count revealed an excessive red cell number (PCV 78%). Thoracic radiographs were unremarkable, blood gas analysis revealed no evidence of hypoxia and her serum erythropoietin concentration was low-normal. The remainder of her diagnostic evaluation was unremarkable. The dog was therefore diagnosed as having primary polycythaemia (also termed primary erythrocytosis). After initial treatment by phlebotomy and replacement fluid therapy, chemotherapy was instituted using single-agent treatment with hydroxurea.

- Hydroxyurea blocks the conversion of ribonucleotides to deoxyribonucleotides, thereby preventing DNA synthesis during mitosis. It is given orally, usually once a day initially before reducing the dose frequency to every other day or every third day depending on any toxicity seen and the clinical efficacy. Following administration it is metabolized by the liver and the metabolites excreted via the kidneys into urine. It is usually a well-tolerated treatment, although some patients will develop gastrointestinal toxicity and myelosuppression. With chronic administration onchodystrophy can also be seen.

The German shepherd in question went into complete remission with no significant side effects. Her PCV remained on the high side of normal (PCV 48–53%) and she remained well for 21 months before she relapsed, at which point the owner elected for euthanasia.

Case 3.7

A 9-year-old neutered male Bichon Frise presented with signs of haematuria without stranguria and was subsequently diagnosed with a transitional cell carcinoma (TCC) located in the body of his urinary bladder. He was taken to surgery and the mass removed before commencing adjunctive chemotherapy with mitoxantrone and piroxicam.

- Mitoxantrone is an antitumour antibiotic (i.e. similar to doxorubicin) that acts by inhibition of topoisomerase II. It has been shown to have activity against many different tumours such as lymphoma and squamous cell carcinoma (SCC), as well as urinary bladder TCC and although frequently effective, the duration of many remissions mitoxantrone generates when used alone is short. It has also been used as a radiation sensitizer in cases of feline oral SCC. It is administered by slow intravenous infusion diluted with 0.9% saline in the same way as for doxorubicin, usually once every 3 weeks for five cycles. Its main toxicity is myelosuppression, but unlike doxorubicin, it does not readily cause allergic reactions, cardiomyopathy, arrhythmias, colitis or tissue damage at the site of extravasation.

- Piroxicam is a non-steroidal anti-inflammatory drug rather than a cytotoxic chemotherapeutic but it has been shown to have an anti-tumour effect in cases of canine TCC. The exact mechanism of action is unclear but it is thought to be through the inhibition of COX-2 (which has been shown to be expressed in a number of tumours including human bladder carcinomas and canine bladder tumours). Prostaglandin E_2 is known to contribute to tumour cell growth, immunosuppression and tumour angiogenesis and studies have shown that combining piroxicam with mitoxantrone may increase the disease-free period in dogs with urinary bladder TCC. Piroxicam is given by mouth once a day with food and the only concern with its use is the (low) potential for gastric ulceration. The other issue in Europe is that it is not licensed for use in animals, but there are other licensed NSAIDs, so its use under the cascade system is at the risk of the prescribing clinician (Fig. 3.19).

The Bichon Frise in this case remained completely well for just over 12 months before the haematuria returned. Abdominal imaging confirmed recurrence of the mass but this time it was located in the bladder neck. Once cytology (sample obtained from a urinary sediment examination) had confirmed the mass to be a relapse of the tumour, the owner declined further treatment and the dog was euthanized.

Case 3.8

A 4-year-old neutered female doberman presented with a 7-day history of progressively worsening lameness on

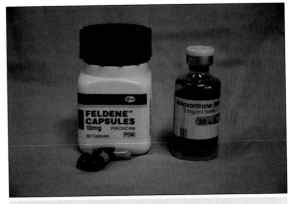

Figure 3.19 Piroxicam is a non-steroidal anti-inflammatory drug rather than a cytotoxic chemotherapeutic

her right foreleg. Radiographs revealed an osteolytic lesion with obvious cortical lysis and significant new bone formation generating a palisading pattern around the lytic lesion. Bone biopsy confirmed the lesion to be an osteosarcoma, so after a full staging process in which no gross metastases were identified, the right foreleg was amputated and the dog then received adjuvant chemotherapy with doxorubicin and carboplatin given alternatively once every 3 weeks for six treatments.

- Carboplatin is a platinum-containing compound that was developed in an attempt to reduce the side effects associated with cisplatin in human medicine. As a heavy metal compound, it binds within and between DNA strands and inhibits protein synthesis and it is therefore cell cycle non-specific. Its spectrum of activity is similar to cisplatin (i.e. primarily canine osteosarcoma, but it also can have some activity against squamous cell carcinoma, pulmonary carcinoma, urinary bladder transitional cell carcinomas, anal sac carcinomas, ovarian carcinomas and mesotheliomas; the author has also anectodally used it in some soft-tissue sarcomas with success) but it has comparably low levels of associated renal toxicity. It is given by intravenous infusion and after absorption its metabolites are excreted in urine, although as carboplatin has a much longer half-life compared to cisplatin, the urinary concentration of metabolites is significantly lower. However, some of the metabolites are still cytotoxic so appropriate care needs to be taken with regard to staff and owner exposure to urine but this risk is substantially lower than in patients who have been give cisplatin. The main toxicity reported is myelosuppression (nadir 11–14 days) although the author has seen a small number of dogs who develop marked gastrointestinal side effects following administration. Nephrotoxicity is rare. Unlike cisplatin (which causes fatal pulmonary oedema in cats) carboplatin is considered safe for use in cats (at 200 mg/m^2 as opposed to a dose of 300 mg/m^2 as used in dogs) and it is generally a very well tolerated, efficacious chemotherapeutic agent if given properly (Fig. 3.20).

- Cisplatin could have been used, either as a sole agent or instead of carboplatin in this case, but it was not used (a) due to the fact it is highly emetogenic and (b) because of the health and safety concerns regarding the toxic urinary metabolites it produces. Following IV injection it rapidly binds to protein and is eliminated via urine in an active form, making collection of urine mandatory for 24 hours during the treat-

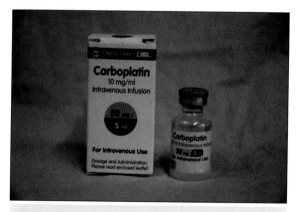

Figure 3.20 Carboplatin is a platinum-containing compound that was developed in an attempt to reduce the side effects associated with cisplatin in human medicine

ment period. The toxicities reported with cisplatin include it being highly emetogenic (many dogs will often vomit within 1 hour of the administration commencing, although the advent of maropitant as a veterinary licensed anti-emetic has reduced this problem) and it is also markedly nephrotoxic, necessitating administration following diuresis that continues after administration.

The dog in this case was also given meloxicam as an analgesic and she remained well for 11 months before the owner presented her due to concern that she had become lethargic and reluctant to exercise. Thoracic radiographs revealed the presence of multiple metastatic lesions so the owners declined further treatment and she was euthanized.

SAFE HANDLING OF CHEMOTHERAPY IN PRACTICE

Please note: The notes in the next section are intended to provide guideline advice only. They in no way are intended to act as a definitive instruction manual as to how to handle cytotoxics in practice. For any clinicians wishing to handle any cytotoxic drugs the author has to recommend they contact their Health and Safety Executive representative to arrange appropriate special CoSHH training. The author and publisher in no way accept any responsibility for injury or harm that results from any colleague using or administering cytotoxic drugs without having received the appropriate training.

The use of cytotoxic drugs in veterinary medicine has to be seen as a serious health and safety issue because these drugs are potentially dangerous. Cytotoxics can have cumulative mutagenic, carcinogenic and terato-genic effects so it is absolutely vital to make every attempt to minimize the exposure of both staff and owners to the drugs and their metabolites. The HSE have strict guidelines as to the handling of these agents for human medicine and these rules apply in veterinary practice too. Therefore, any practices in the UK planning to use chemotherapy must draw up standard operating procedures and local rules of administration in conjunction with the 2002 CoSHH regulations, having undertaken a thorough risk assessment for each agent for which administration is planned. Further guidance on this can be found in Appendix 1 of the CoSHH Approved Code of Practice.

The first thing to consider is when are we most likely to be exposed to the cytotoxic agent we are using? The most common times we could be exposed are considered to be:

1. If a needle is withdrawn from a pressurised vial
2. Drug transfers between various types of equipment
3. When glass ampoules have to be broken open
4. When air has to be expelled from a syringe
5. Equipment that malfunctions, or that has been poorly set-up/maintained
6. The breaking or crushing of cytotoxics in tablet form
7. The excreta (including vomit) from patients receiving cytotoxic treatments.

Exposure is therefore most often through inhalation of aerosolized particles or direct absorption through skin contact as well as by indirect contact from unprotected hand-to-face contact or accidental ingestion from eating/drinking or smoking via hand-to-mouth contact. To ensure this does not occur the following advice should be considered:

1. Full and appropriate training as laid down in the standard operating procedures must be given to all staff involved in the storage, handling and administration of cytotoxic drugs and also to the staff involved in the care of the patients after they have received their treatments
2. Drug storage: All chemotherapeutics should be stored in a separate, secure lockable area away from other medications in a similar manner to that used for controlled drugs. They should be kept away from areas of food/drink preparation and stored in well-labelled, shatter-proof boxes (e.g. lockable

Tupperware). Each open bottle should be separately stored in a zip-lock bag (if multiple use is possible and anticipated) and then kept within the container. Certain drugs need to be dated and the strength marked on the bottle, as once reconstituted, they are only good for a certain period of time. It is vital to read the drug inserts and manufacturers' instructions regarding storage temperature and time and also to obtain the Material Safety Data Sheet (MSDS) from the manufacturer (which is separate to the data sheet usually found in the drug packaging) and details all of the chemical and physical properties of the drug and all of the precautions that should be taken when the drug is handled. All boxes should be labelled with chemotherapy and/or hazard labels (Fig. 3.21).

3. Drug preparation. It is best practice to write down all drug dosage calculations along with your workings even if it is a regular repeat administration. It is also highly recommended to always double-check your dosage, preferably with a colleague. Once the dose has been calculated you must put on appropriate protective clothing. This includes disposable, powder-free gloves (as powder may absorb chemotherapeutics) worn either singly or in a double-gloved fashion, ideally a respirator mask (although much more convenient it is not considered optimal to wear just a surgical mask), an impermeable gown with tight-fitting cuffs (a waterproof surgical gown would be suitable) and safety goggles. The author also wears waterproof over-sleeves (Fig. 3.22). All safety clothing is to be worn by both the clinician and his/her assistant. Staff members who are trying to conceive or may be pregnant, who are breastfeeding or, who are immunosuppressed, should refrain from

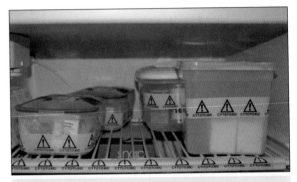

Figure 3.21 The storage of chemotherapeutics in carefully labelled containers in a labelled, safe location

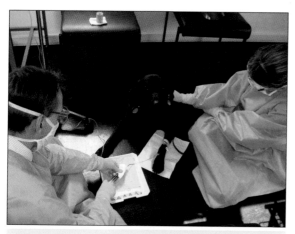

Figure 3.22 The author (RF) and an assistant administering doxorubicin to a Labrador retriever patient, illustrating the chemoprotective clothing worn, the absorbant surface just below the syringe in case of a spillage and the use of an alcohol-soaked swab around the needle

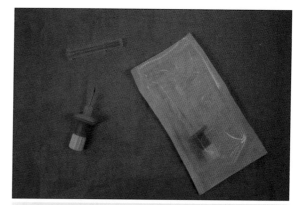

Figure 3.24 Chemo safety-pins, used to reconstitute and withdraw cytotoxics from their vials with reduced risk of aerosol formation

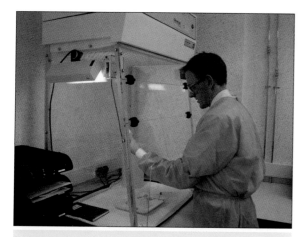

Figure 3.23 The author (RF) drawing up chemotherapy in a laminar flow fume cupboard of the type required to safely handle chemotherapeutics. Note that protective clothing is still worn to ensure protection from drug spillage

handling or being involved in the administration of chemotherapy at any time.

Extreme care has to be used when reconstituting chemotherapy drugs. In theory, all injectable cytotoxic drugs should be prepared in a class II biological safety vertical laminar flow cabinet (fume cupboard) (Fig. 3.23) and it has to be recommended that veterinary surgeons follow this practice. As very few practices other than specialist centres have a fume

cupboard, it may often be more appropriate to refer the patient on to your local oncology specialist, who does have the appropriate facilities to administer the treatments safely. Another alternative possibility is to see if your local general hospital's pharmacy would be happy to prepare all the drugs as required. But as such arrangements can be difficult and not always convenient these notes are intended to enable you to take every precaution to prepare, administer and manage cytotoxic drugs safely.

As a minimum, all clinicians reconstituting chemotherapeutics should wear a full-length waterproof gown, nitrile gloves, perspex goggles and a surgical face mask, or more ideally a respirator. If a mask is worn the mask should be fitted snugly onto the face to ensure that you are breathing through the mask rather than around the edges. It is imperative that mixing should be done in a well-ventilated area, away from draughts caused by vents or fans and away from where others are working. Plastic-backed, absorbent pads should be used to protect work surfaces from contamination. Luer-lock syringes and chemo safety pins are also recommended to reduce the chance of disconnection and aerosolization (Fig. 3.24). A chemo pin, or closed bottle system, is a safety device that is pushed into the top of a vial and provides additional security against excessive pressure within the vial, generating aerosolization and inhalation of the drug.

If a chemo pin is not available, use extreme care in maintaining slight negative to neutral pressure within the vial; never pressurize the vial. Select the syringes used to be as close to the volume required to ensure accuracy and to reduce exposure due to overfilling and spillage. To maintain negative pressure within the drug vial, inject a small amount of diluent if appropriate, followed by removal of a small amount of air. Wrap an alcohol-dampened swab around the top of the vial and needle exit site (Fig. 3.25). If needed, mix gently by swirling or rolling the vial to ensure that all the powder is in solution. Invert the vial and withdraw the drug slowly. Make sure not to push the 'air' out of the syringe; it will still contain small particles of the cytotoxic drug.

4. Injectable drug administration. Firstly, select an appropriately sized intravenous catheter, which has to be placed perfectly and taped in well, as described earlier. It is actually better to use a slightly smaller catheter than usually considered, as this ensures a good blood supply around the catheter and therefore optimal transportation of the drug through the circulation. If there is any suspicion that the catheter has not been placed perfectly (i.e. first time stick without difficulty) which may result in perivascular leakage of the drug, abandon that catheter and use a different leg with a fresh cannula. Once in place, flush the catheter well with at least 5 ml and ideally 10 ml of sterile saline flush to ensure patency and correct placement. The flush should not be heparinized because this may cause precipitation of some

drugs (e.g. doxorubicin). Any extension sets attached must be Leur lock and be tightened properly. The drug must then be administered as instructed, after which the catheter must be flushed well again before it is removed to ensure all traces of the drug are washed off the catheter tip (again, a minimum of 10 ml of sterile saline is recommended). Take care when removing the catheter to avoid splashing either you or your nurse.

If the chemotherapy drug is in a tablet form, such as cyclophosphamide in 'Endoxana' tablets, then the tablets must be kept within their blister packaging until they are needed. The person administering the tablets and any other assistant must wear disposable gloves and the medication given in as stress-free and as rapid a manner for the patient as is possible, ensuring that the tablet has been swallowed whole.

It is important to administer all chemotherapy in a dedicated room or area which is quiet and is not a thoroughfare. Warning signs should be placed on the door into the room indicating that chemotherapy is being administered and that access is restricted until the treatment has been completed (Fig. 3.26).

Place **all** contaminated/potentially contaminated materials (including your gloves) in a labelled cytotoxic waste bag (Fig. 3.27).

This bag must then itself be wrapped in a second, labelled cytotoxic bag, sealed and stored in an appropriate, impenetrable cytotoxic waste container (Fig. 3.28).

The waste must then be incinerated at appropriately licenced premises. Any bedding from the

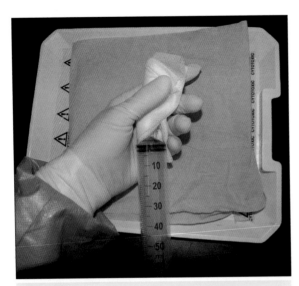

Figure 3.25 Use of an alcohol-soaked swab to help reduce the risk of aerosol leakage when drugs are withdrawn from their vials

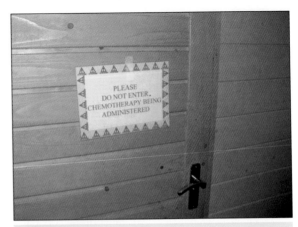

Figure 3.26 The warning sign placed on the outside of the chemotherapy room door whilst a treatment is being administered at the author's hospital

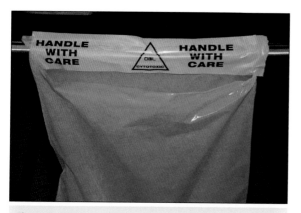

Figure 3.27 Place contaminated/potentially contaminated materials in a labelled cytotoxic waste bag

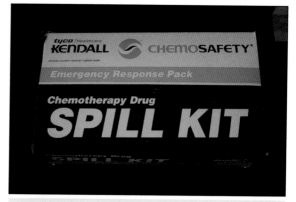

Figure 3.29 A commercially available spill kit, as used in the authors' hospitals

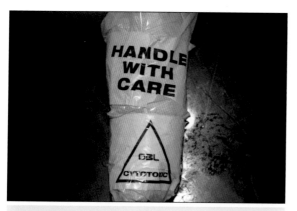

Figure 3.28 The first waste bag must be wrapped in a second, labelled cytotoxic bag, sealed and stored in an appropriate, inpenetratable cytotoxic waste container

patient must be handled whilst wearing gloves and should be washed separately.

5. What to do if there is a spillage?

All practices handling cytotoxic drugs must have a 'clean-up' protocol as part of their local rules, to be used following the accidental spillage of a cytotoxic drug. The protocol should have the following advice:

- Immediately restrict access to the area of the spill to the individual staff member(s) assigned to manage the problem.
- The staff member cleaning the problem should put on full protective clothing as for chemotherapy administration but with the addition of waterproof boots.
- Absorb any liquids using plastic-backed absorbable pads, such as incontinence pads.

- Make every effort not to pierce your gloves, place any broken glass into a puncture proof container (such as a dedicated sharps box).
- Collect any powders on dampened plastic-backed absorbable pads, such as an incontinence pad.
- Place all contaminated material in a properly labelled waterproof bag in the same way as you would at the end of a routine chemotherapy treatment and ensure its correct disposal.
- Carefully rinse all contaminated surfaces with copious quantities of water (remember to be aware of the risk of aerosolization!) then wash them with detergent and repeat this three times.
- Once finished, dispose of all protective clothing in the same way as the contaminated material was disposed of and then wash your hands thoroughly.

6. All practices should also have a 'spill kit' to be used in the event of an accidental drug spillage and this should contain (Fig. 3.29):
   - Four pairs of latex gloves or two pairs of the thicker nitrile gloves
   - A waterproof disposable surgical gown
   - Eye protection glasses
   - Respirator, or at least a face mask
   - Waterproof-backed absorbant pads and disposable paper towelling
   - A disposable scoop to help manage broken glass
   - A puncture-proof container in which to place glass shards
   - Chemo disposal bags and their labels.

7. Owner health and safety. It is imperative to remember that we have a duty of care to prevent accidental exposure of the owners to the chemotherapy follow-

DISCHARGE INSTRUCTIONS FOR PATIENT

X
....

Date ....???...................................

• ....X............... was re-examined today with a view to performing her ....???......... chemotherapy treatment
• Cinical examination revealed her to be ....???.........
• The complete blood count revealed a normal haemogram
• I therefore administered ....?........ mg of ....???................ via her right cephalic vein without incident
• If ....X............... should vomit at any time over the next 5 days, then you have to assume that the vomitus is cytotoxic (i.e. dangerous). Clear the area of anyone else and put on some waterproof gloves. DO NOT TOUCH THE VOMIT WITH YOUR BARE SKIN. Cover the vomit with as much kitchen towel as you can to absorb it. Then cover the kitchen towel with a plastic bag and carefully turn the bag inside out so that it contains the vomit/kitchen paper mass. Place this bag inside another plastic bag for safety. Then clean the floor very slowly and carefully, trying not to be too vigorous and produce an aerosol of any cytotoxic agent that may be left behind. Ideally, use a mop to clean so that you are a distance away from the floor. Once clean, allow to dry naturally and do not allow anyone to touch the floor until it is dry
• Please avoid contact with any bodily fluids (urine, faeces and saliva) from ....X............. for the next 72 hours, as some of the treatment can be excreted via these routes
• I suggest that you also wear a glove to handle any bags you use to pick up ....X........ 's faeces for the next 5 days
• If someone in your family or a friend who will have contact with ....X............... is, or might be, pregnant, then please take every care to avoid contact with bodily fluids as outlined above. Young children need to be protected in a similar manner
• Please can we see her again in ......?...... weeks' time to give ....X........... her next treatment
• Please feel free to call me if you have any questions or concerns whatsoever

Signed ....

Figure 3.30 Discharge instructions for patient X

ing their dog or cat's treatment. We therefore need to counsel owners carefully of the potential risks to them with regard to exposure to potentially cytotoxic metabolites, especially if there are children in the family or if a family member is, or could be, pregnant. The main risks of exposure once the animal is at home come through urine, faeces, saliva or vomitus. It is therefore good practice to send all chemotherapy patients home with special discharge instructions, an example of which is shown in Figure 3.30.

All of the health and safety aspects of chemotherapy administration may seem daunting, but with practice and careful consideration, it is possible to give safe and efficacious treatment in most practice settings. It is definitely advisable to adopt a 'better safe than sorry' approach, but as long as this is undertaken, the safety of the patient, the veterinary staff and the owner will not be compromised. If it is not deemed safe to administer the treatments within the practice then referral to an oncology specialist is highly recommended.

4 Principles of cancer radiotherapy

Radiotherapy is an extremely effective treatment modality in the management of cancer patients, either as a single treatment or as part of a multimodality protocol. Ionizing radiation kills cells via the deposition of energy in, or near to, the cellular DNA, either causing DNA damage directly or via the production of free radicals within the cell. As with chemotherapy, however, ionizing radiation cannot differentiate between normal cells and neoplastic cells, so any proliferating cells will be damaged. Tumour cells are 'selectively' targeted by their increased growth fraction, whereas normal cells that divide more slowly may not be affected so acutely. It is therefore important to realize that radiotherapy can cause both 'early' and 'late' side effects in non-cancerous tissues. Cells that divide rapidly and frequently as part of normal physiology, such as epithelial stem cells, are likely to show the side effects of radiotherapy earlier than tissues comprised of cells that divide more slowly. As with chemotherapy, the total dose that can be given to a patient depends upon the side effects, but with radiotherapy it is very important to always be aware of the possible late side effects that could occur. Early side effects can be minimized by dividing the total dose into a number of 'fractions', administered over a period of time.

In 1975, Withers described the 'Four Rs' of radiotherapy (Repair, Redistribution, Reoxygenation and Repopulation) to explain the fact that giving small doses more frequently seemed to be more effective than giving fewer large doses. In human medicine, most patients will receive at least 20 fractions, often given at daily intervals to enable a higher total dose to be given without the risk of horrendous early side effects (e.g. deep blistering and cutaneous burning). This approach is now being used in canine patients in the USA, where many centres now use a Monday–Friday treatment schedule and give between 18 and 21 fractions over a 3–4-week period, depending upon the tumour type and location. In the UK, however, it has been more commonplace to use a different approach by utilizing what is known as 'hypo-fractionated' regimens, where most patients receive just four or five treatments at weekly intervals, although hyperfractionation is becoming more commonplace. The reasoning behind the use of hypofractionated radiotherapy is several-fold:

- It is often more convenient for owners to come once a week.
- It means the patients only have to receive 4 or 5 anaesthetics, rather than 18–21.
- It keeps the cost reasonable.
- The incidence of acute side effects is generally substantially lower than that seen with hyperfractionated regimens.

In the light of the fact that the incidence of side effects seen by using this approach is very low indeed, it could be argued that this is a more acceptable form of treatment for veterinary patients compared to hyperfractionated regimens, even though it does go against some of the theories in the four Rs. However, in general, the survival times reported by the US veterinary schools is superior to that reported in the UK, so there are two sides to the argument! The newer radiation centres in the UK are moving towards administering more hyperfractionated regimens, so it is likely that more frequent radiation treatments will become the normality in the UK in the near future.

Ionizing radiation can be delivered via an external source (teletherapy or external beam radiation), through placement of radioactive isotopes interstitially (brachytherapy) or by systemic or intracavitary injection of radioisotopes such as ^{131}I. External beam radiation can then be further divided depending upon the energy of the photons involved into orthovoltage or megavoltage therapy, where an orthovoltage machine produces X-rays with an energy of 150–500 keV, whilst a megavoltage machine produces photons with an average energy of over 1 million electron volts (1 MeV). The advantage of megavoltage therapy is that the beam has a much greater penetrating power compared to orthovoltage beams, so deep tumours can be treated. Radiation therapy can also be in the form of an electron beam, which has little penetration power but can therefore be useful in the treatment of some cutaneous tumours such as mast cell tumours.

Tumours which may be amenable to radiotherapy treatment include:

- Oral tumours, such as oral squamous cell carcinomas (SCC), oral malignant melanomas (MM) and fibrosarcomas (FSA). For these tumours, radiation therapy is best used as an adjunct to surgery, although the use of radiation in malignant melanomas sadly does not reduce the incidence of metastases in this very aggressive tumour, even though the primary tumours themselves seem to be quite radiation responsive. Oral SCCs in cats can, theoretically, be treated with radiotherapy, but the location is very important because many of these tumours are sublingual and the risk of radiation toxicity here is high.

- Nasal tumours – radiotherapy is the treatment of choice for these tumours, providing good local control with far less invasive treatment than surgery and interestingly, the addition of surgery to radiotherapy treatment for nasal tumours probably does not enhance life expectancy. Some studies have shown that the use of substances (e.g. cisplatin, doxorubicin) to sensitize the tumour to the radiotherapy is also of benefit in nasal tumours in veterinary patients.

- Brain tumours – many can be successfully treated with radiotherapy, with studies showing median survival times of up to 1 year in dogs and cats for whom neurosurgery is not possible, depending on the tumour type. In particular, the author has had successful experience in treating pituitary tumours causing acromegaly in cats and also in treating pituitary macroadenomas in Cushingoid dogs. However, there can be a concern over delayed radiation side effects in some situations. One problem with the use of radiotherapy in brain conditions is the need to obtain good-quality MRI or CT images with which the therapy can be planned beforehand, but with the rapidly increasing availability of such facilities, this is becoming less of an obstacle than it once was.

- Limb tumours – mast cell tumours and soft-tissue sarcomas can be treated with radiotherapy, almost always following an attempt at surgical resection. External beam radiotherapy can also be useful to shrink mast cell tumours before surgery if the primary tumour is big. There may also be a role for radiation therapy in vaccine-associated sarcomas in cats, although there is considerable risk of spinal cord necrosis as a late side effect, so the usefulness of radiation in these cases is limited.

- Lymphoma – lymphocytes are exquisitely sensitive to radiation, so there are studies showing the usefulness of such therapy as part of the treatment of lymphoma. However, this is rarely (if ever) used in the UK, other than for nasal lymphoma in cats.

- Osteosarcoma – radiotherapy has been used as a palliative treatment to provide analgesia in canine osteosarcoma.

Unfortunately, there are still only four radiotherapy centres for animals in the UK at the time of writing. However, it is likely that there will be others developing in the near future, so radiotherapy is a treatment modality that should be actively considered in appropriate cases, either as a first-line treatment for cases such as nasal tumours, or as an adjunctive treatment following surgical excision of the tumour.

The cancer patient with sneezing and/or nasal discharge

Nasal neoplasia accounts for 1% of tumours in dogs, is considered less common in cats and has also been reported in rabbits. Therefore, although not particularly common in general practice, such cases can generate a diagnostic challenge for practitioners due to the difficulty in directly visualizing the tumour mass. The prevalence of tumour type varies between dogs and cats (dogs: epithelial > mesenchymal > lymphoid; cats: lymphoid > epithelial >mesenchymal; see Box 5.1) and the clinical signs that nasal cancer patients present with can also vary. However, in the majority of cases the clinical signs will be gradually progressive, meaning that patients presenting with recurring or worsening clinical signs warrant further or repeated evaluation. The increasing availability of advanced imaging modalities such as MRI and CT scanning have improved our ability to make accurate and early diagnoses, so the referral of patients to suitably equipped specialist centres with clinical signs that may be attributable to nasal tumours should be considered if possible.

CLINICAL CASE EXAMPLE 5.1 – CANINE NASAL ADENOCARCINOMA

Signalment

9-year-old neutered male Irish setter.

Presenting signs

Right-sided uniliateral serosanguineous nasal discharge which progressed to intermittent epistaxis, and sneezing (Fig. 5.1).

Case history

The relevant history in this particular case was:
- owner first noticed the dog having a runny right nostril compared to the left nostril 2 months previously

- dog then started to sneeze approximately 2 weeks later and the owner also noticed he had started to snore when he was asleep
- the nasal discharge progressed to become thicker and then it became bloody, hence bringing the dog for examination
- otherwise very bright with no other apparent problems.

Clinical examination

The examination revealed:
- Normal facial anatomy and no pain on palpation of the skull
- Obvious haemorrhagic nasal discharge from the right nostril
- No apparent airflow down the right nostril
- No evidence of depigmentation on the nasal planum
- No enlargement of the submandibular lymph nodes
- No intraoral lesions
- Remainder of examination unremarkable.

Differential diagnosis

- Nasal tumour (usually unilateral discharge in early stages, can progress to become bilateral)
- Nasal aspergillosis (can cause unilateral or bilateral discharge)
- Non-fungal rhinitis; bacterial, allergic or idiopathic (usually causes bilateral discharge)
- Nasal foreign body (usually unilateral discharge)
- Systemic coagulopathy (if discharge significantly/ purely haemorrhagic).

Diagnostic evaluation

The dog was anaesthetized and an intraoral radiograph was suggestive of the presence of a soft-tissue mass (Fig. 5.2). The dog was then given an MRI scan, which clearly showed the presence of an intranasal tumour as shown in Figure 5.3.

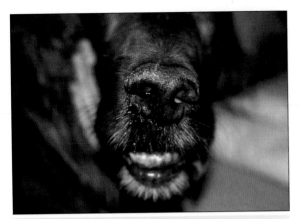

Figure 5.1 *Case 5.1* The dog at presentation, revealing the unilateral epistaxis (courtesy of Nick Bacon, University of Florida)

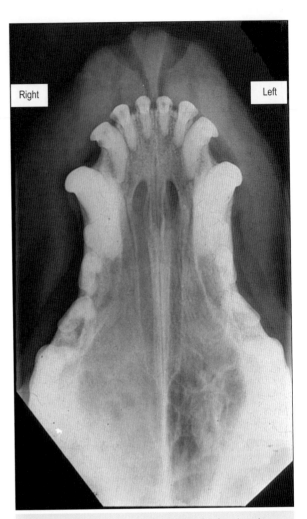

Figure 5.2 *Case 5.1* Intraoral radiograph, showing the loss of turbinate detail and increased radiodensity in the right nasal chamber but no evidence of change in the left nasal chamber

A complete blood count and whole blood clotting time had been assessed and found to be normal before the diagnostic imaging procedure, so whilst remaining under anaesthesia, rigid biopsy forceps were used to obtain several pieces of the tumour for histopathology as shown in Figure 5.4. The histopathology returned to show the mass was an adenocarcinoma.

The dog underwent external beam radiotherapy using a hypofractionated course (i.e. one treatment a week for four consecutive weeks) as described. His clinical signs totally resolved by the third treatment and he remained clinically well for 12 months. He then began to develop unilateral serous nasal discharge again from the right nostril which rapidly progressed to frank haemorrhage and he was euthanized 2½ months after the signs returned.

Theory refresher

Canine nasal tumours are most commonly seen in middle-aged to older dolycephalic dogs but can occur in any breed. Nasal tumours in young dogs would be considered unusual. Medium- to large-breed dogs are more commonly affected and there is some evidence to suggest a possible increase in incidence in dogs living in an urban environment. The initial clinical signs usually involve intermittent unilateral nasal discharge (Fig. 5.5) that progresses over a period typically of 2–3 months to a serosangeous discharge and/or frank epistaxis that may also become bilateral. Occasionally the first presenting sign will be unilateral or bilateral epistaxis or simply a swelling in the region of the nares, nasal planum or frontal sinuses but these signs would be less common

as a primary presenting problem. In cases where the tumour is located in either the frontal sinus(es) or the caudal aspect of the nasal cavity, the presenting complaint may initially be considered as a neurological condition (presenting with dullness, depression, head pressing or possibly seizures) but again this would be a less frequent appearance. More commonly, many owners will report that the dog has developed loud snoring or a gurgling sound when asleep and sneezing is also commonly reported. Otherwise many patients will appear normal to their owners in the early stages of the disease.

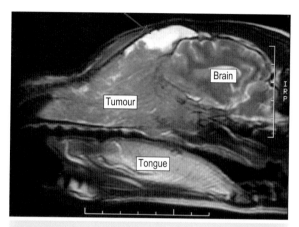

Figure 5.3 *Case 5.1* Sagittal plane T2-weighted MRI scan, revealing a large mass structure filling the right nasal chamber and extending caudally into the rostral portion of the nasopharynx. The scan also reveals the presence of fluid filling the frontal sinus (red arrow) due to obstruction of the frontomaxillary opening by the tumour

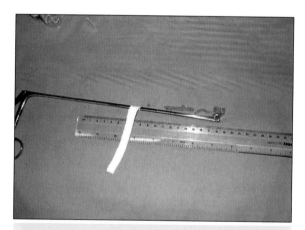

Figure 5.4 *Case 5.1* The rigid forceps used and one of the biopsy samples obtained. The piece of tape was the measurement of length from the medial canthus to the nostril and placement of the tape was to ensure that the forceps were not advanced too far into the nasal cavity, thereby preventing damage to, or penetration through, the cribiform plate

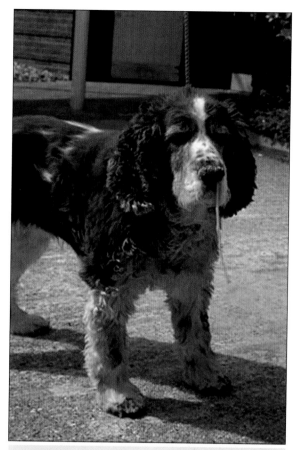

Figure 5.5 An elderly springer spaniel with typical mucoid nasal discharge associated with a nasal tumour. Courtesy of Dr Richard Mellanby, University of Edinburgh

CLINICAL TIP

Any patient, but particularly older dogs, presenting with unilateral nasal discharge, epistaxis or the development of snoring noises should be considered for nasal tumour work-up.

Examination

General clinical examination in a nasal tumour patient is often unremarkable but particular attention should be paid to careful visual examination of the nares and palpation along the entire nasal planum, periorbital region and over the location of the frontal sinuses. Nasal airflow should always be assessed in both nostrils (either by placing a chilled microscope slide near the nostrils, or simply assessing whether there is movement of strands of cotton wool) as there is frequently markedly reduced or absent airflow on the affected side. The presence of unilateral nasal discharge or epistaxis is highly suspicious for a nasal tumour in a middle-aged to older medium- to large-breed dog. Other aspects of the clinical examination to evaluate include careful palpation of the submandibular lymph node chain (local metastases are reported to occur in only 10% of patients at initial diagnosis but these cases need to be identified due to the implications for further evaluation and for the treatment) and a visual oral examination.

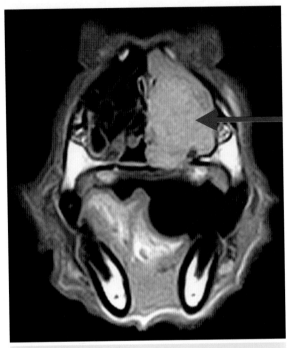

Figure 5.6 The same spaniel as in Figure 5.5, showing the transverse MRI scan of the dog's nose, confirming the presence of a unilateral left-sided tumour (as shown by the red arrow) Courtesy of Dr Richard Mellanby, University of Edinburgh

Box 5.1 Common malignant and benign tumours of the nasal cavity

Common malignant tumours of the nasal cavity	Benign tumours of the nasal cavity
Carcinoma	Fibromas
Adenocarcinoma	Polyps
Squamous cell carcinoma	Low-grade mesenchymal
Sarcomas	tumours (sarcoma)
Fibrosarcoma	
Chondrosarcoma	
Osteosarcoma	
Lymphoma	
Melanoma	

Diagnostic imaging

Nasal radiographs can be useful to reveal evidence of turbinate destruction and the presence of soft-tissue opacity within one or both nasal chambers, but the use of MRI or CT scanning increases the diagnostic sensitivity and gives clear detail regarding the size and extent of the lesion, factors that can prove to be very important when planning treatment (Fig. 5.6). If advanced imaging techniques are not available then the radiographic views that should be obtained are intraoral or open-mouth oblique views to view the nasal cavity and also a skyline sinus view to image the frontal sinus.

CLINICAL TIP

When obtaining nasal radiographs, it is essential to obtain an intraoral view without the superimposition of the mandible in the image.

Biopsy

Direct visualization of a mass may also be possible using either a flexible or rigid endoscope. Identification of a mass via any imaging modality, however, does not generate a specific diagnosis, so tissue biopsy for histopathology is always required for definitive diagnosis. Cytological analysis of nasal wash fluid frequently fails to produce adequate samples and therefore this technique should not be relied on as the sole means of diagnosis and is a practice the authors now rarely use, although it can

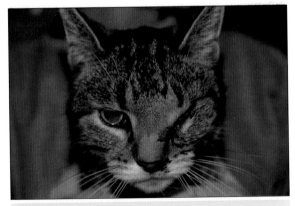

Figure 5.7 An 8-year-old DSH cat with marked nasal swelling and deformation. An MRI scan confirmed there to be a sinonasal tumour present which was confirmed as a carcinoma on histopathology

occasionally prove to be useful. Biopsies can be obtained using flexible endoscopic biopsy forceps (although these only produce small tissue samples), cup forceps or a Volkman spoon. When obtaining biopsies it is essential to ensure the tip of the biopsy instrument is not advanced beyond the medial canthus so as to avoid penetrating through the cribiform plate into the cranial cavity. Obtaining these tissue samples will result in haemorrhage that may seem significant, but this usually stops within a few minutes. It is recommended to assess the platelet count and a whole blood clotting time as a minimum data base before undertaking a nasal biopsy procedure.

> ### NURSING TIP
>
> In case there is haemorrhage when a nasal turbinate biopsy is undertaken, it is advisable to pack the throat with a swab bandage prior to obtaining the biopsies to reduce the possibility of airway compromise and aspiration, but remember to remove this before the animal is recovered!

Whilst attempting to obtain a diagnosis, it is important to undertake clinical staging of the patient to determine the extent of the disease should a tumour be diagnosed. The submandibular lymph nodes need to be carefully palpated and aspirated if enlarged, as cytological evaluation of the lymph nodes is extremely useful to distinguish between a reactive lymphadenopathy and metastatic disease. Canine nasal carcinomas are found to have metastasized to the region lymph nodes in up to 10% of cases. Thoracic radiographs should be considered but they rarely show metastatic disease at initial presentation.

Treatment

Once a definitive diagnosis has been reached, treatment can be planned. Currently the treatment of choice is considered to be external beam radiation therapy with remission times of 8–25 months being reported in the USA following hyperfractionated radiotherapy. In the UK hypofractionated radiotherapy (4 × 8–9 Gy fractions given once every 7 days) is the form of treatment usually available (although hyperfractionated protocols are available) and this also provides good palliative treatment with mean survival times of between 9 and 15 months. One study reported 1-year survival rates of 45% and 2-year survival rates of 15%. Clinical findings that

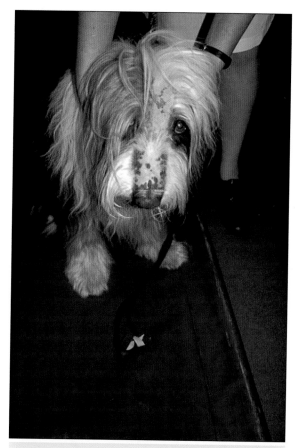

Figure 5.8 'Significant' radiation-induced alopecia in a patient with a nasal carcinoma which underwent otherwise successful hypofractionated treatment

are indicative of a poorer prognosis are the presence of facial swelling, exophthalmos, the identification of bilateral nasal chamber involvement or invasion of the tumour into the oral cavity (unusual). Patients with these more severe clinical signs should still be considered eligible to receive treatment if possible but their response to therapy is less likely to be successful and any remission generated is likely to be for a shorter period of time than patients with a unilateral tumour that is not causing facial swelling or exophthalmos (Fig. 5.7). Surgical removal of the tumours with curative intent is usually not possible and offers no advantages and several considerable disadvantages compared to radiotherapy. In countries where there are no radiotherapy facilities, then the use of chemotherapy with debaulking surgery has been reported with reasonable results. However, the most consistent results are obtained using external beam

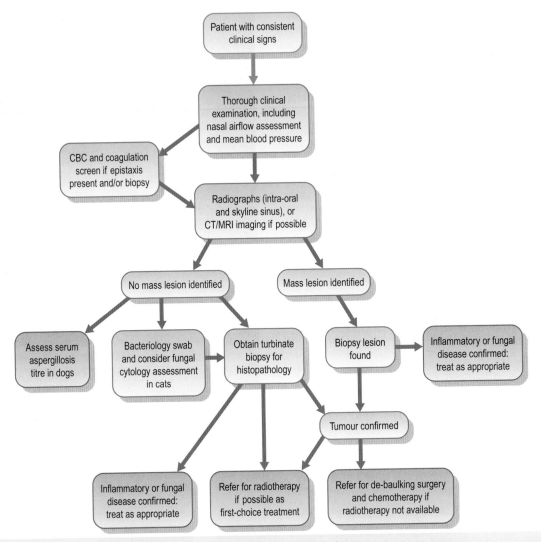

Figure 5.9 Diagnostic plan flowchart for patients with sneezing or nasal discharge

radiotherapy so referral for this treatment should be recommended whenever possible.

Coarse fractionation radiotherapy as used in the UK rarely causes any significant side effects and is extremely well tolerated by the patients. Some dogs experience mild cutaneous erythema, and occasionally alopecia, in the shape of the radiation field as shown in Figure 5.8. A minority of patients will experience oral side effects such as mucositis but these are usually easily controlled with either antibiotics and/or NSAIDs. The clinical signs are also usually very well controlled and many dogs will return to a normal quality of life whilst in remission even though the treatment is rarely curative.

Rabbit nasal tumours

Sneezing and nasal discharges can be seen in rabbits with nasal turbinate carcinoma. The differential diagnoses for these clinical signs include chronic upper respiratory disease and dental disease, so a nasal tumour should be considered in patients in whom these conditions can be ruled out. Establishing a definitive diagnosis is usually by endoscopy and biopsy of the affected nasal tissue. The current treatment recommendation, however, is mainly supportive therapy only, and includes providing analgesia, antibiosis and nebulization. Laser ablation of nasal tissue has been reported as a palliative measure and could be considered where this is available. Other differential diagnoses include osteomyelitis due to dental disease or mandibular osteosarcoma; these can be differentiated by radiography or computed tomography of the head. Hemimandibulectomies have also been reported in the literature if the diagnosis is made of a mandibular tumour.

Conclusions

The diagnostic evaluation plan for any patient with sneezing or nasal discharge is shown in Figure 5.9. The basic approach is to actively pursue a diagnosis of nasal tumour whilst ruling out the other major differential diagnoses, as listed in Box 5.1.

CLINICAL CASE EXAMPLE 5.2 – FELINE INTRANASAL LYMPHOMA

Signalment

8-year-old neutered female domestic short-haired (DSH) cat.

Presenting signs

Sneezing and nasal discharge.

Case history

The relevant history in this particular case was:
- The cat was generally well but had started to sneeze 4 weeks prior to presentation.
- The owner described the cat as having a thick, mucoid nasal discharge which was predominately left sided.
- Since the discharge had developed, her appetite had reduced and she had become picky and less keen to eat.

Clinical examination

The examination revealed:
- Normal facial anatomy and no pain on palpation of the skull
- Thick mucoid nasal discharge from the left nostril
- No apparent airflow down the left nostril
- No evidence of depigmentation on the nasal planum
- No enlargement of the submandibular lymph nodes
- No intraoral lesions
- The remainder of the examination was unremarkable.

Differential diagnosis

- Nasal tumour
- Fungal rhinitis

- Non-fungal rhinitis; bacterial, allergic or idiopathic
- Nasopharyngeal foreign body.

Diagnostic evaluation

A sample of the nasal mucus was assessed cytologically to look for fungal hyphae but this was negative, so the cat was anaesthetized for a more detailed examination and diagnostic imaging. Retroflexed rhinoscopy revealed no evidence of a foreign body within the nasopharynx. Direct rhinoscopy was difficult due to the quantity of mucus present which proved to be tenacious despite extensive lavage. However, it was possible to establish that the turbinates appeared erythematous and irregular. Due to cost constraints, no MRI was undertaken, but intraoral radiographs were obtained, which revealed a generalized increase in opacity in the left nasal chamber. Turbinate biopsies were obtained using gastroscopic grab forceps and histopathology confirmed the diagnosis to be nasal lymphoma.

Theory refresher

Lymphoma is the most common form of nasal tumour reported in cats. In most cases the tumour will exist as a solitary lesion but multiorgan involvement has been reported in up to 20% of cases, including involvement of the brain. It is usually seen in middle-aged to older cats (and these are usually FeLV negative) and causes similar clinical signs to those reported in the dog, namely nasal discharge (again, usually unilateral in the early stages of the disease), sneezing, facial deformity and epistaxis. Some cats will become inappetant, presumably due to bilateral nasal chamber obstruction preventing the cat from smelling and tasting food normally. Aside from lymphoma, adenocarcinomas and sarcomas of various cell types have been reported.

Diagnostic approach

If a cat presents with clinical signs that could be consistent with a nasal tumour, then the diagnostic approach is very similar to that taken in the dog. The main differential diagnoses are inflammatory/allergic rhinitis, fungal rhinitis and tumour disease, so a thorough clinical examination must firstly be performed, especially in the light of the fact that multiorgan involvement has been reported to occur, albeit in a minority of cases. Once this has been completed, investigation of the nasal passages themselves should be undertaken, using intraoral radiographs, CT or MRI imaging, possibly in conjunction with rhinoscopy. Rhinoscopy in cats can be a little difficult due to the limited width of the external nares, but a fine rigid arthroscope can often provide excellent images of a lesion and allow thorough examination of the nasal passages. The authors do not find cytological analysis on nasal flush samples particularly useful to diagnose neoplasia and so do not routinely perform such a procedure, although lymphoma cells are probably more likely to exfoliate than an epithelial or mesenchymal tumour cell population. Cytological evaluation of squash preparations taken from biopsy samples has recently been shown to have a high degree of correlation with the histological diagnosis, so this technique should be considered to enable the clinician to establish whether or not a lesion appears inflammatory or neoplastic as quickly as possible. Cytological analysis of any nasal discharge is often also worth considering, as some cases of fungal rhinitis may be diagnosed this way. Should the imaging be suggestive of a mass lesion, however, then attempting to obtain tissue for histological analysis is essential and for this the authors would consider either using gastroscopy forceps (the larger their diameter, the better!) or a small Volkmann spoon to gather the tissue. Several samples should be acquired having previously undertaken a coagulation assessment (OSPT and APTT measurement) and a complete blood count to help minimize the risk of haemorrhage.

Treatment

Should a diagnosis of nasal lymphoma be confirmed and the disease is only located within the nasal cavity, local treatment can be undertaken using external beam radiotherapy as opposed to systemic chemotherapy. However, if there is any evidence of distant or multiorgan disease, then undertaking systemic chemotherapy has to be considered as the only sensible option. For non-lymphoid tumours, external beam radiotherapy is usually the appropriate first-line treatment in cats, as it is in dogs. Using a coarse fractionation protocol as often used in the UK, one study has shown a median survival time of 382 days for cats with non-lymphoid nasal tumours and a 1-year survival rate of 63%. Cats also appear to tolerate this treatment well, so it should definitely be considered when a diagnosis of a nasal tumour is made in a cat.

CLINICAL CASE EXAMPLE 5.3 – A FELINE NASAL PLANUM CARCINOMA

Signalment

12-year-old neutered male DSH cat.

Presenting signs

An erosive, ulcerated lesion on the nasal planum.

Case history

The relevant history in this case was:
- The cat had been systemically well throughout his life and, other than for routine vaccination and neutering, had had no cause to go to the vet.
- Over the preceding year, the owner had noticed small, black-red-coloured scabs to be present on the pink areas of his nose, which had gradually grown and coalesced to the point where there was one large scab and an underlying ulcer.
- The owner did not think that there was any nasal discharge or sneezing.

Clinical examination

The clinical examination revealed:
- The cat to be in generally good condition
- Obvious darkly pigmented scab with evidence of underlying ulceration of the nasal planum (Fig. 5.10)
- No evidence of enlargement of the submandibular lymph nodes
- No intraoral lesions
- The remainder of the examination was unremarkable.

Differential diagnoses

- Nasal planum neoplasia
  - Squamous cell carcinoma
- Eosinophilic granuloma
- Immune-mediated disease
- Trauma.

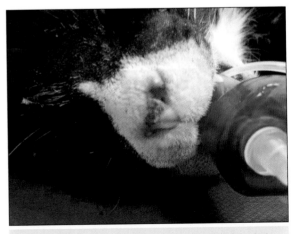

Figure 5.10 *Case 5.3* The cat awaiting biopsy of the lesion

Diagnostic evaluation

In view of the lengthy time course over which the owner reported lesions to have been present and the resulting likelihood of the diagnosis being a squamous cell carcinoma (SCC), it was decided to take a deep wedge biopsy of the affected area without undertaking any further diagnostic imaging. Due to the cat's age, a serum biochemistry profile was undertaken to rule out pre-existing renal disease but once this returned to be normal, the cat underwent the biopsy procedure under a brief general anaesthetic. Histopathological evaluation from a deep punch biopsy of the tissue confirmed the diagnosis to be an SCC with deep infiltration into the underlying dermis. The cat was therefore treated by surgical 'nosectomy' and was alive with no signs of recurrence 12 months later.

'Noesectomies' involve making a 360° skin incision around the skin just caudal to the nasal planum. The surgeon then transects the underlying turbinates to free the nasal planum itself and remove it. Haemostasis should be achieved using digital pressure and swabs as required and overzealous use of electrocautery is to be avoided. Once the planum has been removed, the skin should be sutured to the exposed nasal mucosa using a simple continuous pattern (Figs 5.12–5.14). Good suture placement usually aids haemostasis considerably. Post-operatively the patients must wear a Buster collar to prevent rubbing of the surgical site and early suture removal. Good analgesia is essential and all patients should receive combined opioid and NSAID analgesia both before, during and after surgery. The maxillary branch of the trigeminal nerve can be blocked using either 2% lignocaine or 0.5% bupivicaine, by instilling 0.1–0.3 ml at the intraorbital foramen as the infraorbital nerve exits the foramen. The infraorbital foramen is not easily palpated in the cat, but its location can be established through the normal facial anatomy and the injection made transcutaneously, as shown in Figure 5.11, or transorally.

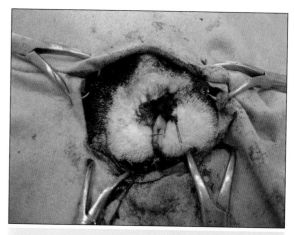

Figure 5.12 *Case 5.3* Intraoperative picture during the treatment surgery showing the appearance once the nasal planum has been removed. Note the use of a simple continuous suture pattern to oppose the skin with the nasal mucosa

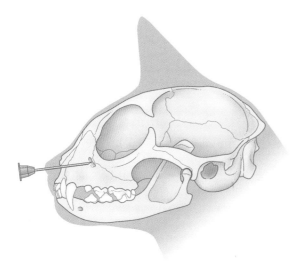

Figure 5.11 Injection site for the infraorbital foramen

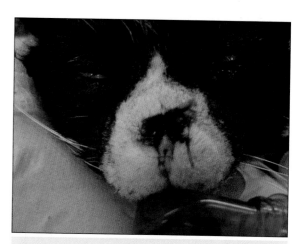

Figure 5.13 *Case 5.3* The appearance of the cat at the end of surgery

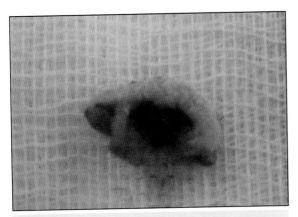

Figure 5.14 *Case 5.3* The excised nasal planum with the tumour clearly visible

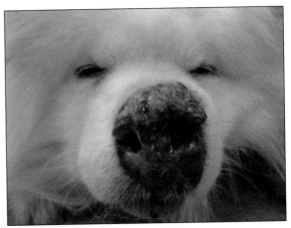

Figure 5.15

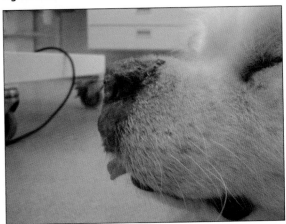

Figure 5.16

Figures 5.15, 5.16 A Siberian husky with a slow-growing, ulcerative and proliferative lesion on the nasal planum. Deep wedge biopsy revealed the diagnosis to be one of squamous cell carcinoma (SCC)

NURSING TIP

Patients who have undergone nosectomy may require some encouragement to eat, so it is certainly worth warming their food and offering the animal's 'favourite' food.

NURSING TIP

Although the nosectomy wound site should be left to heal if possible, some patients do experience significant blockage of the nasal passages by blood clots and inflammatory exudate. Gentle cleaning of the nasal orifice therefore may be required and patients should be monitored closely for this.

Theory refresher

Tumours of the nasal planum are relatively common in the cat, but are considered unusual in the dog. In the cat, the tumours are usually found on poorly pigmented areas of skin (and therefore can also be found on the pinnae [usually tips first] or nictitating membrane) in middle-aged to older white or tortoise-shell-coloured animals. This is thought to be due to increased exposure to ultraviolet light in these cases acting as a transforming trigger factor in animals with a predisposition to the condition created by their pigmentation. Indeed, some owners will think that their cat simply has sunburn on its nose. In dogs, SCC can develop both on the external surface of the nostril or within the nose on the nasal mucosa (Figs 5.15–5.18).

Typically, these tumours are quite slow-growing and start with just a small scab lesion(s) but they will progress over a course of usually at least several months to become ulcerative lesions that may haemorrhage intermittently. They can also appear proliferative. In dogs a significant number will originate intranasally. Frequently, most cats do not appear to be particularly distressed by the presence of the lesion but some dogs appear to find them painful depending on how extensive the lesion is. The tumours are locally invasive and can become

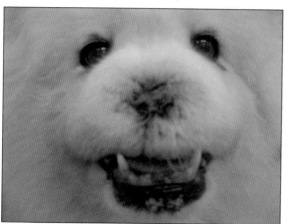

Figure 5.17

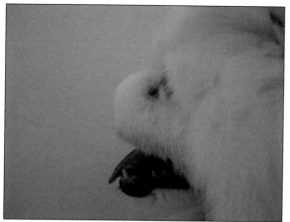

Figure 5.18

Figures 5.17, 5.18 The same dog as in Figures 5.15 and 5.16 6 months following 'nosectomy' surgery, which also involved a rostral maxillectomy due to the extensive nature of the mass. Clinically the dog was very well and was not exhibiting any difficulties following the surgery

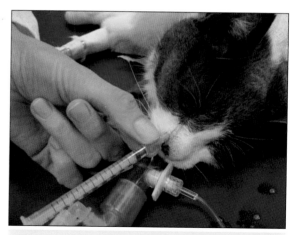

Figure 5.19 Placement of a local nerve block using bupivicaine before a biopsy procedure in a cat with a nasal planum SCC

quite large, but they rarely metastasize and if they do spread, it is usually late in the disease course, meaning that local disease recurrence is of prime concern. Obtaining as definitive a treatment as possible therefore becomes very important to try to effect a curative treatment in these patients.

Diagnosis

In this situation, obtaining a diagnosis by a deep wedge biopsy is the best option as it provides not only a clear histological diagnosis but also indicates the depth that the tumour extends into the tissue. This is very important when deciding which treatment modality will be most appropriate for the patient. Usually, only routine preoperative assessments need to be carried out, as diagnostic imaging rarely provides more useful information in the cat, but in dogs the lesions can often extend significantly caudally, so CT or MRI scanning can be very helpful in this species to indicate how deep the lesion is and therefore help plan definitive surgery. What should definitely be considered is the sensitivity of the skin in this area and much attention should be placed in analgesia both pre- and post-biopsy. In particular, local nerve blocks can be extremely useful to help keep postoperative discomfort to a minimum (Figs 5.11 and 5.19).

Treatment

The answer as to how best to treat these cases depends predominantly on the depth the tumour extends into the underlying tissue, but also whether you are a surgeon or not! In a case series detailing 61 feline cases (including cats with tumours on both the nasal planum and the pinnae), surgery was found to confer the longest disease-free period but treatment has also been described using external beam radiation therapy, cryotherapy, photodynamic therapy and intralesional chemotherapy as alternatives to surgery. Surgery has to be considered as the first-line treatment for both superficial and especially deep lesions because of its success in achieving clean margins and therefore increasing the chance of a good outcome. Superficial tumours may be treated successfully with one of the other modalities listed above. A similar outcome has been reported in dogs. A series of 17 cases of nasal planum SCC in the dog found that surgical resection of the diseased tissue provided the best outcome. Even if the disease is found to be extensive, a more recent study has shown that dogs tolerate nosectomy and rostral maxillectomy up to the level of pre-molar 3 very well and that surgical margins can be obtained using such a technique, leading to low recurrence rates and long disease-free periods. Surgery should always therefore be considered as the treatment of choice.

Photodynamic therapy (PDT) is a technique which utilizes the properties of photosensitive chemicals. These, when exposed to the appropriate wavelength of light, produce a photochemical reaction which produces reactive oxygen species (free radicals) that cause apoptosis if the photosensitizer is present within a cell. Various photosensitizers have been found to be preferentially taken up by neoplastic tissue (either following systemic or local, topical application) and therefore these substances can be utilized as anticancer agents when exposed to the applicable wavelength of light. Because cell death is through apoptosis, the affected tissue heals in a relatively scar-free manner and PDT frequently produces a much more cosmetically acceptable result in the mind of some owners. Topical 5-aminolevulinic acid (5-ALA) cream has been used successfully to treat cats with nasal planum SCC, as this is preferentially taken up and metabolized by malignant epithelial cells into a potent photosensitizer (protoporphyrin IX), meaning that the treatment can be targeted against carcinoma cells whilst being relatively sparing to the surrounding normal cutaneous epithelium. A trial in the UK of this treatment in cats with cutaneous SCC showed a good response rate (96% response rate with a complete response seen in 85% of cases) but 57% of the tumours recurred with a median time to recurrence of 157 days. However, repeat treatment was given to some of the cats and in this group 45% of the cases were disease-free at a median follow-up period of 1143 days. PDT therefore appears to be safe, well tolerated, and effective in the treatment of superficial nasal planum SCCs of cats (Fig. 5.20). It offers an alternative to surgical treatment, but it does not

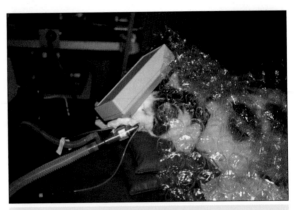

Figure 5.20 A cat receiving PDT using a 635-nm-wavelength laser diode light source following topical 5-ALA cream application to a nasal planum SCC

lead to a durable remission or cure in all cases. Surgical management should therefore always be given strong consideration because surgery is associated with 80% of patients remaining tumour-free at 1-year post diagnosis.

Despite the apparent success of some non-surgical modalities, however, surgery remains the mainstay for treatment of nasal planum tumours for both cats and dogs. Owners therefore need to be carefully counselled as the surgery will significantly affect the appearance of the animal. The complications associated with this surgery are minor and infrequent (stenosis of the new nasal opening is the main concern), so although many owners will seem initially reluctant to allow their cat or dog to undergo this procedure it is very important to explain the good clinical outcomes reported and illustrate how relatively unaffected the animals will appear especially once their hair has re-grown.

In cases with superficial SCC lesions and for whom neither surgery nor an alternative advanced treatment is an option, the topical immune response modifier and stimulant imiquimod marketed as Aldara cream, has been reported to be effective when applied every other day for up to 12 weeks.

The cancer patient with halitosis and/or hypersalivation

Hypersalivation and/or halitosis in a cancer patient are usually signs of an intraoral neoplasm and as such, these clinical signs are frequently accompanied by a poor appetite or complete anorexia, especially in the cat. However, drooling saliva may also be indicative of encephalopathy, especially in the cat, which can be caused by hepatic neoplasia, or possibly by an intracranial mass. Oral cancers are considered to be quite common in veterinary medicine, being reported to be the fourth most common malignancy type seen in clinical practice, accounting for 6% of all canine tumours and 3% of all feline tumours. In dogs, the most common tumour type seen is malignant melanoma, followed by squamous cell carcinoma and then fibrosarcoma, whereas in cats, squamous cell carcinomas are the most common, followed by fibrosarcoma. However, many other tumour types have been reported in the literature and a careful histological analysis is required to ensure an accurate diagnosis is made in every case.

CLINICAL CASE EXAMPLE 6.1 – ORAL SQUAMOUS CELL CARCINOMA IN A DOG

Signalment

7-year-old neutered male Welsh springer spaniel.

Presenting signs

A swelling identified on the lateral aspect of the rostral portion of the nasal bone and oral haemorrhage.

Case history

The relevant history in this case was:
- Owner started to notice blood in the dog's water bowl after he had been drinking 5 weeks previously
- 1 week before presenting he had started to eat more slowly and seemed to tilt his head to the left when prehending food
- Otherwise quite bright and alert.

Clinical examination

Physical examination revealed:
- The presence of a swelling on the lateral aspect of the right nasal bone, just rostral to the upper canine tooth
- Oral examination revealed the presence of a gingival mass (Figs 6.1, 6.2).

Differential diagnosis

- Malignant melanoma
- Squamous cell carcinoma (SCC)
- Fibrosarcoma (FSA)
- Lymphoma
- Basal cell carcinoma
- Epulis.

The submandibular lymph node was enlarged but cytological evaluation of fine needle aspirates revealed this to be due to a reactive lymphadenopathy with no evidence of metastatic disease. In the light of the degree of bony swelling, there was concern that there may be significant tumour invasion into the underlying bone, so an MRI scan was performed (Fig. 6.3). This revealed that the mass had indeed invaded through the nasal bone into the nasal cavity and had actually crossed the midline.

It was felt that the intranasal extension of the tumour indicated that it would not be possible to undertake surgery with curative intent as it would not be possible to obtain clean margins. The oral mass, therefore, was biopsied to see whether or not radiotherapy was a viable treatment option. The histopathology returned to show the mass was a squamous cell carcinoma and as the owners did not want surgery anyway, radiotherapy was offered as the sole treatment. The dog underwent a hypofractionated radiotherapy course as previously described. The swelling reduced in size and the owner's concern with blood in the water bowl stopped for 7 months, but then it returned along with right-sided unilateral serosanguineous discharge and the dog was euthanized 2 months later.

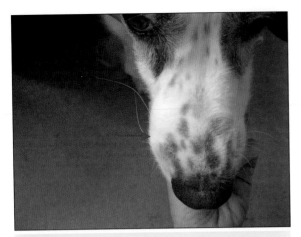

Figure 6.1 *Case 6.1* The dorsal appearance of the nasal bone, showing the swelling on the right lateral aspect (red arrow)

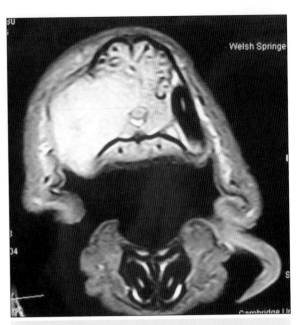

Figure 6.3 *Case 6.1* T2-weighted MRI scan revealing the significant intranasal invasion of the oral tumour

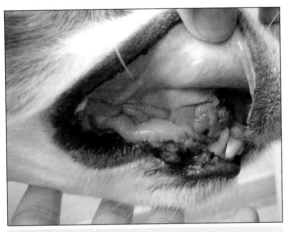

Figure 6.2 *Case 6.1* The intraoral appearance of the tumour

Theory refresher

Many patients with an oral tumour will present because the owner has found a mass within the mouth, but tumours located caudally within the oral cavity or sublingually may be difficult to see. These cases can present with a variety of clinical signs. Drooling saliva that may or may not be blood-tinged, worsening halitosis, dysphagia or progressively worsening inappetance are all potentially consistent with an oral tumour and warrant a careful and thorough oral examination. The index of suspicion may rise further depending on the signalment of the patient; male dogs have a greater risk of developing an oral tumour compared to female dogs and there

are certain breeds (e.g. cocker spaniels, German shepherd dogs, German short-haired pointers, Weimaraners, golden retrievers and boxers) that are reported to have an increased risk of developing oral cancers. Furthermore, large-breed dogs have a higher incidence of fibrosarcomas and non-tonsillar squamous cell carcinomas whilst small-breed dogs show an increased incidence of malignant melanoma and tonsillar carcinoma. Benign lesions such as papillomatosis are more common in younger dogs.

Clinical evaluation

A careful oral examination must obviously be performed, even if this requires sedation or a brief anaesthetic to ensure all areas of the oral cavity (including underneath the tongue and in the fauces) have been visualized and examined. In addition to a careful oral examination, attention must be paid to careful palpation of the submandibular lymph nodes and the general condition of the patient, as many oral tumours will have metastatic potential and the possibility of distant disease must always be considered. Some studies have shown that for highly metastatic tumours such as oral melanoma, a significant percentage of cases will have lymph node involvement despite being palpably normal. So if a melanoma is suspected and the primary mass can be excised, excision of the draining submandibular lymph node(s) is also useful from a staging perspective, although no studies have shown such a procedure generates any favourable prognostic advantage compared to leaving the node behind.

Diagnostic evaluation

In view of the different possible diagnoses and the treatment and prognostic implications of such differences, it is essential to make a definitive histopathological diagnosis by biopsy. Prior to any surgery (biopsy or excision procedure) for an oral mass, left and right inflated lateral thoracic radiographs must be obtained to rule out the presence of visible metastases, as indicated in the section above. Local radiography at the site of the lesion is also strongly recommended to investigate the degree of bony involvement. It is important to remember, however, that an apparently normal radiograph does not rule out bone invasion as there has to be up to 40% bone lysis before a lesion will be visible radiographically. Advanced imaging techniques (particularly CT but also MRI) are more sensitive tools to evaluate the extent of disease and/or the presence of bone lesions and patients should be referred for such investigations when possible or necessary. Being able to accurately plan which treatment or treatment combinations are most appropriate for the patient *before* there has been an attempt at excisional surgery significantly improves the likelihood of success and reduces stress and discomfort, whilst frequently reducing the overall cost of the treatment required.

Once a full staging process has been completed, a biopsy procedure or specific treatment can be planned depending on the outcome of these investigations. The correct treatment may vary depending on the diagnosis and clinical stage reached, so incisional biopsy at surgery remains the first-line method to diagnose the exact nature of most oral tumours (Figs 6.4, 6.5). If it is decided to attempt excisional biopsy, the important fact to remember is that for many oral tumours (with the exceptions of fibrous and ossifying epulides) there is a significant risk of invasion into the adjacent jaw bone, so surgical resection should include bony margins to increase the likelihood of achieving good local control. It is for this reason that it is often sensible to obtain an accurate diagnosis by obtaining an incisional biopsy before attempting excisional surgery. Cats, but especially dogs, generally tolerate partial maxillectomy, mandibulectomy or orbitectomy well and the cosmetic outcomes are good, although this should be discussed with clients carefully beforehand.

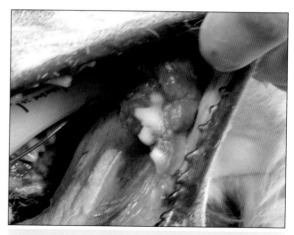

Figure 6.4 An acanthomatous epulis located on the caudal mandible of a dog. Clinical staging indicated that there was no distant disease and the dog was treated with a partial mandibulectomy with good functional results and no tumour recurrence 2 years later

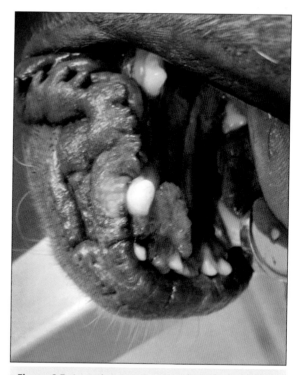

Figure 6.5 An oral squamous cell carcinoma in a great Dane, to illustrate how similar tumours of different cell types appear to the naked eye, hence the need for accurate histopathological diagnosis before a definitive treatment for oral tumours is undertaken

Treatment

With regard to specific treatment, surgery is usually the most appropriate course of action required for oral neoplasia. Exactly what surgical procedure will be required depends upon the tumour type, the tumour size and the tumour location but it is recommended to try to achieve 2-cm margins (including of the underlying bone) if the mass is confirmed to be malignant. Local segmental excision to include the underlying bone is indicated for all small oral tumours (except ossifying and fibromatous epulides) but larger tumours will require more extensive surgery such as hemimandibulectomy, hemimaxillectomy or orbitectomy procedures (Tables 6.1, 6.2).

The immediate postoperative recovery for canine patients who undergo more aggressive or extensive surgery is usually still rapid with most eating well the evening after their surgery and it is, therefore, not usual for feeding tubes to be placed in the dog (Figs 6.6–6.15).

> **NURSING TIP**
>
> Offering soft, gently warmed foods often helps a dog to eat following mandibulectomy/ maxillectomy surgery.

> **CLINICAL TIP**
>
> Enteral feeding tube placement at the time of surgery should be carefully considered in cats, especially in those undergoing a mandibulectomy procedure, as cats have a higher risk of developing postoperative complications compared to dogs.

Table 6.1 Various mandibulectomies (Adapted from Withrow S, Vail D 2001 Withrow and MacEwan's small animal clinical oncology, 4th edn. St Louis, MO, Saunders Elsevier, p 461, reproduced with permission)

Mandibulectomy procedure	Indications	Comments	
Unilateral rostral	Lesions confined to rostral hemimandible; not crossing midline	Most common tumour types are squamous cell carcinoma and adamantinoma that do not require removal of entire affected bone; tongue may lag to resected side	
Bilateral rostral	Bilateral rostral lesions crossing the symphysis	Tongue will be 'too long' and some cheilitis of chin skin will occur; has been performed as far back as PM4 but preferably at PM1	
Vertical ramus	Low-grade bony or cartilaginous lesions confined to vertical ramus	These tumours are variously called chondroma rodens or multilobular osteosarcoma; temperomandibular joint may be removed; cosmetics and function are excellent	
Complete unilateral	High-grade tumours with extensive involvement of horizontal ramus or invasion into medullary canal of ramus	Usually reserved for aggressive tumours; function and cosmetics are good	
Segmental	Low-grade midhorizontal ramus cancer, preferably not into medullary cavity	Poor choice for highly malignant cancer in medullary cavity, since growth along mandibular artery, vein, and nerve is common	

Table 6.2 Various maxillectomies (Adapted from Withrow S, Vail D 2001 Withrow and MacEwan's small animal clinical oncology, 4th edn. St Louis, MO, Saunders Elsevier, p 461, reproduced with permission)

Maxillectomy procedure	Indications	Comments	
Unilateral rostral	Lesions confined to hard palate on one side	One-layer closure	
Bilateral rostral	Bilateral lesions of rostral hard palate	Needs viable buccal mucosa on both sides for flap closure	
Lateral	Laterally placed midmaxillary lesions	Single-layer closure if small defect, two-layer if large	
Bilateral	Bilateral palatine lesions	High rate of closure dehiscence because lip flap rarely reaches from side to side; may result in permanent oronasal fistula	

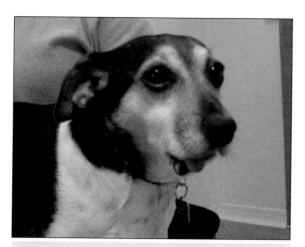

Figure 6.6 One of the more common cosmetic changes in a dog who has undergone a partial mandibulectomy: lateral protrusion of the tongue. Occasionally the jaw will move laterally and may cause the lower canine tooth to impinge on the hard palate

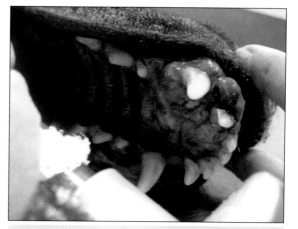

Figure 6.7 A rostral maxillectomy can have a similar effect to that shown in Figure 6.6. The dog here has an osteosarcoma affecting his rostral maxilla

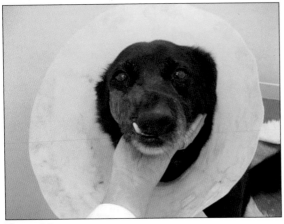

Figure 6.8

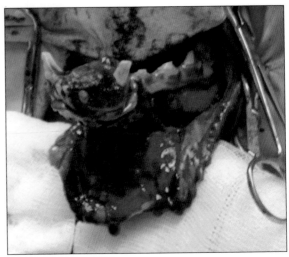

Figure 6.11

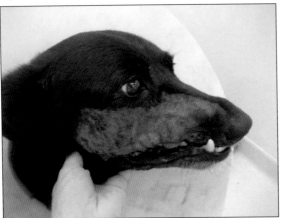

Figure 6.9

Figures 6.8, 6.9 The effects of the removal of the maxilla leave the dog shown in Figure 6.7 with only a mild-moderate facial defect that was actually much harder to see once his hair had re-grown

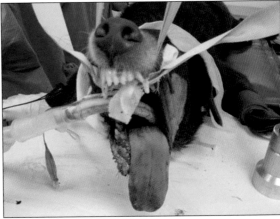

Figure 6.12

Figures 6.11, 6.12 The rostral mandible was then removed, along with the excess soft tissue

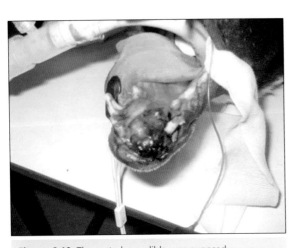

Figure 6.10 The rostral mandible was exposed

Figures 6.10–6.15 An example of how well most dogs do after aggressive surgery. This is the oral SCC in a 10-year-old neutered female Collie cross, immediately before surgery.

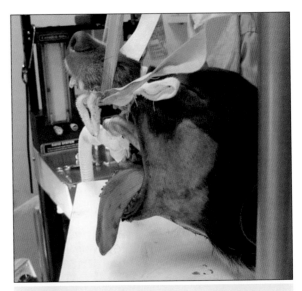

Figure 6.13 Removal of the mandible left an obvious cosmetic defect

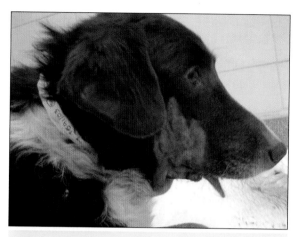

Figure 6.14 However, on recovery the dog looked reasonable

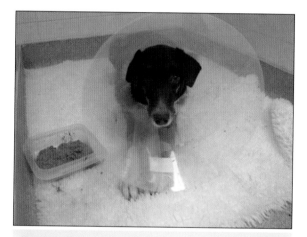

Figure 6.15 From some angles you would not know that she had had surgery!

One study has reported that 72% of the cats which underwent mandibulectomy developed postoperative dysphagia or inappetence and 12% did not regain their ability to eat. However, despite these difficulties, 80% of the owners reported that they were happy with the results of the procedure. This study highlights the importance of careful client counselling and thorough treatment planning before undertaking oral tumour excision, especially in feline patients.

Radiotherapy, either alone or postoperatively, for incompletely excised tumours, is an effective treatment option in tumours with sensitivity to radiation such as canine squamous cell carcinoma and malignant melanoma. Both hypo- and hyperfractionation regimens have been reported, but in the UK currently it would be most common to use a hypofractionated regimen, administering up to 8–9 Gy every 7 days to a total dose of 32–36 Gy. This treatment is usually tolerated extremely well with few if any acute side effects and if a tumour is found to have been incompletely excised, seeking advice from a referral specialist for radiotherapy is certainly advisable. For squamous cell carcinomas 1-year survival rates of up to 70% have been reported with radiotherapy. Radiotherapy given postoperatively has also been shown to increase the response rate and survival times in one study and therefore postoperative radiotherapy should certainly be considered if at all possible in cases of oral SCC if the margins are small or not clean.

Other treatment options

Chemotherapy has little use in helping to control local disease in oral tumours and it only has limited use in some metastatic tumours. Partial responses have been reported using platinum-containing drugs in canine oral malignant melanoma and also with the use of piroxicam in oral squamous cell carcinoma. However, chemotherapy does not currently have a first-line treatment role in oral neoplasia in cats or dogs.

Prognosis

The prognosis for a patient with an oral tumour will vary depending on whether it is a cat or a dog, and the location, type, size, grading and extent of the mass. However, assessment of the literature seems to indicate that there are a few general principles:

- Rostral tumour outcomes > caudally located tumours
- Complete resection outcomes > incomplete resection
- Acanthomatous epulus survival time > SCC survival time > malignant melanoma survival time approximately = fibrosarcoma survival time (depending on location).

Canine oral squamous cell carcinomas have a reasonably good prognosis if located in the rostral oral cavity, but tonsillar and sublingual SCCs are highly metastatic and difficult to excise completely, leading to a guarded prognosis for SCCs in these locations. Sublingual SCC in particular can be very difficult to manage and if the patient is inappetant due to such a tumour, then euthanasia may have to be considered if surgery cannot be performed. Mandibular SCCs have been reported to have 10% local recurrence and 91% 1-year survival rates with surgery alone whilst maxillary SCCs have been reported to have 27% local recurrence and 57% 1-year survival rates with surgery alone. However, anatomical location has a significant bearing on all these figures, with tumours located caudally or sublingually having significantly poorer outcomes.

The prognosis for oral fibrosarcomas is guarded when compared to SCCs due to the locally infiltrative nature of these tumours making it so difficult to obtain completely clean margins, meaning that local recurrence occurs more commonly. However, combination therapy (surgery and radiotherapy) does appear to be advantageous over surgery alone. Without radiation, local recurrence has been reported in up to 59% of dogs compared to 32% in dogs treated with surgery and postoperative radiation.

Future treatments

A possible future treatment will be photodynamic therapy (PDT). A recent study used PDT to treat oral SCC in 11 dogs; eight of the dogs were judged to be cured with no tumour recurrence for at least 17 months and the cosmetic appearance following treatment was considered superior when compared to dogs that underwent surgical excision of their tumour. Although PDT is only available at a few university teaching hospitals in the UK, this may become a more common treatment option in the near future.

CLINICAL CASE EXAMPLE 6.2 – ORAL MALIGNANT MELANOMA

Signalment

9-year-old neutered male black Labrador.

Presenting signs

A 4-week history of progressive inappetance and excessive drooling. The owners had looked in his mouth and found a large mass on his upper jaw.

Clinical examination

Oral examination in this case was possible without sedation and revealed the presence of a large mass emanating from the right mid-maxilla and growing laterally to the left and ventrally. The mass had an irregular surface and was darkly pigmented (Fig. 6.16).

Differential diagnosis

- Malignant melanoma – this is the main differential in the light of the age and breed of the dog and the appearance of the mass
- Squamous cell carcinoma
- Fibrosarcoma
- Lymphoma
- Basal cell carcinoma
- Epulis.

Diagnostic evaluation

As for all oral tumours, once a complete physical examination has been completed it is of the utmost

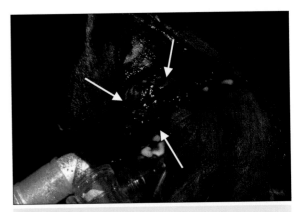

Figure 6.16 *Case 6.2* The mass within the mouth of the Labrador viewed from the left lateral aspect as the tumour extended over the roof of the mouth. The borders of the mass are highlighted by the white arrows

importance to carefully palpate the submandibular lymph nodes and if they are enlarged, to obtain fine needle aspirates for cytology. Secondly, obtaining fully inflated thoracic radiographs under general anaesthesia is essential before any surgical procedure is performed to ensure that there are no pulmonary metastases present.

In this case, the submandibular nodes were moderately palpable but fine needle aspiration revealed no evidence of metastatic tumour cells and the node was deemed to be reactive. The thoracic radiographs were unremarkable.

Treatment

In this case, no oral radiographs were undertaken as the owners declined excisional surgery in the light of the extensive procedure required. A surgical wedge biopsy was therefore obtained which confirmed the diagnosis to be oral malignant melanoma. The owners did, however, opt for external beam radiotherapy so he received 4×9 Gy fractions every 7 days, which produced significant tumour shrinkage with the gross tumour mass almost totally resolving within 6 weeks of treatment starting, although a large area of ulcerated oral mucosa remained (Fig. 6.17).

In this case, following his radiotherapy the dog required intermittent antibiosis and NSAID therapy (meloxicam) to keep his quality of life acceptable, but in the owner's opinion he was normal during this period when on treatment. He then became inappetant again 7 months after his radiation therapy. Oral examination showed moderate regrowth of his tumour and thoracic radiographs revealed the presence of multiple pulmonary metastases, so he was euthanized.

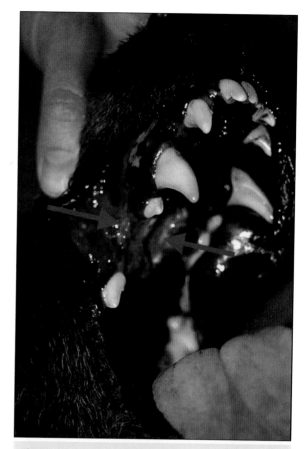

Figure 6.17 *Case 6.2* The appearance of the oral malignant melanoma 2 weeks after the fourth radiation therapy treatment, viewed from the right lateral aspect to show the area of ulcerated mucosa on the hard palate (highlighted by the red arrows)

Theory refresher

Malignant melanoma (MM) is the most common malignant oral tumour reported in the dog. Oral MMs are reported more frequently in smaller breeds of dog and it is generally seen in older animals, the average age of presentation being just over 11 years. They present in a similar fashion to other oral tumours but it is important to note that in approximately 30% of cases the tumour will not appear darkly pigmented (i.e. amelanotic), thereby making it impossible to differentiate it as a melanoma just by visual inspection (Fig. 6.18).

Malignant melanomas generate a guarded prognosis due to their high metastatic potential and 1-year survival rates of less than 35% are reported. The World Health Organization staging scheme for dogs with oral melanoma is based on tumour size, with stage I being a tumour less than 2 cm in diameter, stage II being a tumour measuring 2–4 cm diameter and stage III being a tumour equal to or greater than 4 cm diameter and/or the presence of lymph node metastases. Stage IV disease describes the presence of distant metastasis. The median survival times for dogs with oral melanoma treated with surgery alone are approximately 17 months, $5\frac{1}{2}$ months, and 3 months with stage I, II and III disease, respectively. Surgical excision is usually the first-line treatment and the type of surgery undertaken obviously depends on the location of the tumour, but the standard oncological rules apply, in that if possible a 2-cm margin should be obtained and for a malignant melanoma of the maxilla or mandible (Figs 6.19–6.22), the underlying bone has to be removed to achieve a good local

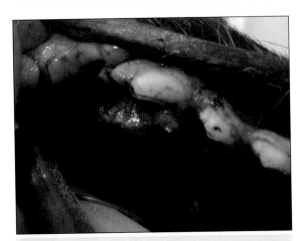

Figure 6.18 An oral malignant melanoma located on the hard palate of a German short-haired pointer, showing that oral MMs are frequently not darkly pigmented

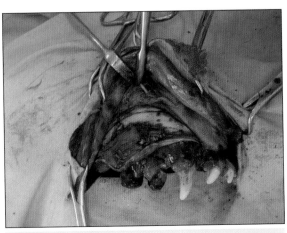

Figure 6.20 The maxilla around the tumour is isolated and incised using a bone saw

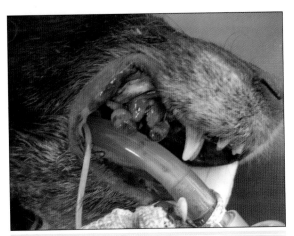

Figure 6.19 The tumour is shown here in situ, originating from the right maxilla and protruding down into the oral cavity

Figures 6.19–6.22 The surgical removal of an oral malignant melanoma.

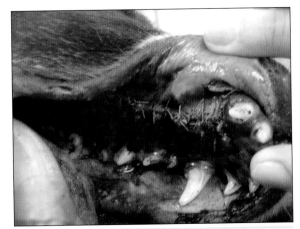

Figure 6.21 The maxilla and tumour are removed and the deficit closed routinely

resection with a partial mandibulectomy or maxillectomy, as described in Chapter 5.

As shown in the main case example, radiotherapy can be useful in the management of oral malignant melanomas. A number of studies have shown that hypofractionated radiotherapy can be used alone in canine cases, with response rates of up to 100% being reported and complete remission seen in up to 70% of cases. However, as well as local recurrence being a problem, metastatic disease is still the cause of death in the majority of dogs treated in this way, with median survival times of up to 7 months reported with radiation therapy alone and 363 days in a report of combined chemoradiation treatment. The decision therefore, whether to use radiotherapy or surgery as the first-line treatment, will depend on individual circumstances and treatment availability.

Chemotherapy only has a very limited role in the management of oral MM. One study has shown that carboplatin generated a 28% response rate (mainly

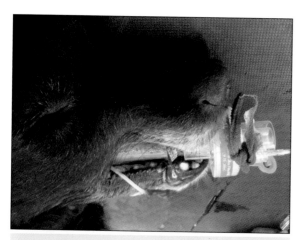

Figure 6.22 Even immediately after surgery, the cosmetic result of a maxillactomy is usually good

partial response defined as a reduction in tumour size by >50%) but the median survival times for this treatment alone were short at 165 days, indicating that sole-agent carboplatin is inferior to both surgery and radiotherapy as a first-line therapy. A second study has shown that 2/11 dogs with oral malignant melanoma responded to a combination of cisplatin and piroxicam. These studies suggest that the platinum-based chemotherapy agents do appear to have some (albeit limited) activity against macroscopic malignant melanoma, so there may be a role for their use as adjunctive, postoperative therapy or in chemo-radiotherapy protocols. However, no large-scale trials to date have shown this to be definitely efficacious when used in this way.

The limiting factor in the survival of malignant melanoma patients is usually not local disease control, but the problem of distant (usually pulmonary) metastatic disease and new therapies are required to reduce the incidence of metastasis. The future for treatment of canine oral MM, however, may lie with the recent development of a xenogenic DNA vaccine which stimulates the production of antityrosinase antibodies and appears to be both safe and efficacious in the treatment of canine oral MM. This treatment is now available in the UK only via oncology specialists, including the authors' hospital, but its development in the US and current on-going trials have generated exciting data indicating that as part of a multimodal treatment approach this new therapy may substantially extend the disease-free period for canine patients with oral MM.

CLINICAL CASE EXAMPLE 6.3 – CANINE SUBLINGUAL FIBROSARCOMA

Signalment

8-year-old neutered male Border collie.

Presenting signs

Halitosis and blood-stained saliva.

Case history

The relevant history in this case was:
- Owner had first noticed halitosis 4 weeks previously
- Noticed dog was eating more slowly than usual but was otherwise bright
- Started to notice blood-stained saliva in the water bowl so went to referring vet thinking dog needed a dental. Referring vet found sublingual mass, so referred him
- Otherwise quite well.

Clinical examination

- Bright and alert but with halitosis!
- Mild-moderate bilateral submandibular lymph node enlargement
- Irregular, erythematous and haemorrhagic mass present on ventral aspect of tongue, attached to the frenulum (Fig. 6.23)
- No other clinical abnormalities were noted.

Differential diagnosis

- Squamous cell carcinoma
- Fibrosarcoma
- Malignant melanoma
- Lymphoma.

Diagnostic evaluation

- Fine needle aspiration of submandibular lymph nodes revealed no evidence of tumour metastasis
- Thoracic radiographs revealed no evidence of pulmonary metastases
- Mandibular radiographs revealed no evidence of bony change
- The decision was made to undertake excisional biopsy.

Diagnosis

- Grade II sublingual fibrosarcoma.

In this particular case, the dog made a rapid recovery from surgery with no complications (Fig. 6.24).

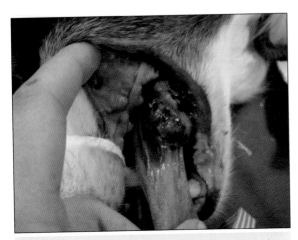

Figure 6.23 *Case 6.3* The appearance of the sublingual mass prior to excisional surgery

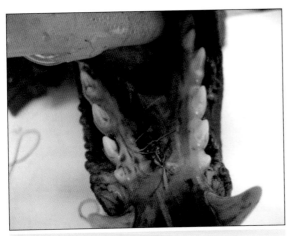

Figure 6.24 *Case 6.3* The immediate postoperative view of the dog with the tumour excised

Theory refresher

Lingual neoplasia is considered rare in veterinary medicine. Sixty-four per cent of lingual masses have been reported to be malignant tumours and approximately half of these cases will be squamous cell carcinomas with a gender predisposition for females and an increased incidence seen in poodles, Labradors and samoyeds. Other tumour types reported in the dog include granular cell myoblastoma, malignant melanoma, fibrosarcoma (most common in Border collies), adenocarcinoma and haemangiosarcoma (most common in golden retrievers). Smaller-breed dogs and especially cocker spaniels show an increased incidence of lingual plasma cell tumours. Lingual neoplasms in the cat are most commonly SCCs and are frequently located on the ventral surface of the tongue near the frenulum (Fig. 6.25).

Diagnosis of lingual neoplasia requires incisional biopsy, which should be preceded by careful palpation of the submandibular lymph nodes and inflated thoracic radiographs to rule out distant metastases before biopsy.

Should the biopsy confirm the presence of a cancerous growth, the recommended treatment is usually surgical excision if possible. However, although partial and even major glossectomy is usually well tolerated with few long-term problems, approximately 50% of lingual tumours are positioned either in the midline or are bilaterally symmetrical, thereby limiting the ability of the surgeon to achieve complete margins without undertaking radical resection, which in turn, is associated with an increased risk of postoperative complications. Referral to a soft-tissue surgical specialist is therefore highly recommended for these cases.

The prognosis for cancer of the tongue depends on the type of tumour, its location, its grade and whether the patient is a cat or a dog. Despite often being large, granular cell myoblastomas have a good prognosis with over 80% of cases being cured with conservative surgery achieving only close margins. As a general rule, rostrally located tumours usually have better outcomes than tumours located more caudally due to their relative ease of removal and possibly their earlier recognition. The histological grade of the tumour is also important. Histological grade I SCCs of the tongue in dogs are reported to have statistically much better survival times following surgical resection than grade II or III SCCs (median survival times 16 months, 4 months and 3 months respectively). There are no studies to the authors' knowledge showing the outcome for dogs with lingual fibrosarcomas, however, although the risk of metastasis is relatively low, there is always a concern regarding local recurrence due to the locally infiltrative nature of sarcomas.

Feline tongue tumours are generally difficult to manage. The long-term prognosis for malignant lingual tumours of the cat is guarded and 1-year survival rates are considered to be less than 25%. Their predilection site on the ventral surface coupled with the fact that they are often sited in the midline attached to the frenulum makes surgical excision problematical. As there is also considerable risk of acute toxicity at this site with external beam radiation therapy, sometimes offering any treatment at all is difficult. Referral to an oncology

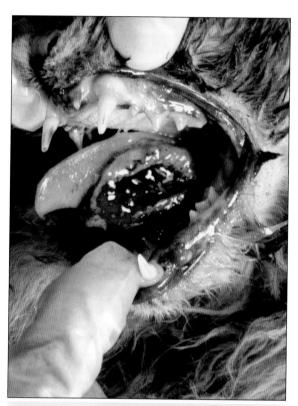

Figure 6.25 The typical appearance of a subligual squamous cell carcinoma in a cat. The position on the frenulum in this case made treatment practically impossible and the cat was euthanized

specialist is definitely recommended for these cases but owners need to be made aware that treatment options may be limited. Photodynamic therapy may be a future option for these tumours and there is also a recent report that the bisphosphonate 'zoledronic acid' has an antineoplastic action against oral SCCs in cats but to the authors' knowledge there are no studies looking at lingual SCCs in particular.

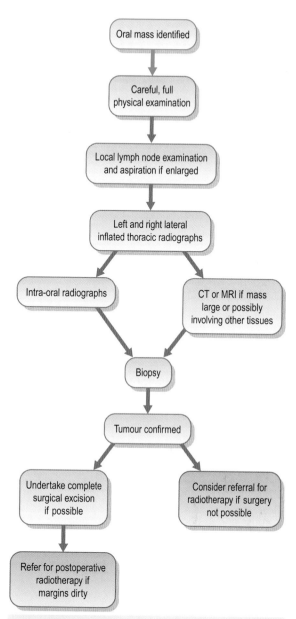

Figure 6.26 Diagnostic plan flowchart for a patient with an oral mass

7 The coughing and/or dyspnoeic cancer patient

Coughing is a clinical sign associated with tracheal or lung pathology and therefore is suggestive of intrathoracic neoplasia in a cancer patient, whilst dyspnoea can indicate pulmonary, pleural, mediastinal, intra- or extra-tracheal or laryngeal pathology. It is therefore important to remember that a coughing or dyspnoeic cancer patient may not simply have lung cancer but may be showing signs that could be caused by a variety of different neoplastic processes:

- Primary lung cancer
- Metastatic (secondary) lung cancer
- Thymic cancer
- Tracheal cancer
- Laryngeal cancer
- Pleural cancer or pleural effusion caused by cancer (e.g. malignant pleural effusion, hepatic cancer causing a coagulopathy, or a splenic tumour causing disseminated intravascular coagulation (DIC))
- Lymphadenopathy in the tracheobronchial lymph nodes due to primary or metastatic cancer.

CLINICAL CASE EXAMPLE 7.1 – PRIMARY BRONCHIAL CARCINOMA IN A CAT

Signalment

14-year-old neutered female domestic short-haired (DSH) cat.

Presenting signs

- 6-week history of progressive coughing
- Owner described cough as soft and slightly moist
- No weight loss noted but cat quieter than normal.

Clinical examination

- Slim body condition and quiet but responsive on examination
- No abnormalities on pulmonary auscultation or percussion

- No dyspnoea or tachypnoea noted
- Otherwise no other abnormalities noted on examination.

Differential diagnoses

- Bronchitis
- Airway foreign body
- Pulmonary neoplasia
  - Secondary metastatic disease
  - Primary.

Diagnostic evaluation

In the light of her clinical history and signs it was decided to undertake thoracic radiographs first. These revealed the presence of a single solitary mass located in the cranial aspect of her right caudal lung lobe. No tracheo-bronchial lymph node enlargement was noted and there was no pleural effusion.

Treatment

In the light of her history and clinical findings, it was decided that the mass required removal, so after pre-anaesthetic blood screens had been undertaken, she was taken to surgery without further diagnostic evaluation and underwent an intercostal thoracotomy, during which a 2-cm diameter mass was identified within the right caudal lung lobe and excision of the affected lobe performed. Careful visual and digital examination of the draining lymph nodes was also undertaken but they were considered to be normal.

The cat was managed postoperatively with opioid and NSAID analgesia and made a slow but steady recovery, being discharged from the hospital 4 days postoperatively. Histopathology revealed the mass to be a moderately differentiated primary bronchial carcinoma. After careful discussion with the owner, no further treatment was undertaken at their request. The cat remained well for 16 months with no sign of recurrence before being lost to follow-up.

Theory refresher

Primary lung cancer in veterinary medicine is considered rare, accounting for approximately 1% of all canine cancer cases and less than 1% of all feline cancer cases. Primary lung cancer cases are usually epithelial in origin (i.e. carcinomas) with adenocarcinomas being the most common subtype reported. A precise diagnosis can be made by subcategorizing the tumour type depending on its location of origin (e.g. bronchial, bronchioalveolar or alveolar) and by the degree of histological differentiation. A clinical diagnosis is usually made by identifying a large, often solitary mass, or possibly multiple masses on thoracic radiographs. Primary lung cancer is more often seen in older animals and whilst there has been no gender or breed predilection shown in dogs, older female cats seem more likely to develop the disease than male cats.

It is also unusual for coughing to be a clinical sign of lung cancer in isolation; rather, many cancer cases which cough will also display signs such as tachypnoea/dyspnoea, lethargy, weight loss, reduced exercise tolerance and poor appetite. Careful questioning of the owner will also frequently establish that these signs have been gradually worsening over several weeks prior to presentation although sometimes the presentation can be acute in nature. Dyspnoea is usually noticed by the owner but any preceding tachypnoea may not be recognized, so again careful questioning to establish the rate of onset of the clinical signs is important. It is also very important to establish the nature of any cough, as many cases of lung cancer will have a non-productive cough and the suspicion for neoplasia will increase in older patients presenting with coughing that is not responsive to antibiotic treatment. However, it is important to remember that many lung cancers can initially be clinically silent, or cause more unexpected clinical signs, especially if the tumour metastasizes to an extrapulmonary site (e.g. to the brain, resulting in neurological signs or to the digits, causing lameness). An example of an unusual manifestation of lung cancer is hypertrophic osteopathy presenting as shifting lameness and warm and/or swollen limbs. The identification of hypertrophic osteopathy (HO) on a radiograph should certainly initiate a search for an underlying neoplastic cause, starting with thoracic radiographs (although HO has also been reported with a variety of other non-pulmonary neoplasms and some non-neoplastic diseases).

Metastatic lung cancer is considered to be much more common than primary lung cancer with almost any

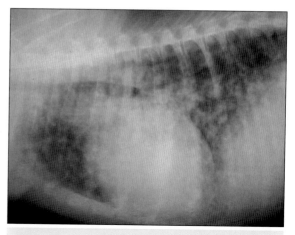

Figure 7.1 Extensive pulmonary metastatic disease in a patient with primary splenic haemangiosarcoma

malignant tumour having the potential to spread to the pulmonary tissue by virtue of the anatomical nature of the vascular supply in the lungs. The identification of lesions on thoracic radiographs that could be consistent with pulmonary metastasis should therefore initiate a clinical investigation as to the location of a possible primary tumour. The tumours most often associated with pulmonary spread are malignant melanoma, osteosarcoma, mammary carcinoma and haemangiosarcoma (Fig. 7.1) but any malignant tumour could theoretically spread to the lung, so a thorough clinical examination and appropriate ancillary tests may be required in such cases.

Diagnosis

Having obtained a careful history, the clinical investigation of a patient suspected to have cancer of the lower respiratory tract begins with a thorough physical examination, looking in particular for signs of abnormal breathing along with careful auscultation of the heart and percussion of all the lung fields, as well as a full systemic evaluation of the animal. However, for patients with pulmonary neoplasia the cornerstone of diagnosis in general practice remains careful thoracic radiography and for this, fully inflated (i.e. obtained under general anaesthesia) left and right lateral thoracic radiographs are still considered to be the minimum standard, whilst obtaining three views provides an optimum radiographic evaluation. Patterns commonly seen vary from discrete nodules or individual masses to poorly defined interstitial patterns. Consolidation of individual lung lobes can also be seen, as can enlargement of the

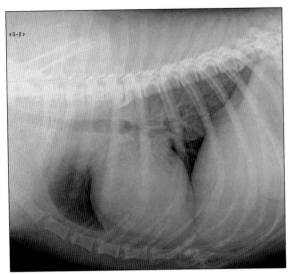

Figure 7.2

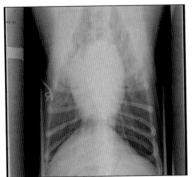

Figure 7.3

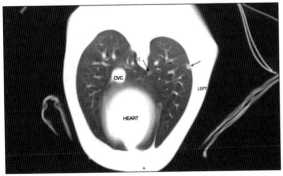

Figure 7.4

Figures 7.2–7.4 Lateral and dorso-ventral (DV) radiographs and a transverse CT scan from a dog with a prostatic carcinoma. The radiographs do not clearly show any metastatic lesions but CT clearly shows the presence of metastatic disease, as highlighted by the two black arrows (Fig. 7.4). Images courtesy of Dr Ani Avner, Knowledge Farm Veterinary Specialist Referral Center, Israel

tracheobronchial lymph nodes if there is nodal metastasis. However, it is important to remember three factors regarding thoracic radiography of neoplasia:

- The radiographic appearance of pulmonary neoplasia can vary markedly depending on the type and stage of the disease.
- Radiographs can be insensitive to detect small metastatic lesions and/or lymphadenopathy, making accurate presurgery staging difficult.
- Radiographs only give the clinician a presumptive diagnosis of a primary lung tumour; histopathology is required to be definitive.

Where available, computed tomography (CT scanning) certainly provides a more sensitive technique for the detection of small lesions, so patients may be considered for referral for this evaluation if possible, especially if a thoracotomy and excisional surgery are being planned and there is uncertainty regarding the clinical stage of the disease. A recent study showed that CT was able to identify enlargement of the tracheobronchial lymph nodes due to the presence of metastatic disease in five cases in which the lymphadenopathy had not been identified on thoracic radiography. However, a different study revealed that although CT provides superior resolution compared to radiography (Figs 7.2–7.4), it is still associated with a significant number of both false-negative and false-positive findings. We have to therefore conclude that we do not have perfect imaging modalities available. So caution must always accompany presurgical evaluation and staging by imaging of a patient with possible lung cancer. However, as the identification of metastatic disease has a significant impact on treatment and prognosis, it is vital to attempt to fully stage these patients and perform the evaluations to the highest possible standards.

Identification of a malignant pleural effusion is generally considered a poor prognostic sign as it indicates diffuse intrapleural disease, although there are reports of successful treatments with intrapleural chemotherapy. The identification of neoplastic cells requires an experienced cytology specialist and samples should be obtained in both plain and EDTA tubes if the samples are being sent to an external laboratory.

Treatment

The first-line treatment for localized primary lung cancer is surgical excision of the lesion by complete lung lobectomy, as illustrated by the cat in this case example. In the light of this, and of the fact that radiographs do not provide a cytological or histological diagnosis, it may be desirable in some circumstances to try to obtain a definitive diagnosis before sending the patient to surgery. Fine needle aspiration of the mass, either by ultrasound guidance or by blind aspiration based on the radiographical position of the mass can be simple and useful. However, there is a risk of iatrogenic pneumothorax and some studies have shown fine needle aspiration of pulmonary masses to have a low diagnostic yield. Bronchoscopy and bronchoalveolar lavage (BAL) can also produce a diagnostic sample and one study has suggested that these are more sensitive techniques than radiography in the diagnosis of pulmonary lymphoma. However, for carcinomas, studies in human medicine have shown that the sensitivity of BAL in reaching a definitive diagnosis varies depending on whether or not the tumour can be visualized, with the diagnostic sensitivity falling when the tumour cannot be seen. It may therefore be best to recommend firstly that a definitive diagnosis before surgery is only sought, if for some reason, it will make a difference to the treatment undertaken, and secondly, that thoracotomy to undertake a complete surgical excision and obtain a histopathological diagnosis is still the optimum treatment if possible. Owners, however, need to be counselled that more extensive disease may be found at surgery even with the most advanced diagnostic imaging investigations having been performed.

for those cases where the tumour is extremely large or where the exact location cannot be identified on radiographs. This approach is not recommended routinely due to the difficulty associated in accessing the hilar vessels and bronchi which are situated dorsally. Moreover, lymph node biopsy is more difficult with this approach. The use of CT to accurately identify the exact location of the tumour and the presence of enlarged local lymph nodes and/or metastatic disease is a useful presurgical imaging tool, however this may not be easily available.

To undertake surgery the patient is positioned in lateral recumbency with the affected lung lobe uppermost. A standard or modified intercostal thoracotomy from the fourth to the sixth intercostal space is usually sufficient to allow access to the lung lobe. Lung lobectomy can be performed either by using standard ligation techniques or by using surgical stapling equipment (TA-55 or TA-90; see suppliers, p. 201). The use of stapling equipment significantly reduces surgical time and allows for a secure lobectomy closure. Before the thoracotomy is closed the area is carefully checked for haemorrhage or leakage of air from the collapsed bronchi. This is achieved by flooding the thoracic cavity with warm sterile saline and submerging the surgical site. Any areas of haemorrhage or air leakages should be meticulously sutured. Local lymph nodes should also be inspected and biopsied if enlarged. A thoracic drain is placed after copious lavage and the thoracotomy site closed routinely.

> **CLINICAL TIP**
>
> Surgical removal of single lung tumours is the treatment associated with the longest survival times and should be considered if possible in all cases.

> **CLINICAL TIP**
>
> This procedure requires considerable expertise from a surgical, anaesthetic and nursing aspect and therefore referral should be seriously considered if any of these three aspects of care is compromised.

An intercostal thoracotomy and lung lobectomy is the procedure of choice if a diagnosis of a solitary lung lobe mass has been made. Other options for removal include excision via thoracoscopy or a median sternotomy. Thoracoscopy removal necessitates specialized equipment with specialist surgeons and anaesthetists and is thus generally available only in certain referral practices. Additionally, due to poor visualization, conversion to a thoracotomy is sometimes required. The use of median sternotomy as an approach to lung lobectomy is reserved

> **NURSING TIP**
>
> Thoracic drains require a high level of nursing and aseptic maintenance. They should be secured well and the patient prevented from interfering with them. In general, if there are no complications and drainage is minimal, then the drain can be removed within 24 hours.

CLINICAL CASE EXAMPLE 7.2 – PRIMARY PULMONARY ADENOCARCINOMA IN A DOG

Signalment

10-year-old female neutered cocker spaniel.

Presenting signs

- 3-month history of progressive coughing
- Coughing worse when lying down or on exercise
- Exercise tolerance reduced
- No weight loss but quieter than normal.

Clinical examination

- Overweight and quiet
- No abnormalities on pulmonary auscultation or percussion
- Soft moist cough noted following walking into the consultation
- No palpable peripheral lymph nodes
- Otherwise the examination was unremarkable.

Differential diagnoses

- Chronic bronchitis
- Congestive heart failure
- Pulmonary neoplasia
  - Secondary metastatic disease
  - Primary.

Diagnostic evaluation

In light of her clinical history and signs it was decided to undertake thoracic radiographs first. These revealed the presence of a large mass just cranial to the heart located in the left hemithorax and a smaller, spherical lesion with a radiolucent centre located in the left dorsocaudal lung field over rib 10 (Fig. 7.5).

An ultrasound-guided fine needle aspirate was obtained from the smaller mass in the left dorsocaudal lung field and the cytology was consistent with a bronchial carcinoma. Careful clinical examination and an abdominal ultrasound examination revealed no evidence of any further focus of neoplastic disease.

Treatment

Although a detailed consultation was undertaken with the owners, during which they were strongly advised to consider a thoracotomy to enable removal of both the larger and smaller lesions, the owners declined surgical management and opted for chemotherapeutic management. The dog therefore received carboplatin at 3-weekly intervals as a dose of 300 mg/m^2. Very pleasingly the dog's cough had resolved within two treatments and she became much livelier. The carboplatin was continued for a further three treatments and the dog remained well throughout. Repeat thoracic radiographs taken after the fifth and final treatment showed a considerable improvement to the appearance of the lungs which matched her clinical improvement (Fig. 7.6).

The dog remained well for 14 months following the diagnosis, but then she re-presented due to a recurrence of coughing and lethargy. Lateral and DV thoracic radiographs revealed the presence of multiple metastases so she was euthanized.

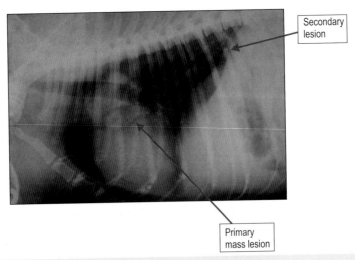

Secondary lesion

Primary mass lesion

Figure 7.5 *Case 7.2* A right lateral radiograph showing the presence of a large primary tumour and a smaller secondary lesion in the dog

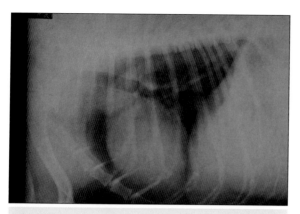

Figure 7.6 *Case 7.2* A left lateral radiograph of the dog after having received five doses of carboplatin by slow intravenous infusion

Theory refresher

As discussed in Chapter 6, the first-line treatment recommendation for primary pulmonary neoplasia in dogs and cats is surgical excision if at all possible, with chemotherapy for lung cancer considered to be a second-line treatment or as postoperative adjunctive therapy at best due to the fact that there is a paucity of data showing consistent efficacy of any particular drug or drug combinations. Chemotherapy cannot therefore be routinely recommended as a sole alternative to surgery. The success of the treatment of the dog in this case example was exceptional but it does show that occasionally, chemotherapy can be extremely useful. Carboplatin has been used in the authors' clinics with some success and there has also been a study indicating that the semi-synthetic vinca alkaloid Vinorelbine has some activity and clinical usefulness in canine lung cancer. Whether or not larger trials will prove a clear role for medical management in these patients remains to be seen. Intrapleural chemotherapy using agents such as carboplatin and mitoxantrone has also been reported to be a useful adjunctive treatment in some cases.

The only pulmonary neoplasm of dogs that has been reported to often respond well to chemotherapy is pulmonary lymphomatoid granulomatosis (PLG). This is a condition reported in several studies and seems to occur in young to middle-aged dogs with no breed or gender predisposition. The dogs generally present with progressive signs of dyspnoea, coughing, exercise intolerance, anorexia, lethargy and occasionally fever and the duration of clinical signs prior to presentation can vary from days to many weeks. Radiographic abnormalities reported include lung lobe consolidation, pulmonary mass lesions, mixed pulmonary patterns of lobar consolidation with ill-defined interstitial and alveolar infiltrates and abnormally large tracheobronchial lymph nodes. A degree of suspicion for this condition can be made by cytological analysis of transtracheal washes or transthoracic fine needle aspirate but definitive diagnosis is by histopathological analysis of surgical biopsies of either a primary lesion or of a tracheobronchial lymph node. In one study, a response rate of 60% was reported to cyclophosphamide and prednisolone with the mean duration of remission being 21 months, although three of the seven dogs in the study did not respond at all. A different study reported a mean survival with treatment of 12.5 months. In the light of this good response to treatment and the risks involved in performing a thoracotomy in a dog with diffuse pulmonary disease, it may be acceptable in some cases to use the response to treatment as a diagnostic tool in a dog with radiographs that may be consistent with PLG (as it would be very unusual for any other diffuse neoplastic conditions of the canine lung to resolve/substantially improve with basic chemotherapy).

Radiotherapy is of very limited use in canine lung cancer, as the sensitivity of the pulmonary tissues to radiation makes it difficult to administer efficacious doses without causing significant side effects. Radiation therapy therefore is rarely recommended for pulmonary neoplasia in small animal patients in the UK.

Metastatic cancer is usually not treated surgically unless there is only a large, single metastatic lesion, but there are reports to indicate that for certain cases, pulmonary metastatectomy can augment survival times and disease-free periods. However, as survival times are generally still poor, such invasive surgery cannot be routinely recommended. Referral to a surgical oncology specialist is definitely recommended if a patient may be considered to be a candidate for such treatment.

Prognosis

The prognosis for patients with primary lung cancer depends upon the clinical stage of the disease and also on the tumour type, so referral to the WHO classification scheme is useful (Box 7.1). A recent study from the UK showed that dogs with papillary adenocarcinoma that had stage T1N0M0 disease had the longest survival times, with a median survival time (MST) of up to 555 days. These data are supported by other studies which indicate that approximately 50% of dogs with a single pulmonary adenocarcinoma measuring less than 5 cm in

Box 7.1 The World Health Organization classification scheme for canine primary lung cancer

T1	Solitary tumour surrounded by lung or visceral pleura
T2	Multiple tumours of any size
T3	Tumour invading neighbouring tissue
N0	No evidence of lymph node involvement
N1	Neoplastic lymph node enlargement
M0	No evidence of metastases
M1	Metastases present

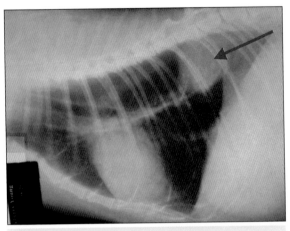

Figure 7.9 A radiograph of the thorax of the cat in Figures 7.7 and 7.8 in which a single, large mass was identified in the left caudodorsal lung field (red arrow). Aspiration of this also revealed carcinoma cells and it was considered most likely that the pulmonary lesion was the primary with the facial and toe lesions being secondary metastases. The cat was euthanized

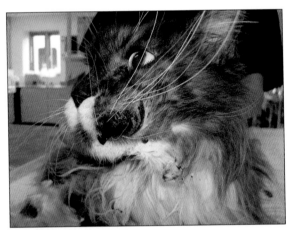

Figure 7.7

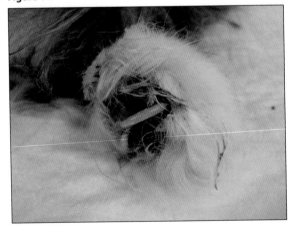

Figure 7.8

Figures 7.7, 7.8 A 9-year-old domestic long-haired (DLH) cat which presented with a non-healing wound on his face and left fore foot. On examination the non-healing wounds were found to be due to mass lesions, aspiration of which revealed the masses to be carcinomas

diameter will be alive 1 year after surgery and their mean survival time is approximately 20 months but that this mean survival time drops to only 8 months if the lesion is greater than 5 cm in diameter. Dogs with pulmonary squamous cell carcinomas also have a worse prognosis when compared to dogs with pulmonary adenocarcinomas (mean survival time of 8 months compared to 19 months in one study). The histological grade certainly impacts on the outcome; dogs with low histological grade adenocarcinomas have on average more than twice the life expectancy of dogs with high histological grade adenocarcinomas (MST 16 months compared to 6 months in one study).

In cats, it appears that the histological grade of the tumour is the only important prognostic factor, with high-grade tumours having a poor survival when compared to moderately differentiated tumours (2.5 months compared to 23 months respectively in one study). An additional anomaly in cats is the atypical condition in which they develop a primary pulmonary carcinoma that metastasises to the digits (and often to other unusual sites too, such as skeletal muscles, skin and kidney) (Figs 7.7–7.9). These patients usually present with painful digital swellings and lameness and, unfortunately, the condition seems very poorly responsive to treatment with average survival times of 1–2 months being reported. Primary pulmonary carcinoma therefore needs to be considered as a possible differential diagnosis in lame cats, particularly if multiple digital swellings are identified.

The presence of metastases and/or a pleural effusion also, as seems logical, have prognostic significance, with patients presenting with metastatic lesions and/or a pleural effusion having significantly poorer outcomes with mean survival times often being as short as 1 or 2 months. However, there are two papers that describe the use of intracavitary chemotherapy as a way of treating animals with malignant effusions and this is now a technique that is used regularly and successfully in the author's (RF) clinic (Fig. 7.10). See also Clinical Case Example 7.3.

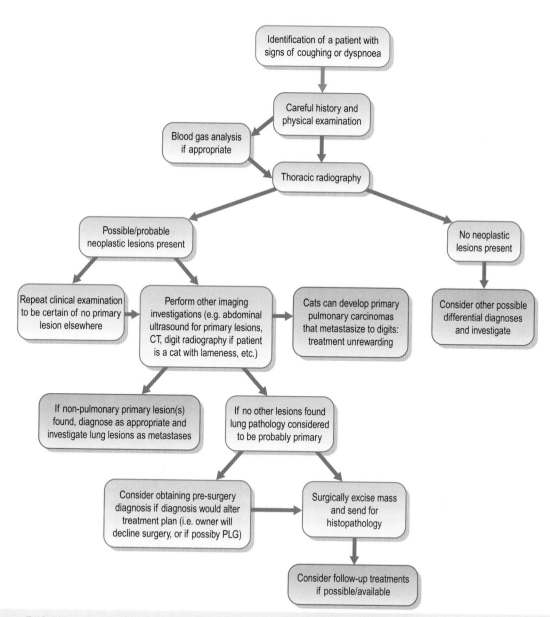

Figure 7.10 Diagnostic plan flowchart for a patient presenting with coughing and/or dyspnoea

CLINICAL CASE EXAMPLE 7.3 – MALIGNANT PLEURAL EFFUSION IN A DOG

Signalment

8-year-old entire female Irish setter dog.

Presenting signs

- A 5-day history of lethargy, inappetance, coughing and progressively worsening abdominal distension.

Clinical examination

- The dog was quiet but moderately alert
- Thin body condition
- Increased breathing rate with increased respiratory effort
- Percussible fluid line and poorly audible breath sounds in the ventral third of the thorax
- Obvious abdominal distension with a palpable fluid thrill.

Diagnostic evaluation

- Thoracic radiographs confirmed the presence of a pleural effusion but no intrathoracic cause was noted
- Abdominal ultrasound confirmed the presence of ascites and revealed marked bilateral ovarian enlargement, with an irregular outline to both ovaries and a heterogeneous appearance
- Abdominocentesis and therapeutic thoracocentesis revealed the presence of a malignant effusion containing malignant epithelial cells (i.e. carcinoma cells) (Fig. 7.11).

Treatment

- Once the pleural effusion had been drained the dog was taken to surgery for exploratory laparotomy. At surgery both ovaries were found to be markedly enlarged, irregular and friable, so the dog underwent ovariohysterectomy. In addition, small white nodular plaques were identified on the peritoneal surface, so these were biopsied.
- Histopathological analysis of the ovaries confirmed the diagnosis to be bilateral ovarian carcinoma. The peritoneal nodules also returned to be consistent with a metastatic carcinoma, thereby explaining the secondary malignant effusions.

Diagnosis

- Metastatic ovarian carcinoma with carcinomatosis and secondary malignant pleural and abdominal effusions.

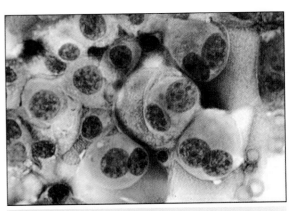

Figure 7.11 The microscopic appearance of neoplastic epithelial cells within an effusion. Note the large nuclei with multiple nucleoli, some multi-nucleated cells and the degree of variation of the cell and nuclear shape and size. Courtesy of Mrs Elizabeth Villiers, Dick White Referrals

Further treatment

The pleural effusion was managed initially postoperatively with surgically placed chest drains but once the diagnosis was made, intrapleural chemotherapy was initiated using 300 mg/m^2 carboplatin, given once every 3 weeks for five treatments. The first treatment was given through the previously placed chest drains but all subsequent treatments were administered via a 21 gauge latex catheter with the dog under medetomidine and butorphanol sedation. The pleural and abdominal effusions resolved within 5 days of starting the intrapleural chemotherapy and the dog's demeanour improved considerably. She exhibited no side effects from the treatment and remained well for 13 months before she re-presented with recurrence of the pleural effusion. Thoracocentesis confirmed recurrence of the carcinoma, so she was euthanized.

Theory refresher

As previously mentioned, malignant effusions represent a significant disease burden as not only do they significantly compromise the patient's quality of life, they represent the possibility of serosal metastasis in every location that has contact with the fluid and as such, are an indicator of a poor prognosis. Any malignant tumour theoretically has the potential to cause a malignant effusion and the appearance and nature of the effusion found can vary due to the fact that malignant effusions can develop due to a variety of (and differing combinations of) pathological mechanisms, namely:

- Increased vascular permeability
- Obstruction of lymphatic vessel flow
- Increased hydrostatic pressure
- Reduced plasma oncotic pressure.

Neoplastic effusions are usually modified transudates or exudates, but it is possible for:

- Transudates to exist if the underlying neoplastic disease causes hypoalbuminaemia
- Septic exudates to be present if an intestinal tumour results in intestinal perforation
- A chylous effusion to be caused by a tumour obstructing lymphatic return.

It is also important to remember that the number of neoplastic cells present within an effusion will vary and their appearance can be altered by their presence within an effusive fluid, so working with a good clinical pathologist to diagnose these cases is essential.

Neoplastic effusions are most commonly seen secondarily to lymphoma, metastatic carcinomas and mesotheliomas, so the identification of potentially malignant epithelial cells in an effusion should alert the clinician to the presence of an actively metastasizing cancer, as was the case in the dog reported here. Treatment of the effusion initially involves identification of the site of the primary lesion and then secondarily assessing the patient for the presence of gross metastases (which may themselves be the cause of the effusion). If there is no gross secondary disease and the primary tumour can be treated successfully (usually by excision), then this may provide symptomatic relief, albeit temporarily. However, neoplastic effusions are themselves a form of metastasis, so further treatment has to be recommended. There are two published reports regarding the use of intracavitary chemotherapy and both report good success using cisplatin, carboplatin or mitoxantrone to treat the effusions. In the author's (RF) clinic a retrospective study has shown that dogs with a carcinomatous malignant pleural effusion treated with intracavitary carboplatin had a median survival time of 295 days and that the treatment was very well tolerated. Furthermore, the largest published study relating to intracavitary chemotherapy showed that without treatment the MST for affected dogs was 25 days compared to an MST of 322 days with treatment. Both in the study in the author's clinic and also in the published studies, the drugs have all been administered at the doses recommended for intravenous administration (i.e. 300 mg/m² for carboplatin) and the incidence of toxic side effects is small. The recommendations from these studies are that the number of

treatments given is dictated by how long it takes for the effusion to clear, with the treatments being given regularly until the effusion resolves, after which, one further treatment is administered. In the author's clinic a standard dose of 300 mg/m² carboplatin is diluted with normal saline to a 5 mg/ml solution before being injected as a bolus into the thorax via an injection cannula. This cannula is then flushed with 10 ml of sterile saline before removal. If both sides of the thorax are being treated, then the dose is divided equally into each hemithorax. This protocol is repeated every 3 weeks until resolution of the pleural effusion is achieved, after which just one more treatment is administered as explained above. The rationale of giving chemotherapy in an intracavitary manner is that the exposed cell surface layers receive a dose 1–3 logs higher than that achieved with intravenous administration.

The response to treatment seen in the Irish setter reported here was significantly better than expected in the light of her disease burden, but illustrates the potential benefit of this simple technique in canine medicine.

Ovarian tumours are not a common problem in dogs or cats, probably due to the high number of female animals who undergo ovariohysterectomy in the UK, although they are a well-recognized problem in rabbits. Ovarian tumours can be classified depending on their cell of origin into one of three types, namely epithelial cell tumours (which include carcinomas), primordial germ cell tumours (such as teratomas) and sex cord stromal cell tumours (such as granulosa cell tumours). Tumours from the epithelial cell tumour group account for approximately 50% of the canine clinical cases reported and, of these, ovarian adenocarcinomas are often associated with extension through the ovarian capsule and into the peritoneum leading to extensive peritoneal implantation and the development of a malignant effusion. Sex cord tumours are the second most common form reported in the dog and these tumours differ from the epithelial group in that they are endocrinologically active in approximately 50% of cases. In cats, sex cord stromal tumours are the most common form reported and in this species they are also often endocrinologically active.

In both dogs and cats, ovarian tumours are more commonly reported in middle-aged to older animals but the clinical signs will vary according to the cell of origin of the tumour. Epithelial tumours can be clinically silent until the effect of a space-occupying mass becomes evident, either due to the physical presence of the tumour itself or due to the effects of any secondary effusions. Stromal sex cord tumours, however, frequently produce excessive amounts of oestrogen resulting in clinical signs of vulval enlargement, vulval discharge, recurrent oestrous activity, alopecia or aplastic anaemia. If the tumour is a progesterone-producing neoplasm, then cystic endometrial hyperplasia and/or pyometra can result. Stromal sex cord tumours in cats are often associated with oestrogen production causing clinical signs of persistent oestrous activity and alopecia.

The first-line treatment for ovarian neoplasia is surgical excision of the tumour and generally ovariohysterectomy is recommended. Careful exploration of the abdomen and especially a careful visual inspection of all the serosal surfaces is recommended at the time of surgery to evaluate the patient for the presence of serosal metastases. If no metastases have developed and complete excision is possible, then the prognosis is considered to be good. However, the presence of metastatic disease carries a guarded prognosis. The use of intracavitary chemotherapy is to be recommended if it is possible but survival times of less than 1 year are to be expected if tumour spread is found.

OTHER RESPIRATORY TRACT TUMOURS

Thymic neoplasia can cause coughing by both direct bronchial compression, or due to aspiration pneumonia caused as a result of paraneoplastic megaoesophagus. The diagnosis and management of thymomas are considered in more detail in Chapter 8. When considering a patient with a possible tracheal tumour it is important to note that there are other non-neoplastic conditions that can cause intraluminal mass lesions or nodular changes that are visible radiographically, such as tracheal parasites, granulomas and inflammatory polyps, so establishing a definite diagnosis is essential, especially as tracheal and laryngeal cancers in dogs and cats are considered to be uncommon. In one review of 78 cases there were 16 canine tracheal tumours, seven feline tracheal tumours, 34 canine laryngeal tumours and 24 feline laryngeal tumours. The review found that epithelial malignancies were most common in the feline trachea and the canine larynx whilst osteochondroma was most common in the canine trachea and lymphoma, the most common feline laryngeal malignancy. Patients were middle-aged to older and presented with signs consistent with upper airway obstruction or dysphonia.

Tracheal tumours may be able to be biopsied via either flexible or rigid endoscopy and if possible, it is

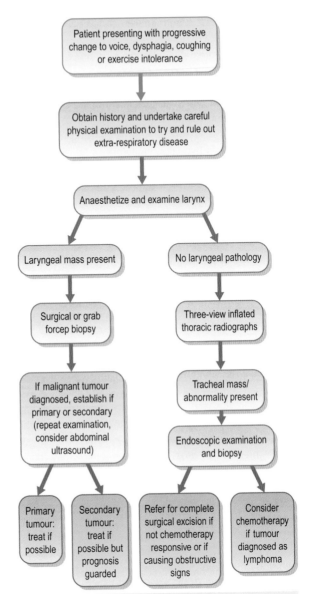

Figure 7.12 Diagnostic plan flowchart for patients presenting with dysphonia, dysphagia and/or coughing

worth attempting to reach a definitive diagnosis before considering surgery in case the tumour is lymphoid in nature and therefore potentially chemotherapy responsive. However, the majority of tracheal tumours will require surgical resection, which is easily possible if up to only four tracheal rings require removal and an end-to-end anastomosis is performed. Larger resections carry a significant risk of postoperative dehiscence and due to the potentially difficult surgery and postoperative care required for these patients, referral to a soft-tissue surgery specialist is recommended for any tracheal resections. However, the prognosis is considered good if complete resection can be achieved and the lesion is benign, although it is important to note that benign tracheal tumours in cats are considered to be rare. There are no large-scale studies available reporting the success of malignant tracheal tumour resection in small animals.

Laryngeal tumours are frequently malignant and locally invasive (Fig. 7.12). Rhabdomyomas in the dog are an exception to this and although they can often be large, they are minimally invasive and do not appear to metastasize. Aside from this, many different tumour types have been reported to develop in the canine larynx (osteosarcoma, chondrosarcoma, fibrosarcoma, squamous cell carcinoma, adenocarcinoma and mast cell tumour) whilst the most common tumour of the feline larynx is lymphoma. Secondary tumours metastasizing to the larynx (and trachea) have also been reported. It is therefore important to obtain good-quality biopsies from a laryngeal tumour, although careful consideration must be given to airway patency following the procedure. Treatment will depend to some degree on the tumour type present. Rhabdomyomas can usually be excised completely whilst retaining normal laryngeal function but malignant tumours may be difficult to manage, as complete laryngectomy (as used in human medicine) is rarely considered in veterinary medicine. Radiation therapy or chemotherapy may be possible and effective depending on the tumour type but malignant laryngeal cancer in cats and dogs carries a guarded prognosis.

8 The dysphagic/gagging/ regurgitating cancer patient

Dysphagia is defined as painful or difficult swallowing and can usually be subclassified as oral dysphagia, pharyngeal dysphagia and cricopharyngeal dysphagia. Dysphagia, therefore, generally refers to pathology within the oral cavity and/or the pharyngeal region. Gagging is defined as the reflex part of swallowing/vomiting, involving elevation of the soft palate followed by reverse peristalsis of the upper gastrointestinal tract and it is often accompanied by retching, which is the involuntary and ineffective attempt to vomit. Regurgitation is defined as the passive, retrograde expulsion of gastric or oesophageal contents and as such is a sign of oesophageal disease. Cancer patients with some or all of these clinical signs therefore could have neoplastic disease in one or more than one of several locations:

- Oral cavity
- Tonsils
- Pharynx/parapharyngeal tissues
- Oesophagus
- Mediastinum (thymus, tracheobronchial lymph nodes or heart base)
- Inner ear
- Central nervous system.

CLINICAL CASE EXAMPLE 8.1 – TONSILLAR CARCINOMA IN A DOG

Signalment

10-year-old neutered male Labrador dog.

Presenting signs

Inappetance, difficulty drinking and excessive salivation.

Case history

- No previous pertinent medical problems
- Two weeks previously, the owner noticed that the dog was starting to become reluctant to eat and

seemed to have difficulty swallowing both food and water. He would go to his bowl and appear interested, take the food into his mouth and then move his head forward in small jerking movements and would extend his neck. This had progressed to him dropping food out of his mouth and then walking away
- The dog was becoming quieter than normal, reluctant to exercise and had lost weight
- In the 5 days prior to presentation he had started to make a sound as if he was trying to clear his throat.

Clinical examination

- The dog was quiet and not particularly responsive
- Resentment when an attempt was made to open his mouth for oral examination
- Palpable swelling in the retropharyngeal region, mainly on the left
- Normal pulmonary auscultation
- No cranial nerve abnormalities, except an inability to assess gag reflex.

Diagnostic evaluation

In this particular case, as the dog would not allow a thorough oral examination, it was decided to undertake a more detailed evaluation under sedation. Careful oropharyngeal examination revealed the presence of an ulcerated mass lesion originating in the region of the left tonsil but extending dorsally and enlarging over the palatine region to the right tonsillar crypt (Fig. 8.1).

Differential diagnosis

- Tonsillar carcinoma
- Tonsillar lymphoma
- Malignant melanoma.

Further evaluation

The dog was anaesthetized and inflated thoracic radiographs were obtained. These revealed no metastatic

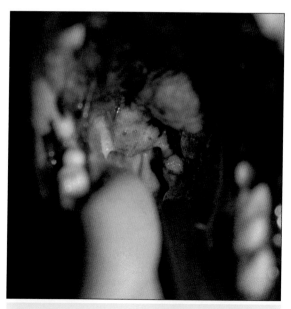

Figure 8.1 *Case 8.1* Intraoral appearance of the significant tonsillar mass extending over the entire palatine arch

lesions. The lesion was then biopsied with rigid grab forceps and haemostasis was achieved by direct pressure using sterile swabs. Prior to biopsy the laryngeal area was packed with a swab bandage to absorb any excessive haemorrhage. The swelling in the retropharyngeal region was assessed by ultrasound. This revealed two large, homogeneous structures consistent in appearance with the retropharyngeal lymph nodes. Fine needle aspirates of these were obtained for cytology.

Diagnosis

- Tonsillar carcinoma with metastasis to the retropharyngeal lymph nodes

In the light of the diagnosis and staging of the tumour, no treatment was recommended other than NSAIDs and antibiotics. The dog was euthanized 5 days later.

Theory refresher

Patients presenting with dysphagia, gagging or retching firstly require a careful history to be obtained in order to attempt to establish exactly what the clinical sign(s) is (are). Oral dysphagia may present as difficulty prehending the food, or as an abnormal movement when swallowing, such as a head tilt or a more violent 'head-throwing' action as if to force the food down, whilst patients with pharyngeal dysphagia often prehend their food normally but then exhibit frequent attempts to swallow, often expressed as frequent flexing and stretching of the neck. Once the presenting problem and history have been established, a careful clinical examination is essential. This should include a thorough neurological evaluation to identify any neuropathy or neuromuscular pathology. Careful visual examination of the oral cavity and oro-pharynx is also required, which may necessitate the use of sedation or even a brief general anaesthetic as some tonsillar tumours will be painful. The aims of the clinical examination are to identify: (a) the primary disease location if possible, (b) the extent of any disease process, (c) the presence of any complicating secondary problems such as aspiration pneumonia and (d) the suitability of the patient for treatments (i.e. Are they currently too ill for major surgery? How will post-surgical nutrition be delivered?).

Tonsillar tumours can present with progressive dysphagia, inappetence, oral/pharyngeal pain, cervical swelling or possibly blood-stained hypersalivation. Diagnosis is made by direct visualization of a tonsillar mass (which often appears reddened, ulcerated and haemorrhagic) and then incisional or excisional biopsy. In the light of the risk of haemorrhage, excisional biopsy is usually considered to be best practice for this condition. Unfortunately, however, the prognosis for patients with primary tonsillar tumours is guarded. Primary tonsillar cancers in cats and dogs are almost always malignant; with squamous cell carcinoma (SCC) being the most common tumour type reported but tonsillar lymphoma has also been described. Other tumour types reported within the tonsils are metastasizing oral neoplasms, especially malignant melanoma.

Tonsillar carcinomas are usually seen in older dogs (mean age 10 years in one study, range 2–17) and are considered highly metastatic tumours, with 10–20% having pulmonary metastasis identified at initial presentation and 77% having distant metastasis identified on post-mortem. No specific breeds have been identified as having a particular predisposition to this disease but some studies have reported a significantly higher incidence of the condition in dogs living in urban environments compared to rural locations. Tonsillar carcinomas display rapid growth, significant invasion into surrounding tissues and early metastasis to regional lymph nodes and then lungs and/or other distant organs. Treatment therefore is difficult, as although tonsillectomy may help to alleviate the presenting clinical signs in the short term (and such a procedure may also be required to achieve a definitive diagnosis), it can never be considered to be a procedure undertaken with curative intent. The efficacy of tonsillectomy with postoperative radiotherapy has been studied and this approach does appear to offer better control of local spread and increases the average survival times compared to surgery alone. But the 1-year survival rates are still very low at 10% and the mean survival time reported in one study was only 151 days. Sole-agent chemotherapy does not appear to have any reasonable activity against tonsillar carcinomas. In one study, various chemotherapy combination treatments were assessed and the mean survival times were only approximately 100 days despite treatment. Combining external beam radiation therapy with chemotherapy (doxorubicin and cisplatin) does appear to generate significantly longer survival times (mean 306 days) but disease progression and the development of distant metastasis is still the major obstacle to longer-term survival times. Currently therefore, the treatment associated with the longest life expectancy for patients with carcinoma of the tonsil would be surgical excision followed by combination radiation and chemotherapy. However, in many cases, advising that no further treatment would be fair for the animal is certainly acceptable if the disease is extensive and the primary tumour is causing significant clinical problems.

CLINICAL CASE EXAMPLE 8.2 – AN OESOPHAGEAL PLASMACYTOMA IN A DOG

Signalment

12-year-old female neutered golden retriever dog.

Case history

Presented for investigation of a 2-week history of regurgitation, haemorrhagic diarrhoea, melena and regenerative anaemia.

Physical examination

- Quiet and lethargic but otherwise examination was unremarkable.

Diagnostic evaluation

- Modest hypoproteinemia (53 mmol/l)
- Regenerative anaemia (HCT 22%, reticulocyte count 287 × 10^9/L)
- Coagulation times (APTT, OSPT) were within normal limits, as was her platelet count

- Thoracic radiography demonstrated a soft-tissue density (approximately 2 × 3 cm) in the caudal oesophagus at the sixth intercostal space. Upper gastrointestinal contrast studies highlighted the mass further. Abdominal ultrasound revealed no significant abnormalities. Upper gastrointestinal endoscopy revealed a mass within the oesophagus just caudal to the heart base, emanating from the right lateral oesophageal wall, measured 5 cm in length and occupying approximately a third of the oesophageal diameter. On the dorsocaudal surface there was a clearly friable area that was haemorrhaging (Figs 8.2–8.4)
- The remainder of the upper gastrointestinal tract was unremarkable.

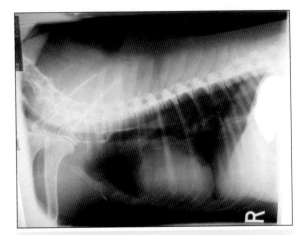

Figure 8.2 *Case 8.2* The initial barium oesophogram

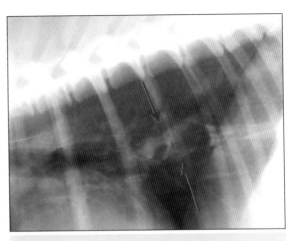

Figure 8.3 *Case 8.2* The intraoesophageal mass highlighted by the arrows

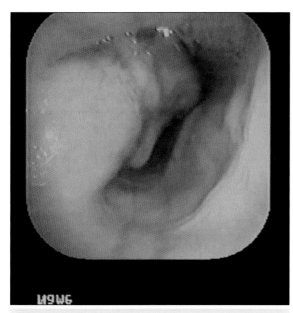

Figure 8.4 *Case 8.2* The endoscopic appearance of the mass

Treatment

- The mass was removed surgically via an intercostal approach and oesophagotomy. The patient was positioned in right lateral recumbency to facilitate an eighth intercostal thoracotomy approach. The left caudal lung lobe was packed cranially with moistened laparotomy sponges. The oesophagus was visualized and the vagal branches bluntly dissected free. The oesophagus was elevated with umbilical tapes and palpation of the oesophagus permitted localization of the intraluminal mass. The oesophagus was incised on its lateral aspect and fluid material was aspirated from the lumen. The mass was found to have a pedicle attachment and was dissected from the muscularis layer with wide local margins. The defect in the muscularis/mucosa was closed with single interrupted sutures of 4/0 polydioxanone The oesophagotomy site was further closed with a second layer of single interrupted sutures using polydioxanone. The thoracic wall was routinely closed and a 6.7-mm diameter thoracic drain tube was positioned caudal to the thoracotomy wound. The pleural space was aspirated via an underwater seal and the drain removed 12 hours later.

Diagnosis

- Histopathology confirmed the mass to be an IgG-positive plasmacytoma.

The dog made a rapid and uneventful recovery from surgery and her anaemia totally resolved within 10 days, thereby confirming this to be due to blood loss from the tumour. Six months after her surgery, she underwent a further oesophagoscopy which confirmed no evidence of regrowth of the mass and the dog remained well.

Theory refresher

Patients who regurgitate can be difficult to initially identify as many owners will perceive the clinical signs as being vomiting rather than regurgitation. Regurgitation is a passive event during which the oesophageal contents are expelled either very soon or possibly minutes to hours after feeding. It is usually possible to differentiate from vomiting by the lack of strong abdominal contractions and also regurgitation should not normally have yellow-green bile staining. Regurgitated food may have a 'sausage shape' and should certainly appear undigested but this alone is not pathognomonic. Many animals may also regurgitate large volumes of viscous white froth which, if there is significant intraoesophageal pathology, may be blood-stained. Some patients will be quiet or dull before regurgitating, especially if they are experiencing significant oesophageal discomfort as a result of the underlying pathology and/or because of the resulting oesophageal distension. Regurgitating patients may also often present with secondary inhalation pneumonia (manifested as dullness, pyrexia, tachypnoea/dyspnoea and a moist productive cough) which obviously can generate complications in that these patients will be significantly sick because of their infection as well as from the cause of their regurgitation and their poor nutritional status. If it proves difficult to establish from the history whether a patient is regurgitating or vomiting, observing them attempting to eat a test meal can be extremely useful.

Oesophageal cancer is rare, accounting for less than 0.5% of all canine and feline tumours. In dogs the most frequently identified tumour type is a carcinoma, although sarcomas secondary to *Spirocerca lupi* infestation would be considered more common in indigenous regions (Africa, Israel, and south-east USA). Occasionally, more unusual tumours such as osteosarcoma or plasma cell tumours have been reported within the oesophagus. Paraoesophageal tumours of the heart base, thyroid and thymus can also invade into the oesophagus resulting in oesophageal signs but this is unusual. In cats, squamous cell carcinomas are considered to be the most frequently recognized primary oesophageal tumour. Interestingly they are reported to occur more frequently in females and are most often located just caudal to the thoracic inlet. Neoplasia can also affect the oesophagus in the form of a thymoma inducing myasthenia gravis, causing megaoesophagus. It is reported that up to 66% of canine thymoma cases will present with myasthenia gravis, which may be focal, oesophageal or generalized and patients with either form often present with clinical signs of regurgitation, although patients with the generalized form of the disease will also display the characteristic signs of weakness on exertion, etc.

Following the history and clinical examination, further evaluation of a patient that is regurgitating and may therefore have an oesophageal neoplasm is made by undertaking thoracic radiographs, initially with plain films but possibly also by undertaking a barium contrast series. Barium studies need to be undertaken with caution in patients which have aspirated in the past, as aspiration of barium will result in the long-term presence of the contrast agent within the bronchi. Should a stricture or mass be identified within the oesophagus, oesophagoscopy should then be undertaken and grab biopsies of the mass obtained at the same time if the mass is present within the lumen. Attempting to reach a diagnosis without resorting to surgery is advisable, if possible, for patients with primary oesophageal tumours, because the prognosis varies considerably depending on the tumour type. Malignant oesophageal tumours are often not resectable due to the frequently advanced stage of the disease by the time they present and the surgical difficulties encountered by undertaking extensive oesophageal reconstruction. In addition, malignant oesophageal tumours commonly show a high incidence of metastatic disease. However, although there are no large-scale studies describing the use of chemotherapy as a sole-treatment modality in canine oesophageal tumours, one report describes the use of doxorubicin following partial oesophagectomy in six dogs that had *Spirocirca lupi*-associated oesophageal sarcomas and the median survival time in these dogs was 267 days. Adjunctive chemotherapy may therefore have a role to play in combination with good surgical management of these tumours but further studies in this area are required. The use of radiotherapy is restricted to the extrathoracic oesophagus due to the poor tolerance of the surrounding intrathoracic tissues. Referral therefore, of patients with an oesophageal malignancy to a soft-tissue/surgical oncology specialist for further evaluation and excision, if possible, is highly recommended, but the prognosis for these patients is often guarded. Conversely, benign lesions such as leiomyomas or plasmacytomas often have a reasonable prognosis as long as their size does not preclude complete surgical excision.

Cranial mediastinal tumours may cause signs of regurgitation or gagging due to a direct mass effect resulting in oesophageal compression, oesophageal invasion (unusual) or due to the development of myasthenia gravis as a paraneoplastic syndrome. Heart base tumours are rare in dogs and even more unusual in cats and it would be considered unusual (although possible) for them to affect the oesophagus. There is also one case report of a gastric carcinoma extending cranially along the distal oesophagus into the cranial mediastinum causing recurrent dysphagia. The tumour within the cranial mediastinum that most commonly affects the oesophagus, however, is thymoma. The presence of a thymoma causing secondary oesophageal dysfunction was first described in the dog in 1972 and since then there have been many studies showing that thymomas can be associated with an autoimmune paraneoplastic syndrome characterized by megaoesophagus and polymyositis. The incidence of megaoesophagus varies depending on the report; one study showed that 47% of dogs with a thymoma had megaoesophagus, whilst a second study indicated that 66% of cases were affected. It is therefore possible to conclude that a significant number of dogs with a thymoma will develop megaoesophagus and this has a very important prognostic value, as the presence of megaoesophagus has been shown to reduce the chances of a successful outcome.

CLINICAL CASE EXAMPLE 8.3 – A MEDIASTINAL LYMPHOMA IN A DOG

Signalment
6-year-old neutered male Labrador dog.

Presenting signs
- Progressive history over the preceding 3 weeks of gradually worsening appetite with associated weight loss, tachypnoea and retching.

Clinical examination
- Quiet and poorly responsive
- Tachypnoeic with increased respiratory effort
- No audible lung sounds in the ventral third of the thorax and thoracic percussion in this area was dull
- Reduced thoracic compressibility
- No other abnormalities detected.

Diagnostic evaluation

- A right lateral thoracic radiograph revealed the presence of a large cranial thoracic mass and a DV thoracic radiograph confirmed the mass to be within the cranial mediastinum (Fig. 8.5)
- Thoracic ultrasound confirmed the presence of a mediastinal mass
- Fine needle aspirates of the mass were highly suggestive of lymphoma (Fig. 8.6)
- A B-cell lymphoma was confirmed as the diagnosis by undertaking flow cytometric analysis of aspirate samples.

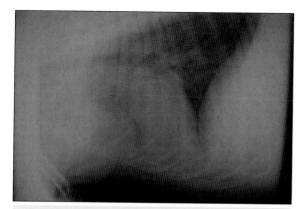

Figure 8.5 *Case 8.3* A right lateral thoracic radiograph showing the presence of a large cranial thoracic mass

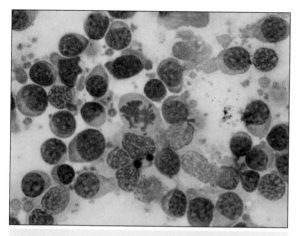

Figure 8.6 *Case 8.3* The appearance of a fine needle aspirate sample (Giemsa stain, x100), showing the presence of large lymphoblasts containing variable numbers of variably shaped nucleoli. Note also the mitotic figure in the middle of the image

Treatment

- After careful discussion with his owners, the dog was started on a modified Madison-Wisconsin multidrug chemotherapy protocol (see page 195) which he received for 25 weeks.
- The dog went into complete remission (Fig. 8.7) and remained healthy for 14 months before relapsing.
- The owners declined using doxorubicin as a rescue agent on cost grounds, so the dog was treated with oral CCNU. This generated a partial remission, in that he became well in himself again but the mass did not totally resolve radiographically. He remained well for just under 5 months on CCNU and then he deteriorated and was euthanized.

Theory refresher

Cranial mediastinal tumours are most likely to be either a thymoma or lymphoma. Thymomas originate from the thymic epithelium, but due to the cellular nature of the thymus the tumour is often significantly infiltrated by lymphocytes thereby making cytological differentiation between thymoma and lymphoma sometimes very difficult. They are not considered to be common tumours and they generally occur in older animals. No breed predilections have been proven, although medium- to large-breed dogs may be reported disproportionately more often. There are three histological types of thymoma (epithelial, lymphocyte-rich and clear cell) but there seems to be no clinical or prognostic value in differentiating between them. What is more important from a surgical point of view is whether the thymoma is well-encapsulated and not invading surrounding tissues

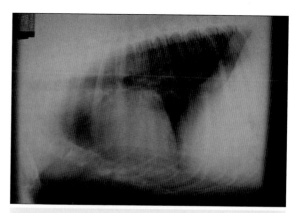

Figure 8.7 *Case 8.3* A right lateral thoracic radiograph from the dog at week 9 of his chemotherapy protocol, showing complete resolution of the cranial mediastinal mass

(so-called 'benign' thymoma) or whether it is attached to and invading surrounding structures such as the pericardium and cranial vena cava (so-called 'malignant' thymomas). The use of the terms 'benign' and 'malignant' are misleading as they do not relate directly to the histological appearance of the tumours or their behaviour and metastasis from a 'malignant thymoma', although reported, is rare.

Although thymomas can cause regurgitation and gagging, most patients will present with clinical signs more attributable to the respiratory system, with coughing, tachypnoea and exercise intolerance frequently reported. On physical examination, careful auscultation and percussion of the thorax may reveal reduced/absent breath sounds in the cranioventral thorax and caudal displacement of the heart sounds, whilst thoracic palpation frequently reveals reduced compressibility of the chest. Radiographs of the thorax reveal either a clear soft-tissue density cranial to the heart, or possibly the presence of a pleural effusion, in which case, ultrasonography will be useful to identify the presence of a cranial mediastinal mass.

Making a definitive diagnosis by cytology is worth attempting but can be frustrating due to the high number of small lymphocytes that are usually found in thymomas, creating difficulty differentiating thymoma from lymphoma (Fig. 8.8). This can be complicated by

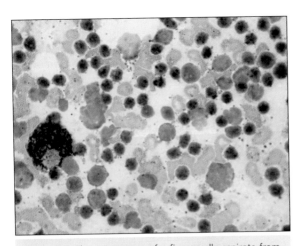

Figure 8.8 The appearance of a fine needle aspirate from a patient with a thymoma. There is a mixed population of lymphoid cells and scattered mast cells. Epithelial cells have not been harvested in this aspirate (this happens not uncommonly). The mast cells are a characteristic of thymomas and the lymphoid cells are mixed but mainly small. Courtesy of Mrs Elizabeth Villiers, Dick White Referrals

the fact that a minority of thymomas will be hypercalcaemic on serum biochemistry analysis, a feature more commonly associated with lymphoma.

Although the signalment of the patient may help (lymphoma is more usually seen in younger cats and dogs whilst thymoma generally occurs in older animals), other ways of obtaining a definitive diagnosis often need to be considered. Tru-cut biopsies are an option but these too, do not always lead to a definitive result, especially if the mass has a significant cystic component to its structure. Good biopsy samples are usually obtained using thorascopic biopsy techniques but this is not readily available outside referral centres. A recent study, however, showed that flow cytometry analysis of aspirate samples can be extremely useful, as thymomas appear to generally have more than 10% of their lymphocytes co-expressing CD4 and CD8 whilst almost all lymphomas will have fewer than 2% of the CD4+ CD8+ lymphocytes. At the time of writing, only the University of Cambridge veterinary diagnostic laboratory offers flow cytometry as a routine test within the UK to the authors' knowledge but this is certain to change over the next few years. Aspirate samples are obtained as usual but are placed into phosphate-buffered saline rather than onto a microscope slide and submitted along with other standard slide samples for microscopic analysis. If possible, cytology and flow cytometry on ultrasound-guided aspirates remains the author's diagnostic method of choice, coupled with the ultrasonographic appearance of the mass, as a study from 1991 suggested that lymphoma usually appears as a homogeneous, often hypoechoic mass, whilst thymoma usually has a heterogeneous appearance. If this does not lead to a definitive diagnosis the author recommends undertaking thoracoscopy and thoracoscopic biopsies, reserving surgical thoracotomy and attempted excisional biopsy only if the other techniques fail to reveal the diagnosis.

If a definitive diagnosis cannot be reached, it may be acceptable in some situations to see if the mass will shrink with chemotherapy. However, the authors' experience of this is inconsistent, probably because many lymphomas do not respond quickly enough to vincristine and L-asparaginase and the clinical deterioration in many cases prompts surgical intervention. It is also ethically questionable to give a dog without a proven lymphoma drugs such as doxorubicin in the light of the possible side effects some dogs will experience. Surgery therefore sometimes becomes both a diagnostic and therapeutic tool, as the definitive treatment for thymoma is complete surgical excision and in cases where a presurgical

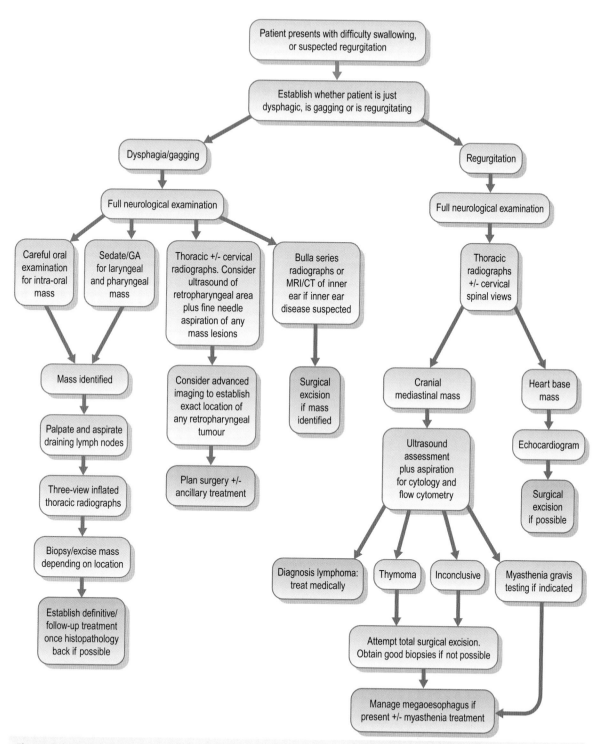

Figure 8.9 Diagnostic plan flowchart for patients presenting with dysphagia, gagging or regurgitation

diagnosis has been elusive, undertaking exploratory thoracotomy becomes the only realistic option. If possible, the mass should be excised completely, but this may be difficult in cases of undiagnosed lymphoma and also in malignant thymomas. If excision is deemed impossible, then large wedge biopsies should be taken to ensure that representative samples can be analysed histopathologically.

The prognosis for benign thymomas in dogs and cats that can be excised is generally very good, especially if there is not a concurrent megaesophagus present. Eighty-three per cent 1-year survival rates have been reported for such cases in dogs whilst one study showed that 10/12 cats had no recurrence of their tumour following excisional surgery, although two did die in the immediate postoperative period. Cases that present with megaoesophagus are more challenging; as it is currently not possible to predict whether or not the oesophageal dilatation will resolve and many cases do not. One paper suggests that removal of the thymoma led to an improved response to anticholinesterase treatments, but management of megaoesophagus remains a considerable medical challenge and many patients will succumb to aspiration pneumonia.

Thymoma in the rabbit is associated with dyspnoea, bilateral exophthalmos and facial oedema. It is considered rare, but there are a number of reports and reviews in the literature. Metastasis is occasionally reported both within the thoracic cavity and abdominal cavity. Diagnosis is by radiography, ultrasound-guided fine needle aspiration and MRI that reveal the presence of a cranial mediastinal mass. The treatment of choice is surgical excision by median sternotomy. Chemotherapy and radiation therapy have been considered as adjunct therapy after surgical resection. However, radiation therapy provides only short-term control of disease progression and chemotherapy has limited utility.

There are a large number of differential diagnoses for dyspnoea in rabbits and these include respiratory and cardiac disease. Other neoplastic causes for dyspnoea include secondary metastasis of a uterine adenocarcinoma or lymphoma. Both of these are considered extremely common neoplastic diseases of the rabbit.

9 The vomiting and/or diarrhoeic cancer patient

Vomiting is the active expulsion of material from within the stomach and/or upper small intestine. Vomiting should always be differentiated from regurgitation either by careful history evaluation or by direct observation. Vomiting usually causes a prodromal nausea (characterized by salivation, lip licking, appearing anxious or pacing) and then usually proceeds to retching, whilst a regurgitating patient does not usually exhibit these features. Vomiting also usually involves visible contraction of the abdominal muscles whereas regurgitation usually does not. Analysis of the vomitus itself usually reveals a pH less than 5 (regurgitated fluid should not be acidic) unless there is bile present, in which case the pH will often be alkaline. Assessment of the vomitus for the presence of bilirubin (either based on the yellow-green colour or by using a simple urine dipstick) can therefore sometimes be helpful too.

Vomiting can be caused by disease in many areas of the body and therefore from an oncological point of view, may indicate the presence of a tumour in locations other than the stomach. It is helpful to adopt a logical body-systems-based approach to the investigation of a vomiting cancer patient, by considering where and what type of tumour may be present as shown in Box 9.1.

CLINICAL CASE EXAMPLE 9.1 – GASTRIC ADENOCARCINOMA IN A DOG

Signalment

9-year-old neutered male Labrador dog.

Presenting signs

Persistent vomiting.

Case history

The relevant history in this particular case was:
- No pertinent previous history relating to the gastro-intestinal system.

- The dog started to vomit intermittently 5 weeks previously but initially seemed well. However, over the preceding 2 weeks, the vomiting had progressed from occurring after some meals, to occurring after every meal, leading to inappetance and loss of condition.
- Vomiting had continued despite the poor appetite, with vomitus consisting mainly of viscous white froth that in the 3 days prior to examination had contained small flecks of blood.

Clinical examination

- Quiet and disinterested in his surroundings
- Thin body condition
- Mild discomfort on palpation of cranial abdomen
- No other specific abnormalities.

Differential diagnosis

- Gastrointestinal disease
  - Severe gastritis
  - Foreign body
  - Gastric neoplasia
    - Adenocarcinoma
    - Lymphoma
  - Intestinal neoplasia
  - Pancreatitis
- Hepato-biliary disease
  - Hepatitis
  - Cholangitis
  - Hepatic neoplasia
    - Hepatocellular carcinoma
    - Lymphoma
- Metabolic disease
  - Renal failure
  - Electrolyte disturbances.

Diagnostic evaluation

- Serum biochemistry ruled out major metabolic disease

- Diagnostic imaging (plain thoracic and abdominal radiographs and abdominal ultrasound) revealed no significant abnormalities
- Gastroscopy revealed the presence of an ulcerated lesion on the lesser curvature located on the pyloric aspect of the angularis inscisura (Fig. 9.1)
- Biopsies from the periphery of the ulcer revealed a gastric adenocarcinoma.

Theory refresher

Gastric cancer is thought to account for less than 1% of all malignancies and is seen less often in cats compared to dogs. It is generally a disease seen in older dogs and the most common form is gastric adenocarcinoma (approximately 75% of all cases) although leiomyosarcoma, lymphoma, mast cell tumour, extramedullary

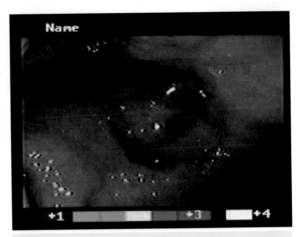

Figure 9.1 *Case 9.1* A video endoscopic image from the dog, showing a large, erythematous ulcerated area on the pyloric side of the angularis incisura

---

Box 9.1 Types of tumour that could be associated with causing vomiting

Gastric tumours
Adenocarcinoma
Lymphoma
Gastrointestinal stromal tumours (GISTs)
Mast cell tumour
Extramedullary plasmacytoma
Fibrosarcoma
Malignant histiocytosis
Histiocytic sarcoma

Intestinal tumours
Lymphoma
Adenocarcinoma
GISTs
Carcinoid
Mast cell tumour
Extramedullary plasmacytoma
Extraskeletal osteosarcoma
Haemangiosarcoma

Abdominal tumours
Pancreatic adenocarcioma
Hepatocellular carcinoma
Hepatic lymphoma
Biliary carcinoma
Alimentary lymphoma
Haemangiosarcoma

Tumours causing metabolic dysfunction
Hepatocellular carcinoma
Gastrinoma
Urinary bladder transitional cell carcinoma (causing ureteric or urethral obstruction)

CNS tumours

---

plasmacytoma and fibrosarcoma have all been reported. In cats, the stomach is the least common part of the gastrointestinal tract to be affected by tumours, but, if present, lymphoma is the most likely tumour type to be identified. The clinical histories in affected patients can be quite vague, although as in the case example, most cases will present with a progressively worsening history of vomiting, and frequently, dogs with gastric tumours will present appearing generally unwell, although depending on the duration of the history, some cases will present in good condition. The presence of fresh blood or 'coffee ground' haematemesis is only suggestive of the presence of gastric ulceration but this raises the index of suspicion for gastric neoplasia in an older dog.

Initial diagnostic evaluation, as in the clinical case example, can frequently appear unremarkable. Positive contrast radiographic studies may reveal a lesion within the gastric lumen, or be suggestive of gastric ulceration, but ultrasound may often not reveal the presence of a lesion unless it is located within the distal third of the stomach due to the difficulties of imaging the cranial areas of the stomach, unless it is fluid-filled. However, ultrasound can be very useful to assess the gastric and mesenteric lymph nodes and if these are found to be enlarged, to enable ultrasound-guided fine needle aspiration to be performed. Many gastric tumours are diagnosed late in the clinical stage of the disease, by which time, metastasis to the local lymph nodes or other surrounding organs may have occurred, so such assessment

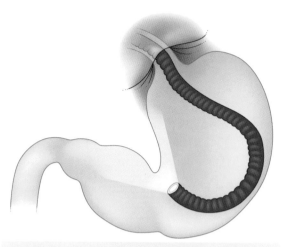

Figure 9.2 The 'J-manoeuvre'; adapted from 'Veterinary Endoscopy for the Small Animal Practitioner', Timothy C McCartney, Elsevier-Saunders 2005, p. 294

is essential in the clinical staging of the disease. Ultrasound can also reveal the loss of layering of the gastric structure that may be seen with an infiltrative condition such as lymphoma.

Flexible endoscopy is very useful to identify intraluminal lesions but it is vital that a logical, stepwise examination technique is adopted to ensure that all the gastric mucosa has been thoroughly visualized. Although the majority of gastric tumours in the dog will be located on the lesser curvature or within the antrum, it is important to remember that a 'J-manoeuvre' must be performed to ensure that the cardiac area has been fully examined, as it is possible for small tumours to exist just behind and above the gastro-oesophageal junction and these are easy to miss on simple aboral evaluation if the endoscope is not retroflexed (Fig. 9.2).

If the stomach contains a significant volume of gastric juice, then this should either be suctioned out through the endoscope, or the dog turned from one lateral recumbency to the other to ensure that all areas of the mucosa have been visualized. Some authors recommend premedication of gastroscopy patients with anticholinergics, as these can help reduce the volume of gastric secretions and the degree of gastric motility, but their use is obviously one of personal preference. The authors generally do not find the use of anticholinergics necessary and prefer to undertake gastroscopy with the dog lying in left lateral recumbency, as this allows a clear view of the antrum and pylorus without the risk of fluid obstruction in this area.

Biopsying lesions with endoscopic grab biopsy forceps needs to be undertaken carefully, especially if gastric ulceration is identified. It is not advisable to attempt endoscopic biopsy of the ulcerated tissue itself, as this (a) will likely only yield necrotic tissue of little or no diagnostic use and (b) carries a greater risk of perforation of the gastric wall. Rather, it is better to biopsy the tissue adjacent to the ulcer, as this is much more likely to produce tissue of diagnostic use whilst carrying no greater risk than normal of causing accidental perforation. Obtaining multiple biopsies is essential to increase the representative nature of the samples obtained. It is also important to remember that if one lesion is found and biopsied, a complete gastric examination is still essential in case there is more than one lesion present.

Unless the histopathology confirms the diagnosis to be lymphoma, the only treatment commonly utilized for gastric tumours in cats and dogs is surgery, but this needs to be performed with full owner knowledge that in many cases, even with complete resection, the prognosis has to be considered to be guarded. Gastric adenocarcinomas are usually aggressive tumours that metastasize to the local lymph nodes, liver and finally lungs if left untreated. Many cases present late in their disease course and the possibility of microscopic metastasis existing before the macroscopic form of the disease has been identified has to be considered, so undertaking surgery with curative intent is difficult. However, if a lesion is found to be solitary, then partial gastrectomy can be considered. The problem with such surgery is that as a wide resection is usually required, reconstruction often entails a gastroduodenostomy (Billroth I) and referral to a soft-tissue or oncological surgical specialist is recommended for these patients. The other concern is that the prognosis, even with radical surgery is often poor with survival times in excess of 6 months being uncommon and some studies citing mean survival times as short as 2 months. No chemotherapy has been shown to be efficacious for gastric adenocarcinomas in dogs or cats and its use is not recommended.

Other benign or lower-grade malignant gastric tumours may be more amenable to surgical excision, thereby illustrating the importance of attempting to obtain a presurgical diagnosis if possible. Leiomyomas appear to be found more frequently in the proximal third of the stomach and can usually be removed via a midline laparotomy. Partial gastrectomy has been greatly facilitated in recent years by the use of surgical stapling equipment such as the TA-55 and TA-90 (p. 201). At the time of surgery it is important to examine and biopsy local lymph nodes and any suspicious areas on the surface of the liver or within the omentum.

CLINICAL CASE EXAMPLE 9.2 – DIFFUSE HEPATOCELLULAR CARCINOMA IN A DOG

Signalment

9-year-old neutered female golden retriever dog.

Presenting signs

Persistent vomiting.

Clinical history

- Two weeks of mild lethargy but generally well
- 4 days prior to presentation vomiting and very dull.

Physical examination

- Quiet but responsive
- Mild jaundice
- HR 140 bpm
- No obvious liver enlargement.

Diagnostic evaluation

- ALT 446 iu/L
- ALP 250 iu/L
- TBil 45 mmol/L
- PCV 33%
- Postprandial bile acids 87 μmol/L
- Abdominal and thoracic radiographs unremarkable
- Ultrasound revealed a diffuse, heterogeneous echotexture throughout all liver lobes. No other abnormalities noted (Fig. 9.3)
- Coagulation profile (one-stage prothrombin time, activated partial thromboplastin time) and complete blood count were checked before fine needle aspiration of the liver was undertaken
- Cytology revealed pleomorphic polygonal cells in a chaotic pattern. The cells had large round nuclei with variably prominent and variable numbers of nucleoli. The cytoplasm was sparse and grainy
- Diagnosis: diffuse hepatocellular carcinoma.

Theory refresher

This case illustrates how a tumour outside of the gastro-intestinal tract (and this could therefore also apply, especially to pancreatic tumours) can cause significant gastric signs of disease. The exact reasons why liver disease causes vomiting often cannot be identified, but portal hypertension, hepatic encephalopathy and an altered cytokine environment may all play a part. This case also

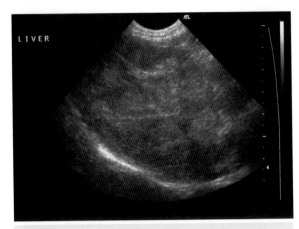

Figure 9.3 *Case 9.2* Ultrasound picture revealing the diffuse, heterogeneous echotexture identified throughout all liver lobes

illustrates that diffuse hepatic disease can cause quite specific clinical signs and it must be remembered that the same type of tumour could cause different clinical signs in different patients.

Considering canine hepatocellular carcinoma specifically, the tumour can exist in three main forms:

1. Single, 'massive' tumour
2. Multiple nodular tumour
3. Diffuse tumour.

The prognosis varies considerably between these different types. If a single massive tumour can be excised without difficulty and there is no evidence of metastatic disease, then average survival times of more than 1400 days have been reported and although these tumours do carry a metastatic potential, the rate of tumour spread clinically appears to be low. Massive hepatocellular carcinomas on the right-hand side of the liver carry a more guarded prognosis with respect to surviving surgery due to the increased risk of intraoperative vena cava trauma, but once removed, their prognosis is the same as for massive hepatocellular carcinomas arising from the left-hand side of the liver. However, the prognosis for both the nodular forms and the diffuse forms is extremely guarded, as surgical excision is usually not possible due to the extensive nature of the disease and many hepatocellular carcinomas appear to be inherently chemotherapy-resistant. The dog in the case example was not considered a candidate for surgery due to the diffuse nature of her tumour affecting every liver lobe, so she was euthanized.

Other forms of hepatobiliary tumour can cause vomiting and also certainly inappetance along, possibly, with other signs such as ascites and polydipsia. Neoplasia can develop within the biliary tree, and especially in cats, bile duct adenomas are frequently reported. Benign tumours such as these generally only cause clinical signs to become apparent when they grow to such a size as to exert a local mass effect. However, malignant biliary neoplasia in the form of a biliary carcinoma, which is reported to be the most common malignant hepatobiliary tumour of cats and the second most common hepatobiliary malignancy in dogs in some studies, cause clinical signs due to their aggressive behaviour. Malignant biliary tumours can form within the gall bladder, within the hepatic biliary tissue or within the extrahepatic bile ducts. Metastasis with biliary carcinoma is frequently found at presentation with spread being seen both locally to the draining lymphatics and also potentially to distant sites. In cats, spread along the peritoneal surface can develop, leading to carcinomatosis in many cases. The treatment for each case therefore depends upon firstly whether the tumour is benign or malignant. Biliary adenomas are usually amenable to surgical excision, although this may require a liver lobectomy, and the prognosis for these cases can be considered to be good. Surgery is obviously advisable for cases of biliary carcinoma as long as the preoperative staging did not identify any metastatic disease. However, even in patients who have no distant disease noted on staging, survival times of greater than 6 months following surgery are unusual, due to the development of distant metastatic disease. No efficacious chemotherapeutic regimens have been described for this disease in cats or dogs, so the use of medical cytotoxic therapy cannot be recommended at the time of writing.

Hepatic 'carcinoids' are a form of neuroendocrine tumour that develop from the neuroectoderm cells within the liver and are therefore not a form of carcinoma, despite their name. However, these also behave in an aggressive fashion with metastatic disease frequently being identified on clinical staging procedures. No efficacious chemotherapeutic regimens have been described for this disease in cats or dogs, so the use of medical cytotoxic therapy cannot be recommended at the time of writing.

Epithelial pancreatic tumours such as pancreatic carcinoma can certainly produce vomiting, lethargy and weight loss. These tumours can be small and difficult to visualize on ultrasound but their aggressive behaviour frequently means that the metastatic disease is identifiable on clinical staging. No efficacious chemotherapeutic regimens have been described for this disease in cats or dogs, so the use of medical cytotoxic therapy cannot be recommended at the time of writing, meaning that surgical excision is the only treatment advisable. If a partial pancreatectomy is to be performed, considerable thought has to be given as to the postoperative management, as it is quite likely that the patient will develop pancreatitis as a result of the surgical handling of the pancreas. Placement of a jejunostomy tube should therefore be considered. The problem with placing a more simple gastrostomy tube is that feeding through a G-tube is often just as likely to induce vomiting as feeding per os, but at least if a G-tube is placed then there is a chance to feed the animal if it is inappetant post-surgery. Elective postoperative placement of a naso-oesophageal feeding tube in an animal that is vomiting is not generally encouraged due to the possibility of the animal repositioning the tube during a vomiting or retching episode which could include the tube passing into the trachea. Should this occur and it not be detected before feeding then takes place, the resulting aspiration pneumonia is likely to be disastrous.

CLINICAL CASE EXAMPLE 9.3 – A CAT WITH INTESTINAL LYMPHOMA

Signalment

13-year-old neutered female domestic short-haired (DSH) cat.

Presenting signs

A 4-week history of gradually worsening inappetance, weight loss and diarrhoea.

Clinical history

The relevant clinical history for this case was:

- Usually healthy, fully vaccinated and wormed regularly, fed premium-brand dry cat food
- Over the preceding 4 weeks, she had become gradually more lethargic and withdrawn. Her appetite was reduced and she was losing weight
- Her faecal consistency had been progressively worsening, from being pasty through to very watery over the period of her illness. In the week prior to presentation the owner described the faeces as being like 'watery paste'.

Clinical examination

- Quiet and lethargic, poor hair coat quality and poor body condition

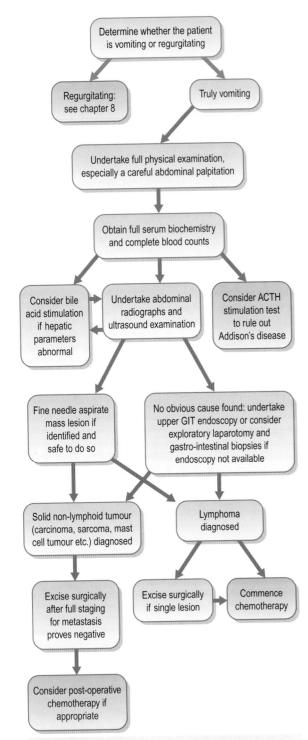

Figure 9.4 Diagnostic plan flowchart: vomiting and regurgitation

- No palpable masses on abdominal palpation
- No palpable peripheral lymph nodes.

Diagnostic evaluation

- Serum biochemistry revealed hypoalbuminaemia (19 g/L) and mild elevations in ALT and ALP. Bile acid stimulation was normal
- FeLV/FIV negative
- Urinalysis was unremarkable
- Abdominal ultrasound revealed a complete loss of layering and thickening of the intestinal wall within the small intestine, along with a mild mesenteric lymphadenopathy
- Fine needle aspiration of the mesenteric lymph nodes was non-diagnostic
- Flexible endoscopy revealed a normal appearance to the gastric mucosa but the duodenal mucosa appeared thickened, granular and pale in appearance (Fig. 9.5).

Diagnosis

- Grab biopsies of the duodenal mucosa confirmed the diagnosis to be lymphoma.

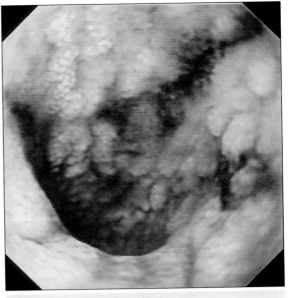

Figure 9.5 *Case 9.3* The endoscopic appearance of the duodenal mucosa in the cat revealing the irregular, almost nodular appearance of the intestinal surface. Courtesy of Dr Alex German, University of Liverpool

Treatment

- The cat was treated with a high-dose COP protocol and improved clinically within 5 days of commencing treatment, in that the owner described her as less lethargic and her appetite improved. Her diarrhoea stopped 8 days after treatment commenced and the cat improved considerably. Repeated ultrasound 4 weeks after the treatment had started showed none of the abnormalities previously identified to be present, thereby indicating that the cat had gone into complete remission
- She remained well for 15 months before being lost to follow-up.

Theory refresher

Intestinal neoplasia accounts for up to 10% of all canine and feline tumours reported in the veterinary literature and as with gastric neoplasia, many different tumour types have been reported to arise within the intestine but the main two are lymphoma and adenocarcinoma. Malignant epithelial tumours (adenocarcinomas) will more commonly arise in the small intestine of cats and the colon or rectum in dogs. Other, non-epithelial tumour types that have been reported include GISTs (gastrointestinal stromal tumours), leiomyomas (some of which are not included as a type of GIST), adenomatous polyps (usually found in the rectum of dogs) and carcinoids, which are tumours that histologically resemble carcinomas but actually arise from endocrine tissue and are frequently aggressive in behaviour.

The incidence of intestinal neoplasia increases with age, with the mean reported age for intestinal neoplasia in the cat being between 10 and 12 years whilst the mean age of occurrence in the dog is reported as being between 6 and 9 years of age. Interestingly, most reports indicate a slight male predilection to the development of intestinal neoplasia in both species and certain breeds appear to be over-represented in the literature; Siamese cats seem particularly predisposed to developing intestinal neoplasia whilst medium- to large-breed dogs (particularly collies and German shepherd dogs) are reported to develop disease more frequently than small-breed canines. With the exception of the role of FeLV and/or FIV in intestinal neoplasia in cats, there are no known causes for intestinal neoplasia.

The clinical signs that an intestinal neoplasm can produce will vary between patients and it is important to remember that the intestine has a large functional compensatory reserve, meaning that the development

Box 9.2 General signs of small and large intestinal diarrhoea

General signs of small intestinal diarrhoea	General signs of large intestinal diarrhoea
Watery diarrhoea	Mucoid diarrhoea
Large volumes passed with almost normal frequency	Small volumes passed often with a significant degree of tenesmus
Usually little, if any, defecatory tenesmus	Increased frequency of defecation
No fresh blood seen	Fresh blood often noted
Weight loss often noted	Weight loss not usually a feature until late in the disease

of diarrhoea indicates a sufficient degree of disease to cause breakdown in the compensatory mechanisms. Some animals with intestinal neoplasia will exhibit concurrent vomiting; others will display just diarrhoea along with weight loss and usually a progressively worsening nature to the clinical signs. In cases with diarrhoea, it is important to attempt to localize the clinical signs to be predominantly of small intestinal origin or of large intestinal origin (Box 9.2).

Serum biochemistry profiles may show hypoalbuminaemia due to a protein-losing enteropathy along with other, non-specific indicators of intestinal function such as high serum urea if there is proximal small-intestinal haemorrhage and mild to moderate elevations in ALP and sometimes also ALT (as a reflection of a secondary hepatopathy in response to the intestinal disease). The presence of a protein-losing enteropathy can be confirmed by simply ensuring that there is no excessive urinary protein loss by assessing the urinary protein : creatinine ratio and also by undertaking a bile acid stimulation test to ensure that the liver function is normal. With regard to other possible biochemical abnormalities, some more unusual cases report hypoglycaemia in cases with smooth muscle tumours, but this is uncommon.

Abdominal radiography, and especially positive contrast radiographs may help identify the presence and location of an intestinal tumour, but ultrasound is frequently the most useful diagnostic imaging tool to turn to for investigation of these patients as it is highly sensitive and specific for the identification of intestinal mass lesions. Any solid mass lesions or enlarged lymph nodes that are identified should be considered for fine needle aspiration to investigate the possibility of primary neoplastic or secondary metastatic disease, whilst diffuse thickening of a section of intestinal wall along with a loss of the normal 'layered appearance' to the intestine is suggestive of a diffusely infiltrative primary intestinal neoplasm. Definitive diagnosis requires tissue biopsy in many cases (but not in all cases if fine needle aspiration is clearly diagnostic) and again, ultrasound can be helpful to determine whether this can be achieved with a flexible endoscope or not. In cases where the lesion(s) cannot be reached by endoscope, obtaining biopsies either by laparoscopy or exploratory laparotomy has to be considered. These cases present particular surgical problems, in that they are frequently malnourished as a result of their disease and they may be hypoalbuminaemic, thereby increasing the risk of breakdown of the surgical wound, in particular of any enterotomy or enterectomy sites. Meticulous attention must therefore be given to closing these wounds properly. If a single mass lesion has been found then excisional biopsy should obviously be attempted but the surgery must firstly include a careful visual and digital exploration of the abdomen to ensure that there is no other distant disease that may not have been detected by the diagnostic imaging. If the lesions are found to be extensive and diagnosis is required quickly, undertaking impression smears (obtained from the cut surface of the tumour) or some fine needle aspirates from several of the masses for cytological analysis can be a very quick and simple technique that is certainly worth undertaking before closure of the laparotomy site.

Once a diagnosis has been made, unless lymphoma has been confirmed, the treatment of choice is almost always surgical excision if possible and if it was not carried out in the biopsy process. Depending to some degree on the type and grade of the disease, the prognosis for intestinal tumours is generally considered to be better than that for tumours of the stomach due to the relative ease with which complete excision can be achieved with minimal morbidity for the patient. In patients where no metastatic disease can be found and complete excision is achieved the prognosis is reasonable. Studies have shown, for example, that for intestinal adenocarcinomas the mean survival time is approximately 15 months with 1- and 2-year survival rates being approximately 40% and 33% respectively. For mesenchymal tumours/GISTs the figures regarding outcome in cases without evidence of metastatic disease are more encouraging still, with 1- and 2-year survival rates of 80% and 67% being seen for small intestinal disease and 83% and 62% for caecal tumours. The prognosis, however, is considerably worse for patients in whom metastatic disease is detected, with survival times of approximately 3 months described for patients with intestinal adenocarcinomas. Part of the reason for this poor outcome is that there are no clear recommendations regarding the use of chemotherapy in dogs or cats in non-lymphoid neoplasia of the intestine. There is a report of improved survival times in cats with intestinal adenocarcinomas given doxorubicin but this finding has not been reported elsewhere. Therefore, at this stage it is difficult to recommend routine adjuvant chemotherapy following surgical excision of any tumour except lymphoma.

Alimentary lymphoma can present quite differently in dogs and cats; cats often present having a single solid mass that is frequently palpable, with diffuse disease being less common. However, dogs much more commonly have multifocal, diffuse disease infiltrating the submucosa and lamina propria, sometimes affecting several areas of the intestinal tract. Chemotherapy is the first-line treatment of choice for an alimentary lymphoma, although surgical excision of a single malignant mass before commencing treatment may be considered if there is no evidence of distant disease in the diagnostic staging process. However, one study in cats showed that there was no advantage in undertaking surgical excision of a single lymphoma mass with follow-up chemotherapy treatment compared to treatment with chemotherapy alone. The degree of success seen with chemotherapy can vary widely and the substage of the patient before treatment starts appears to be especially important; animals that appear significantly poorly with alimentary lymphoma frequently do not respond well to treatment. The specific subtype of lymphoma seen in the cat probably also significantly affects outcome; cats with lymphocytic lymphoma appear to respond much more favourably than cats with lymphoblastic lymphoma.

Once the staging process has been completed and a diagnosis of lymphoma has been reached, the choice of protocol to use comes down to one of personal preference based on experience, cytotoxic drug-handling facilities and the available finance for the client (Fig. 9.6). In the UK, COP is still most often used in primary practice, although many specialists will recommend using a doxorubicin-containing protocol such as CHOP, the Madison-Wisconsin protocol or CVT-X. The reason for this is that although there are no large-scale, randomized comparison studies comparing the response to treatment with COP against a doxorubicin-containing pulse-therapy protocol, the literature in general suggests that the use of a multidrug, pulse-therapy protocol containing doxo-

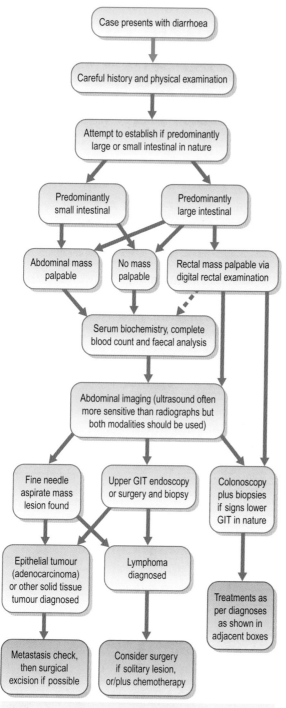

Figure 9.6 Diagnostic plan flowchart: diarrhoea

rubicin in general produces a higher chance of generating a complete remission, that the length of first remission is longer than when compared to animals receiving COP and the 1- and 2-year survival figures are superior if doxorubicin is administered. However, doxorubicin is relatively expensive, needs to be handled with care to avoid operator exposure and extravasation absolutely has to be avoided due to the extensive perivascular soft-tissue damage that can result. There have also been two reports of successful treatment for feline alimentary lymphoma with just chlorambucil and prednisolone with good success rates (average survival time of 704 days in one study) and this is also a protocol that the author now frequently utilizes. As a general rule, cats usually tolerate chemotherapy very well. Remission rates of between 56–80% have been reported with average first remission times of approximately 7 months, although 2-year survival rates of up to 34% are reported in one study. A different study suggested that the general response to COP in feline alimentary lymphoma was poor with a median survival of just 50 days being reported. However, this study also showed that a subset of cats responded extremely well to treatment, suggesting that average survival times may be skewed by a minority of patients who respond in a much more positive manner than the majority. The prognosis for alimentary lymphoma patients also appears to be dependent on whether or not a complete remission can be achieved, as patients that only achieve a partial remission generally have significantly shorter survival times. In summary therefore, chemotherapy is always worth attempting in cases of feline alimentary lymphoma unless the cat is significantly unwell but it is difficult to be very accurate regarding the probable outcome. However, in general many cats will enjoy a good quality of life with chemotherapy, so its use should not be discounted.

10 The haematochezic or dyschezic cancer patient

Haematochezia describes the presence of what appears to be fresh blood on the surface of, passed concurrently with, or admixed into faeces. This is obviously different to melena, which describes dark, usually black-coloured, tarry stools caused by the presence of digested blood within the alimentary tract. Haematochezia may or may not be accompanied by dyschezia (which describes the difficult or painful passing of faeces) and/or diarrhoea, but it usually indicates disease within the colon, rectum or anus. Dyschezia commonly indicates disease within the anal or perianal tissues, so it may be possible by careful observation of the clinical signs to narrow down the location of the underlying pathology but as with any other suspected condition, a thorough clinical examination and diagnostic evaluation must always be performed to accurately locate the pathology. When considering these patients from the point of view of possible neoplastic causes, the differential diagnosis list for a patient with haematochezia and/or dyschezia is shown in Box 10.1.

CLINICAL CASE EXAMPLE 10.1 – A DOG WITH AN ANAL SAC ADENOCARCINOMA

Signalment

10-year-old neutered male Labrador-cross dog.

Presenting signs

Dyschezia and occasional fresh blood on otherwise normal faeces.

Clinical history

- 4-week history of progressively worsening difficulty in defaecating, in that he would strain considerably to pass faeces, his defaecatory frequency had increased considerably and his faeces appeared thinner than normal, with occasional fresh blood also being noted on the stools.

- The dog was also drinking more and becoming inappetant.
- He was initially lively but had become relatively lethargic in the 10 days prior to his examination.

Diagnostic evaluation

- Actually quite bright and in good body condition
- No abnormalities noted apart from swelling in the left perineal region (Fig. 10.1)
- Digital rectal examination revealed a solid, irregular mass to be present within the left anal sac
- Serum biochemistry revealed significant hypercalcaemia (total 3.9 mmol/L, ionised calcium 1.98 mmol/L) with low-normal phosphate (1.05 mmol/L). No other abnormalities were detected.
- PTHrP was significantly elevated, confirming the hypercalcaemia to be a hypercalcaemia of malignancy
- Thoracic and abdominal radiographs and abdominal ultrasound revealed no evidence of lymph node metastases
- Ultrasound of the swelling revealed an irregular mass to be present in the region of the anal sac.

Treatment

- The dog was taken to surgery and the mass was excised (Fig. 10.2)
- Histopathology confirmed the mass to be an anal sac adenocarcinoma, which was then classified as being stage 2 disease (see Table 12.1, p. 123).

Outcome

The dog made a rapid and excellent recovery and his signs of dyschezia resolved. The dog was monitored by clinical examination and abdominal ultrasound 3 and 6 months postsurgery but no evidence of metastatic disease was noted. Fourteen months after his surgery he developed chronic renal failure but he sadly did not respond well to treatment for this, so he was euthanized.

Box 10.1 Differential neoplastic diagnoses for a dog or cat presenting with haematochezia or dyschezia

Differential neoplastic diagnoses for a dog or cat presenting with haematochezia	Differential neoplastic diagnoses for a dog or cat presenting with dyschezia
Ileocaecal tumour (carcinoma or lymphoma most commonly) Colonic tumour (carcinoma or lymphoma most likely) Rectal polyp Anal sac adenocarcinoma Perianal adenoma	Anal sac adenocarcinoma Rectal polyp Prostatic, urinary bladder or urethral neoplasia Extraintestinal pelvic canal neoplasia (e.g. soft-tissue sarcoma or haemangiosarcoma arising within the pelvic musculature) Sacral or coccygeal neoplasia

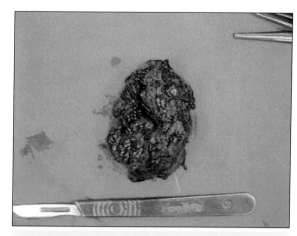

Figure 10.2 *Case 10.1* The appearance of the mass following its resection

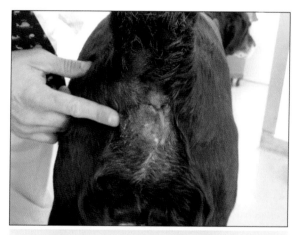

Figure 10.1 *Case 10.1* The perineal swelling found in the Labrador

However, abdominal ultrasound and thoracic radiographs revealed him to still be free of metastatic disease.

Theory refresher

There are many possible neoplastic differential diagnoses for a patient presenting with haematochezia or dyschezia as Box 10.1 illustrates. It is, therefore, vitally important for the attending clinician to obtain a detailed history and undertake a thorough physical examination in every case to ensure that a correct diagnosis is reached.

Perianal adenomas (also known as 'hepatoid tumours') are the most common form of perianal tumour but they are usually asymptomatic and, more often than not, are found by the owners. These tumours are benign, usually being seen in older dogs, especially intact males. This gender predisposition is thought to be due to the tumour development being sex-hormone dependent in that testosterone can stimulate their development and oestrogens suppress their development (so affected females have usually been neutered). These tumours grow slowly, unlike their potentially malignant counterpart, perianal adenocarcinomas which although similar in appearance, generally grow more rapidly and therefore can cause dyschezia if they reach a reasonable size. Perianal adenomas usually respond well to castration with or without mass removal (usually recommended if there is any ulceration) with over 90% cure rates being reported. However, perianal adenocarcinomas rarely respond to castration, meaning that careful surgery attempting to obtain clean margins is required for these tumours. However, obtaining margins can be difficult due to the locally invasive nature of these tumours and also the fact that they are frequently located close to the anal sphincter. There is no clearly efficacious chemotherapy for perianal adenocarcinoma, so good surgical excision is the only recognized treatment for these tumours. In one American study, the clinical stage of the tumour had a clear prognostic significance for perineal adenocarcinoma; 60% of cases with primary tumours less than 5 cm in diameter were alive for at least 2 years after surgery but dogs with lymphatic involvement or distant metastatic disease had a median survival time of only 7 months.

Apocrine gland adenocarcinomas of the anal sacs are tumours seen relatively frequently in general practice, with their incidence being quoted as 17% of all perianal tumours and 2% of all canine skin tumours (as opposed to the tumour being considered rare in cats with apocrine gland adenocarcinoma of the anal sac only being reported in two cats). Although more common in older dogs, these tumours have been reported to occur in dogs as young as 5 years old, so a careful digital evaluation of the anal sacs is highly recommended in any dog presenting with signs of dyschezia, haematochezia or in whom perianal swelling is identified. Metastatic disease can also cause pelvic obstruction presenting as obstipation.

The main concerns for 'anal sac carcinomas' are their metastatic potential and also their ability to cause hypercalcaemia (approximately 25–50% of cases). Studies have suggested that between 50 and 80% of cases will have metastatic disease at the time of presentation with the iliac and sublumbar lymph nodes being the main predilection site for secondary disease. Late metastasis to the liver and lungs is a possible feature. It is also important to remember that small primary tumours can still give rise to large secondary tumours so careful disease staging is definitely required before contemplating surgical excision for this condition. Lateral abdominal radiographs and abdominal ultrasound (to evaluate the sublumbar lymph node chain and the liver and spleen in particular) really should therefore accompany left and right inflated lateral thoracic radiographs in all cases suspected to have an anal sac adenocarcinoma. If a patient is found to be hypercalcaemic, this will obviously require treatment and stabilization before surgery can be considered.

Surgical excision is the first-line treatment for anal sac adenocarcinomas but the disease-free period and survival times may be increased if adjunctive radiotherapy with or without chemotherapy is also employed. Several studies have indicated that the median overall survival time for these patients is approximately 18 months, but the TNM staging of each tumour has significant prognostic significance (see Table 12.2). Animals with metastatic disease that cannot be treated surgically have a substantially poorer prognosis than those in whom no macroscopic disease is left behind.

Postoperative chemotherapy has certainly been described and studies have looked at using both platinum-containing drugs (cisplatin and carboplatin) and also melphalan. In studies using the platinum drugs, partial remission was achieved using medical therapy alone but the response rate was low at approximately 30% and the median survival time was 6 months.

However, this suggests that platinum-containing compounds do have some activity against anal sac adenocarcinomas. The work using melphalan was undertaken in Australia and describes using melphalan postoperatively (at which sublumbar lymphadenectomy was undertaken if metastases were present) with survival times of approximately 2 years being reported. However, in the author's (RF) experience of using postoperative melphalan, survival times this long in patients with metastatic disease that even undergo metatastecomy is unusual. There may be a breed bias to these figures too, so further work is required to establish the role for chemotherapy postsurgery in anal sac adenocarcinomas but it is certainly worth considering.

CLINICAL CASE EXAMPLE 10.2 – A DOG WITH A RECTAL POLYP

Signalment

10-year-old neutered female bearded collie dog.

Presenting signs

Haematochezia and frank rectal haemorrhage.

Clinical history

The clinical history in this case was:
- Progressive 6-month history of soft faeces admixed with fresh blood and sometimes just fresh dripping anal haemorrhage which had not improved with courses of oral sulfasalazine or metronidazole
- The dog did not exhibit defaecatory tenesmus or mucoid faeces, she had not lost significant amounts of weight and her demeanour and exercise tolerance remained good.

Diagnostic evaluation

- Appeared bright and alert
- No abnormalities noted apart from the presence of fresh blood on the glove following rectal examination
- Serum biochemistry and complete blood count normal (no evidence of anaemia but mild polychromasia noted on blood film examination)
- Lateral and VD abdominal radiographs were unremarkable
- Abdominal ultrasound revealed an irregular, concentric colonic wall thickening measuring up to 8.2 mm and extending over several centimetres. In this area the mucosa was significantly thickened but appeared homogeneous

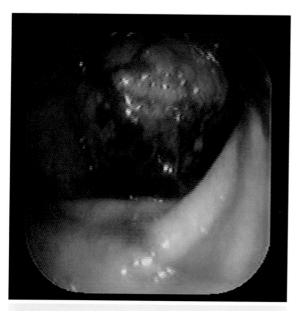

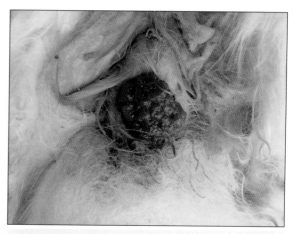

Figure 10.4 A rectal papilloma in a rabbit

Figure 10.3 *Case 10.2* The appearance of the mass within the colon showing the surface haemorrhage that was responsible for the dog's clinical signs

- Colonoscopy revealed a large, irregular haemorrhagic mass to be present on the ventral surface of the colon, approximately 20 cm proximal to the anus. The mass was very haemorrhagic and appeared ulcerated on the surface. The remainder of the colonoscopy appeared normal (Fig. 10.3)
- Grab biopsies were suggestive that the mass was a colorectal polyp. In the light of the location of the mass, the dog was taken to surgery and the mass removed via midline laparotomy and partial colectomy. She made a good recovery and developed no further problems. The mass was sent for histopathology and this confirmed that it was an adenomatous polyp with no evidence of malignancy present.

Theory refresher

Colorectal polyps are the most common form of benign intestinal tumour and in one case series, collies were the most common breed affected. Other than adenomatous polyps, leiomyomas and fibromas of the rectum have also been reported. As with most intestinal neoplasia, middle-aged to older animals are more likely to be affected and there appears to be no gender predisposition for this condition. The polyps are usually single in nature, but multiple lesions have been described, so a thorough evaluation of the entire colon should always

be undertaken to ensure that when found, one single polyp is the only pathology present. It has been suggested that polyps may represent a premalignant lesion, especially when they are large (> 1 cm in diameter), and they can certainly undergo carcinomatous change, so they need to be removed if possible and sent for histopathology to confirm the diagnosis. Obtaining a grab biopsy of the surface may sometimes give a misleading diagnosis as only a superficial piece of tissue will be obtained, so confirmatory histopathology analysis post-excision should be considered essential. If the mass was found to be malignant, colorectal adenocarcinomas are the most common form of malignant neoplasia reported in the dog whilst colorectal lymphoma is the most common form of malignancy reported in the cat. Lymphoma in the dog is more likely to be rectal as opposed to colonic in nature.

The most common form of rectal mass in the rabbit is rectal papilloma (Fig. 10.4), which is a virally induced tumour of the anorectal junction and has a classic cauliflower appearance. They can regress spontaneously, although surgical removal could be performed if it is causing the rabbit clinical difficulties. Diagnosis of these tumours can be made by fine needle aspiration, surgical biopsy or removal and histopathology. Radiography of the chest is indicated if a malignant tumour is suspected.

Regardless of the species of animal presenting, a thorough clinical examination is required in all cases in which the clinical signs could be consistent with a rectoanal tumour, including undertaking a careful digital rectal examination if possible, as one study showed that in over

60% of dogs with adenocarcinoma, a mass was palpable on digital palpation. If no mass can be identified, then careful diagnostic imaging is often useful and ultrasound is usually more useful than radiography, although double-contrast colonography can be used and may in some situations (such as a colon containing significant amounts of gas and therefore making it difficult to perform an ultrasound) be very helpful. CT and MRI scanning, if available, will also provide accurate diagnostic information but are rarely needed to make a diagnosis. One problem with ultrasound is that the presence of gas within the colon can often interfere with the image acquisition meaning that an intraluminal mass may not be visible. However, ultrasound is certainly useful to identify the presence of enlarged colonic lymph nodes in cases of malignant tumours with metastatic disease and if the colonic lymph nodes are found to be significantly enlarged then ultrasound-guided fine needle aspiration should be performed if possible. Ultimately, however, direct visualization of the lesion and a tissue biopsy will be required and the simplest and least invasive way of obtaining this will be via endoscopy. Flexible endoscopy, in particular, is extremely useful to examine and biopsy the rectum and colon but it is of paramount importance to prepare the patient properly first, particularly if the lesion is located proximally, as the colon has to be clean to prevent faecal matter obscuring the optical surface of the endoscope, thereby preventing a thorough examination of the mucosal surface. The authors generally stop all food for 24–48 hours prior to the procedure but allow access to oral rehydration solutions. The patients then receive multiple warm water enemas starting 8–12 hours before the endoscopy is due to begin, giving 20–30 ml/kg on each occasion. The end of the enema tube should be well lubricated and gently advanced as far as it will pass without being forced in any way. The use of soapy water enemas should be avoided, as these can be associated with mucosal irritation and inflammation. An alternative approach to this is to use an oral gastrointestinal lavage solution such as 'Klean-Prep', which causes marked osmotic diarrhoea. Usually the solution is administered two or three times, 1–3 hours apart, 12–18 hours before the colonoscopy is planned. A warm water enema is then usually administered 1 hour before the procedure is due to start to ensure the colon is clean.

Flexible endoscopy also offers a treatment solution, as it is now possible to obtain endoscopic loop diathermy devices, which can be placed around the base of a mass. An electrical current is then passed through the loop, cutting and cauterizing the mass as the loop is constricted. To be effective the mass ideally has to have a 'neck', but a UK study showed that this was an effective technique to help manage benign rectal growths that were not amenable to conventional surgery. There is a risk of rectal perforation so it is not a technique to be undertaken lightly. However, the use of endoscopic loop diathermy has now also been reported in the author's hospital for the successful removal of a gastric mass in a dog and this is a technique that may develop more in the coming years.

The prognosis for colorectal polyps is generally good if they are treated early and with complete excision with disease-free periods of 2 years or more usually being reported. As previously explained, the concern regarding these benign tumours is that they can undergo malignant transformation if they are left untreated, so a digitally palpable 'polyp' should never be left untreated if possible. They usually exist as solitary lesions but can occasionally be multiple. If the mass is located in the caudal part of the rectum then it may be possible to remove it via a 'pull-through' procedure (Fig. 10.5). Many different techniques for this have been described but one common technique involves the caudal retraction of the rectal mucosa through the anus using stay sutures until the lesion is exposed and then removing the mass with a 2-cm margin before closing the mucosa. Alternatively some authors describe caudally retracting

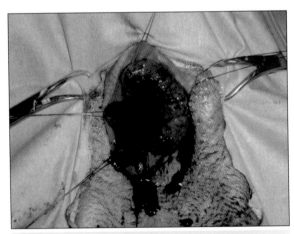

Figure 10.5 An example of a rectal pull-through procedure, using stay sutures to retract the rectal mucosa caudally to exteriorize a mass which can then be excised, the mucosa sutured and then returned to its normal position. Courtesy of Dr Hervé Brissot, Dick White Referrals

the rectum through a circumferential perianal incision by the use of stay sutures until again, ideally, a 2-cm margin of normal tissue can be seen. The rectal mass can then be excised and an anastomosis performed but this technique is significantly more invasive and when possible, the authors recommend the more simple pull-through technique described firstly.

If masses are located more proximally, or within the colon, then a ventral laparotomy will be required to facilitate removal. However, before considering such surgery it is important to plan the antibiosis requirement for the patient. The colon contains a very large number of a mixed bacterial flora and many authors advocate commencing antibiosis before the surgery takes place, although at the authors' hospitals it would be routine to administer a broad-spectrum bactericidal treatment such as a clavulanate-potentiated amoxicillin at induction and then combine this treatment with metronidazole for up to 10 days postsurgery. For the surgery itself, colectomy is indicated for tumours that are confined only to the colon. A colectomy may be total or subtotal (where the ileocaecocolic valve is preserved) depending on the extent of the tumour. For tumours entering the distal colon or proximal rectum a pubic osteotomy or pubic symphysiotomy can be performed, although in most cases of isolated colonic polyps or tumours that are not located so far distally, these procedures are usually not necessary. The colectomy is carried out using a similar technique to a small-intestinal end-to-end anastomosis with the exception that:

- A single-layer simple interrupted appositional suture pattern is recommended for colonic suturing rather than a continuous pattern
- It is preferable to ligate the vasa recta of the left colic and caudal mesenteric arteries rather than the main vessels themselves. This is so that as much blood supply to the colon as possible is preserved.

Mechanical staples have also been shown to be effective in the closure of colectomies in dogs. It is important to note that whatever technique is used for the anastomosis, clean gloves and instruments should be used for the closure (to help prevent tumour seeding should the mass return to be malignant) and the wound closed routinely.

The prognosis for a dog with a malignant colorectal tumour depends largely on the tumour type. Canine colorectal adenocarcinoma cases have been reported to have median survival times of 22 months following surgery but dogs with GISTs generally have longer survival times. The prognosis for malignant colonic masses in cats appears to be significantly worse than the dog, with one report detailing 46 cases reporting survival times of 3.5 months for lymphoma cases, 4.5 months for adenocarcinoma cases and 6.5 months for mast cell tumour cases.

11 The anaemic cancer patient

Anaemic animals can have many underlying conditions causing the problem, so it is vital that a logical, stepwise clinical approach is taken to ensure an accurate diagnosis is reached. The first question to ask once a patient is diagnosed with anaemia is whether the anaemia is regenerative or non-regenerative, as the differential diagnoses to be considered and the diagnostic evaluations to be undertaken will differ once this question has been answered. The determination as to whether a patient has regenerative anaemia or not can be indicated by the presence of polychromasia and anisocytosis on blood smear examination, but the most accurate way is made by assessing the reticulocyte count using a supravital stain such as a new methylene blue (NMB) on a freshly made blood smear. To undertake a reticulocyte count, the clinician should:

1. Mix a fresh EDTA-blood sample with an equal volume of NMB stain made up to a concentration of 0.5% in normal saline
2. Leave this mixture to stand for 20 minutes
3. Mix the solution again and make a blood smear in the usual way
4. Examine the blood smear under a microscope at 100X in the monolayer region and record the number of reticulocytes seen after counting at least 300 cells (Fig. 11.1).

Absolute reticulocyte counts are generally the most useful assessment to make, as percentage reticulocyte values will always be affected by the total red cell count (already low in an anaemic patient). The corrected reticulocyte percentage can help determine whether or not the degree of regeneration is appropriate for the degree of anaemia but this is not always a reliable assessment. The reticulocyte production index, likewise, is a tool to help determine whether or not the degree of response seen is appropriate (Box 11.1).

If the clinician does not have a supravital stain available a regenerative anaemia can also be assessed by simply looking at a normally stained blood smear and looking for anisocytosis and polychromasia. Routine blood smears are also very useful to look for other erythrocyte changes, such as microcytosis or hypochromasia, both of which may suggest iron deficiency and therefore a possible chronic blood loss problem. However, the presence of polychromasia or anisocytosis does not truly define whether an anaemia is regenerative or not, so an absolute reticulocyte count should be obtained in all anaemic animals.

CLINICAL CASE EXAMPLE 11.1 – A HAEMORRHAGING SPLENIC MASS IN A DOG

Signalment
4-year-old entire male Labrador dog.

Presenting signs
Acute-onset collapse the previous day and pale mucous membranes.

Clinical history
The relevant history in this case was:
- The dog had no history of any previous problems, was up to date with routine vaccination and worming and had not travelled outside of the UK
- The day prior to presentation, he had collapsed whilst returning home from exercise. His collapse had been characterized by acute-onset hind-limb weakness, muscle flaccidity and tachypnoea but he had not lost consciousness or exhibited any overt seizure activity. He remained recumbent for approximately 10 minutes before gradually being able to stand and the owner had noted very pale oral mucous membranes. However, he had improved overnight and seemed quite bright in the owner's opinion at presentation.

Physical examination
- The dog was relatively bright and alert and was exhibiting no mucous membrane pallor on examination

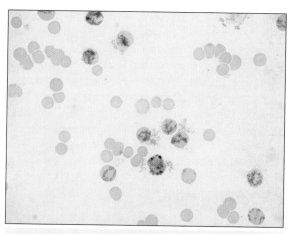

Figure 11.1 The appearance of reticulocytes in a sample of blood taken from a dog and stained with NMB. Courtesy of Mrs Elizabeth Villiers, Dick White Referrals

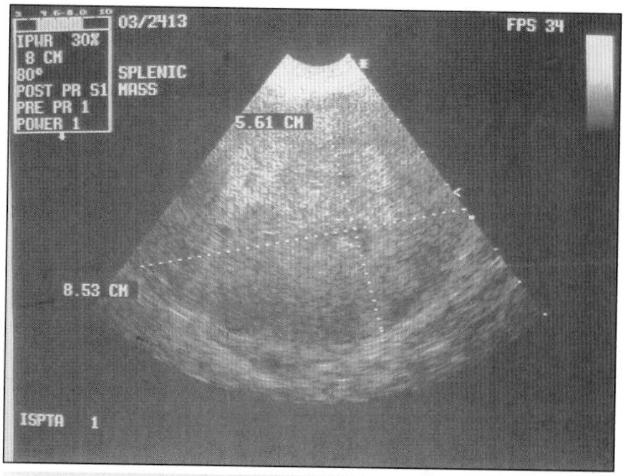

Figure 11.2 *Case 11.1* An ultrasound image of the splenic mass revealing its heterogeneous appearance

---

Box 11.1 The reticulocyte production index

- Absolute reticulocyte count (×10⁹/L) = % of reticulocytes observed on blood smear × red blood cell count (×10¹²/L)
- Corrected reticulocyte percentage

$$= \frac{\text{reticulocyte} \% \times \text{patients PCV}}{\begin{array}{c}\text{Average PCV for that}\\ \text{species (45\% dog, 37\% cat)}\end{array}}$$

- Reticulocyte production index = corrected reticulocyte percentage × reticulocyte maturation time

The reticulocyte maturation time varies depending on the degree of anaemia the patient is experiencing. The values are based on human data and therefore may be inaccurate for veterinary medicine but are given as 1 day for a PCV of 45%, 1½ days for a PCV of 35%, 2 days for a PCV of 25% and 2½ days for a PCV of 15%

- He was slightly tachycardic (HR 110 bpm) with a good-quality femoral pulse
- Pulmonary auscultation and percussion were unremarkable
- Abdominal palpation revealed splenomegaly but no balotable free-fluid.

Diagnostic evaluation

- A full CBC revealed a slightly subnormal PCV (33%) with evidence of polychromasia, anisocytosis and an absolute reticulocyte count of 94 × 10⁹/L (normal < 50 × 10⁹/L). No spherocytes were identified and no auto-agglutination was noted
- A coagulation screen was normal

- Thoracic radiographs were unremarkable but abdominal radiographs confirmed the splenomegaly
- Abdominal ultrasound revealed the presence of a heterogeneous mass in the body of the spleen along with a small volume of free abdominal fluid (Fig. 11.2). Aspiration of this fluid revealed it to be blood
- Echocardiography showed there to be no cardiac lesions.

Treatment

- In the light of his history and the clinical findings, acute haemorrhage from the splenic mass was considered the most likely differential diagnosis to explain his collapse but the presence of a regenerative response suggested that previous episodes of haemorrhage had taken place (as the regenerative response can take up to 5 days to be seen), so the dog was taken to surgery for exploratory laparotomy and splenectomy. Only the spleen was found to be abnormal so it was removed entirely without difficulty and the histopathology subsequently confirmed the mass to be a haemangiosarcoma.
- Once the dog had recovered from surgery, he received doxorubicin at 30 mg/m² once every 2 weeks for a total of five cycles.

Outcome

- The dog remained well for 12 months after the surgery, after which time he started to lose weight and become lethargic. He was re-examined and thoracic radiographs confirmed the presence of multiple metastatic lesions, so he was euthanized.

Theory refresher

Haemangiosarcoma (HSA) is a malignant mesenchymal tumour that arises within the vascular endothelium and most commonly develops (in dogs) within the spleen where it accounts for approximately half of all splenic neoplasms. The other predilection sites include the right atrium, skin, pericardium, liver, lungs, kidneys, oral cavity, muscle, bones, the urinary bladder and peritoneum. The predilection sites in cats are different in that there is an approximately even incidence of 50% occurrence between the visceral form (which includes disease in the spleen, liver and/or intestines) and the skin form.

HSA is a tumour generally seen in older animals, with most studies reporting a mean age of occurrence of between 8 and 13 years of age. However, as the case reported here illustrates, the tumour can occur in much younger animals. Large-breed dogs appear to be overrepresented with the German shepherd dog seemingly the most commonly affected breed and some studies suggest that male dogs may be more frequently affected than females. Non-cutaneous HSA in dogs is usually associated with having aggressive metastatic behaviour, probably somewhat in part due to the close approximation of the tumour cells with the vasculature and patients presenting with signs that could be consistent with a splenic mass should always undergo careful clinical staging prior to excision of any mass whenever possible. Splenic HSAs that bleed are also at risk for developing serosal metastasis, as the primary tumour is often very friable and many cases appear to have bled before the problem is diagnosed, meaning that metastatic disease can develop in places such as the omentum, mesentery and diaphragm as well as the more expected locations such as the liver and lungs. HSA also has a relatively high rate of metastasis to the brain and has been cited as the mesenchymal tumour most likely to spread to the CNS in dogs, with an incidence figure of 14% being reported in one study. Visceral HSA in cats can also behave aggressively, but the cutaneous form in either species is usually not so aggressive.

HSA patients can present with variable clinical signs depending upon the location and size of the tumour. Common signs include (episodic) weakness, pallor, weight loss, abdominal distension and signs of right-sided heart failure due to the presence of a pericardial effusion. In particular, a history of note is a large-breed dog that presents with signs of acute collapse that seems to correct spontaneously, as was described in this case. It is thought that in such cases the collapse is caused by acute hypotension following a haemorrhagic episode which then corrects as the red cells are reabsorbed into the circulation. Collapse could also be due to the presence of a tumour within the heart, causing either a physical obstructive effect to right-sided cardiac output, the development of a cardiac arrhythmia or cardiac tamponade caused by haemorrhage within the pericardial sac. However, some cases will simply present with vague signs of waxing and waning lethargy, or simply of abdominal distension.

> ### CLINICAL TIP
>
> Any dog presenting with a short recent history of intermittent collapse, especially young to middle-aged, medium- to large-breed dogs, should have HSA on their differential diagnosis list and need to undergo a careful clinical evaluation to ensure that one is not present.

Cutaneous HSA presents as discrete firm, raised, dark red to purple papules or nodules, or possibly also subcutaneous haemorrhaging masses.

> ### CLINICAL TIP
>
> Many cases will also be mild-moderately anaemic and in theory this anaemia should be regenerative in nature but this is to a degree, time-dependent, as it usually takes 3–5 days for a regenerative response to be seen.

The diagnosis is therefore usually made based on a combination of clinical history, clinical examination findings and diagnostic imaging findings. If a mass is found within the spleen, then it is often best to recommend not obtaining fine needle aspirates, as if the mass proves to be an HSA, then the act of aspiration itself is likely to cause haemorrhage, thereby substantially increasing the risk of seeding tumour cells throughout the abdomen and establishing metastatic lesions. It is very important to remember that there is a long differential diagnosis list for masses within the spleen (haematoma, haemangioma, splenic nodular hyperplasia, leiomyosarcoma, lymphoma, malignant fibrous histiocytoma) and some studies have suggested that up to 45% of splenic masses may NOT be malignant, so obtaining biopsies for histopathology is mandatory. The mainstay of treatment therefore is complete surgical splenectomy, performed via a midline celiotomy but prior to surgery it is prudent to undertake a full coagulation profile (manual platelet count, one-stage prothrombin time and activated partial thromboplastin time or an activated clotting time if available in an emergency, and a d-dimer assessment) as HSA is a tumour that is associated with paraneoplastic coagulopathies such as disseminated intravascular coagulation (DIC). The reason for this is that the blood vessels within the tumour itself are anatomically abnormal, which causes platelet aggregation and also significant shear-stress to the red cells as they pass through, which results in erythrocyte damage, such as the formation of schistocytes and/or acanthocytes. In addition to these structural changes, the blood vessels within the tumour often have incomplete endothelial linings, thereby exposing underlying collagen and stimulating the coagulation cascade. All of these changes can lead to inappropriate coagulation and the eventual deregulation of the cascade, causing DIC. A full coagulation assessment therefore is vital. However, once this has been found to be normal, surgery can proceed. The incision should be large (extending from the xyphoid to the pubis) to allow removal of very large splenic tumours and also provide access for a full abdominal exploration which must include the liver, mesentery and local lymph nodes. Any suspicious lesions in these areas should be either aspirated or biopsied at the time of surgery as well. A complete splenectomy rather than a partial splenectomy is indicated with either suspected or confirmed malignant neoplasia.

CLINICAL TIP

Surgical suction is extremely useful when performing a splenectomy as many will be haemorrhaging already or start to haemorrhage during surgery due to the friable nature of splenic masses. Also many anaemic patients may benefit from a blood transfusion preoperatively or require one during surgery if blood loss is excessive so preparation for this is advised. However, autotransfusion of the haemorrhaging blood from the abdomen is not recommended for patients with splenic neoplasia.

Splenectomy can be performed either by ligating individual hilar vessels close to the spleen as they enter the parenchyma or it can be performed by ligation of the major splenic vessels (including the short gastric arteries).

The latter technique is a much faster and simpler technique and has been shown not to compromise the vascular supply to the stomach. Omental adhesions to the spleen can be bunch ligated and divided (Fig. 11.3). Ligation of the splenic artery and vein is best achieved using a double-ligation technique. A suture material that has good handling properties (e.g. silk) or forms secure ligatures is appropriate for performing this surgery.

An alternative to suture material is to use vascular clips or a mechanical stapler. The ligating dividing stapler (LDS) is a device that simultaneously places two clips (made of stainless steel or titanium) on a vessel as a blade cuts between them. Each cartridge contains 15 pairs of 'U'-shaped staples. Vessels that need to be double ligated need to have a single ligature placement before the LDS is applied (Fig. 11.4). This device decreases

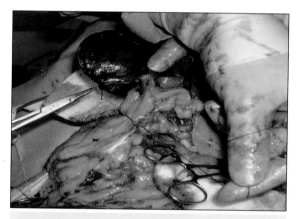

Figure 11.3 The use of suture material to mass ligate small vessels within the omental attachments

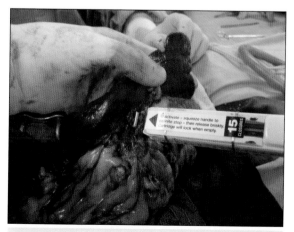

Figure 11.4 The application of an LDS for occluding and cutting between the hilar vessels in a total splenectomy

surgical time by performing rapid vascular occlusion and is extremely useful in splenectomies.

After the splenectomy is complete and exploratory laparotomy performed, the abdominal cavity is lavaged and closed routinely. If possible the entire spleen should be submitted for histopathology; however, if this is not feasible then a representative sample should be submitted and the remainder stored in formalin in case the need for further sample submission becomes necessary.

NURSING TIP

The most common complication following splenectomy is haemorrhage and this can occur as an immediate or late complication, most commonly as a result of suture or staple failure. Regular assessment for evidence of haemorrhage (vital parameters, girth circumference) is important for early recognition and intervention.

CLINICAL TIP

Any dog undergoing a splenectomy is prone to the development of ventricular arrhythmia in the 24–48-hour postoperative period, so close postoperative monitoring is to be recommended. If an arrhythmia was to cause significant haemodynamic instability then it should be treated but they usually resolve on their own.

Postoperative chemotherapy has been considered in many studies and the general conclusion of these is that adjunctive chemotherapy using a doxorubicin-containing protocol definitely improves the outcome for all cases except for small, simple cutaneous tumours for which the prognosis is good anyway. The prognosis for all other forms of haemangiosarcoma is still guarded even with good chemotherapy. Doxorubin has been administered as a single-agent treatment given either at 2- or 3-weekly intervals or in combination with vincristine and cyclophosphamide (the so-called 'VAC' protocol) and survival times of between 172 and 250 days are reported, compared with other publications reporting postoperative survival times of 65 days or less without adjunctive chemotherapy. What does become apparent on reading these reports is that the tumour burden and clinical tumour stage are the most important prognostic

---

Box 11.2 TNM classification and clinical staging for haemangiosarcoma

T_1 Tumour < 5 cm in diameter and confined to primary site
T_2 Tumour > 5 cm in diameter and/or ruptured and/or invading the subcutaneous tissues (if a cutaneous tumour)
T_3 Tumour invading adjacent tissues

N_0 No local lymph node involvement
N_1 Positive local lymph node involvement
N_2 Distant lymph node involvement

M_0 No evidence of distant metastasis
M_1 Evidence of distant metastasis

Stage I disease T_0 or T_1, N_0, M_0
Stage II disease T_1 or T_2, N_0 or N_1, M_0
Stage III disease T_2 or T_3, N_0, N_1 or N_2, M_1

---

factors, so as with the other tumours described in this text, it is good clinical practice to establish the clinical stage of the disease using the TNM system (Box 11.2).

The study which evaluated the use of doxorubicin given every 2 weeks for a total of five cycles showed that clinical stage related to median survival times in the following manner: stage I disease, 257 days; stage II disease, 210 days; stage III disease, 107 days. The prognosis for dogs with non-cutaneous HSA is therefore guarded and even with adjunctive chemotherapy and surgery the 1-year survival rate is no better than 10%. The prognosis for visceral HSA in cats is also generally poor. However, the prognosis for the cutaneous form of the disease is a little better. If the tumour is restricted solely to the dermis without deeper invasion, a study of 25 dogs showed that the median survival time was 780 days, compared to a median survival time of 172 days if the tumour was invading into the subcutaneous tissue. Good histopathology is therefore required in these cases, as adjunctive therapy should certainly be considered in invasive dermal HSA but not necessarily for superficial dermal HSA if complete margins have been achieved.

CLINICAL CASE EXAMPLE 11.2 – A HAEMORRHAGING INTESTINAL MASS IN A DOG

Signalment

7-year-old neutered female Labrador dog.

Presenting signs

Progressively worsening lethargy and weight loss.

Clinical history

The relevant history in this case was:

- The dog had no history of any previous problems, was up to date with routine vaccination and worming and had not travelled outside of the UK
- Over approximately a 6-month period prior to being examined, the dog had started to 'slow-up' in the owner's opinion. They had sought the advice of their own veterinary surgeon when they felt she was becoming notably lethargic and also tachypnoeic. The referring veterinarian found her to be anaemic so referred her for evaluation.

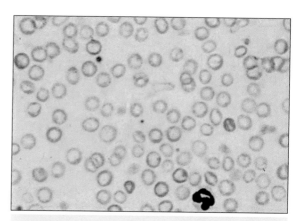

Figure 11.5 *Case 11.2* The appearance of the red cells on blood smear from the patient. Note the somewhat small erythrocytes, their thin outer rim and large area of central pallor, characteristic in appearance of an iron-deficiency anaemia. Courtesy of Mrs Elizabeth Villiers, Dick White Referrals

Physical examination

- The dog was moderately bright and alert but rapidly became quiet during the consultation. In addition she was exhibiting obvious mucous membrane pallor on examination
- She was moderately tachycardic (HR 145 bpm) with a good-quality femoral pulse
- Pulmonary auscultation and percussion were unremarkable
- Abdominal palpation revealed no abnormalities
- Her hair coat appeared dry and dull.

Diagnostic evaluation

- A full CBC revealed a significantly subnormal PCV (15%) with a hypochromic, microcytic appearance to the blood film consistent with an iron-deficiency anaemia in which the iron stores had been exhausted (Fig. 11.5)
- Serum biochemistry revealed mild elevations in ALT and AlkP consistent with an anaemic patient and a mild hypoalbuminaemia (albumin 17 g/L). However, a bile acid stimulation test was unremarkable
- Urinalysis (on a free catch sample) was unremarkable
- A coagulation screen (one-stage prothrombin time and an activated partial thromboplastin time) was normal
- Thoracic radiographs were unremarkable
- Abdominal ultrasound revealed the presence of a small, discrete mass within the wall of the mid-jejunum with no local lymphadenopathy or other abnormalities noted. Fine needle aspirates of the mass were attempted but unfortunately they were non-diagnostic.

Treatment

In the light of this history and the clinical findings (in particular the absence of apparent urinary tract haemorrhage and there being no evidence of hepatic dysfunction), chronic haemorrhage from the intestinal mass was considered the most likely explanation for the anaemia, which would obviously be completely consistent with a blood-loss anaemia. To confirm this, the dog was fed a cottage cheese and potato diet for 3 days before a faecal sample was collected and tested for faecal occult blood. This test returned to be positive. The decision was therefore taken for the dog to undergo exploratory laparotomy and local enterectomy to remove the mass, which was successful and uneventful (Figs 11.6, 11.7). The mass was submitted for histopathology which revealed the mass to be a low-grade leiomyosarcoma with marked mucosal ulceration and haemorrhage. No further treatment was recommended.

Outcome

- The dog made a full recovery from the surgery and at her 21-day check up her anaemia had substantially improved with her PCV having risen to 32%. One week later it was up to 35% and the dog appeared very well. She then remained well for 16 months after the surgery before being lost to follow-up.

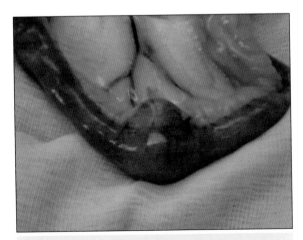

Figure 11.6 *Case 11.2* The appearance of the mass at surgery, located on the mesenteric border of the jejunum

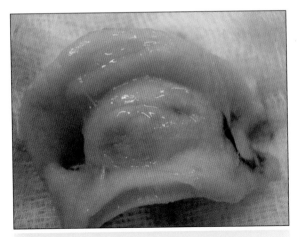

Figure 11.7 *Case 11.2* The cut surface of the mass following its excision, revealing an irregular, ulcerated surface

CLINICAL TIP

This case illustrates the fact that the presence of only a small intestinal tumour can lead to quite marked anaemia and that this can also occur without the development of any other gastrointestinal signs. Do not therefore rule out the possibility of an intestinal tumour because there are no other classic intestinal clinical signs or because a mass cannot initially be identified on a cursory abdominal ultrasound scan.

Theory refresher

As illustrated in Figure 11.11, the presence of a regenerative anaemia indicates that the patient is either bleeding somewhere or has haemolysis and if a patient has a regenerative anaemia that is thought to be due to haemorrhage then identifying the site of the haemorrhage is the first priority. Suspicion for haemolysis is raised by the identification of spherocytes on a blood smear in the presence of a regenerative anaemia picture whilst suspicion for gastrointestinal haemorrhage is increased by the identification of a regenerative anaemia with thrombocytosis and hypoalbuminaemia, possibly with a microcytic, hypochromic appearance on blood smear, most of which were reported in this case. GIT haemorrhage patients are usually negative for spherocytes. It is also important to remember that chronic haemorrhage can lead to iron deficiency, so if the causal problem has been longstanding in nature the anaemia will eventually become poorly regenerative or non-regenerative in nature as haemoglobin production is reduced. Gastrointestinal haemorrhage can be as a result of oesophageal, gastric, small intestinal or large intestinal lesions which may be malignant, benign or non-neoplastic (such as parasitic or inflammatory) in nature. It is also important to remember that gastroduodenal ulceration can develop secondarily to non-intestinal disease such as a severe hepatopathy, so although unusual, a diffuse hepatic tumour with very poor hepatic function or a liver failure patient may present as a blood-loss anaemia case.

Other possible sites into which a patient can haemorrhage are the urinary tract and so-called 'third-space' sites, which basically means the abdominal and thoracic cavities. Accurate identification of the site of haemorrhage is therefore essential and can be done by:

1. Undertaking a full and detailed clinical examination, including thoracic percussion and auscultation, abdominal palpation and digital rectal examination
2. Implementing a full coagulation screen assessment (one-stage prothrombin time, activated partial thromboplastin time, a manual platelet count and buccal mucosal bleeding time)
3. Performing a dipstick and sediment analysis on a free-catch urine sample
4. Requesting a faecal occult blood assessment after the patient has been fed a meat-free diet (e.g. cottage cheese and potato) for 72 hours
5. Obtaining good-quality thoracic radiographs and abdominal ultrasonography
6. Carrying out a bile acid stimulation test.

Once the location of the haemorrhage has been established, identification of the underlying cause is the next priority. Neoplasia can cause haemorrhage either directly at the site of the tumour but also possibly by causing a systemic coagulopathy such as DIC, although these patients are usually very ill. Identifying local sites of haemorrhage usually relies on high-quality diagnostic imaging, as was undertaken in this particular case. If an intestinal mass is found or suspected then the treatment of choice for intestinal tumours is surgery (with the exception of the majority of lymphoma cases) and a full exploratory laparotomy should be performed to inspect the entire gastrointestinal tract, liver, spleen and mesenteric lymph nodes. Any areas suspicious for metastasis should be aspirated or biopsied. The area of intestine to be resected is isolated and the surrounding region packed with laparotomy sponges to reduce contamination. The extent of resection should include margins of a minimum of 4 cm either side of the tumour and any enlarged local mesenteric lymph nodes included in the resection. The intestine can be isolated using either an assistant's fingers or with non-crushing forceps such as Doyens after contents are milked away from the surgical site. The mesenteric vessels supplying the segment of intestine are ligated in addition to the arcades supplying the mesenteric border of the intestine. Once the vessels are divided the intestine is sharply incised using a scalpel and submitted entirely for histological examination. Anastomosis is best achieved using either a single-layer simple interrupted approximating suture pattern or a simple continuous suture pattern (author's [JD] preference). Both patterns are best started by first placing sutures at the mesenteric and antimesenteric borders. For the simple continuous pattern, two separate sutures of swaged-on material are used and each in turn is advanced circumferentially in opposite directions and tied to the end of the other. The advantages of the simple continuous pattern are less mucosal eversion, more precise apposition of the submucosal layer and a shorter surgical time. The suture material of choice is often a matter of the surgeon's preference, however, synthetic absorbable materials are generally recommended and the authors' choice is a monofilament absorbable material such as polydioxanone (Figs 11.8, 11.9).

An alternative method of end-to-end anastomosis is using mechanical stapling equipment. This provides a more rapid anastomosis although it is more expensive. There are many choices of intestinal staplers including the thoracoabdominal 30 stapler, the end-to-end anastomosis stapler and gastrointestinal anastomosis stapler.

Recently the gastrointestinal stapler has been shown to give excellent results in 15 clinical cases of end-to-end anastomosis, however, surgeon experience is likely to be an important factor with the success of this technique. Additionally, skin staplers have been trialled experimentally and have been shown to provide a safe and rapid means of closure.

After closure the area should be copiously lavaged and suctioned and a leaf of omentum can be wrapped or loosely sutured around the suture line. The deficit in the mesentery should also be suture closed to avoid the possibility of incarceration. It is advisable that a new set of gloves and instruments be used for routine abdominal closure to avoid the possibility of both tumour seeding and spread of contamination.

CLINICAL TIP

Whichever means of anastomosis is selected the risk of failure is minimized with the application of careful surgical techniques to avoid ischaemic damage to the surgical site. Leakage from the suture line immediately after anastomosis should be evaluated and this can be achieved using a slow injection of saline adjacent to the incision into the intestinal lumen with an assistant's fingers in place and observation of the suture line for leakage (Fig. 11.10).

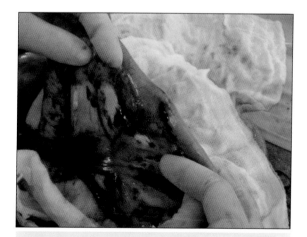

Figure 11.8 An intestinal adenocarcinoma in a cat prior to resection

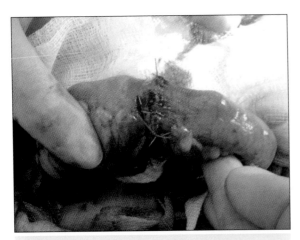

Figure 11.9 The appearance of an end-to-end anastomosis using approximating simple interrupted sutures after excision of a small intestinal adenocarcinoma

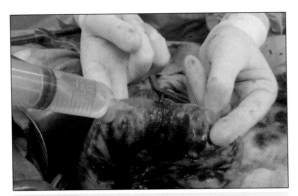

Figure 11.10 Saline being used to test for the presence of leakage at the surgical site postoperatively

NURSING TIP

The key to successful nursing with these cases is early enteral nutrition. It is not advised to withhold food in any patients that have undergone gastrointestinal surgery so early postoperative feeding should be encouraged to enhance wound healing. The metabolic energy requirement (MER) of the patient should be calculated (as shown in Appendix 4) and then the calorie requirements should be met. If the patient has been inappetant for a number of days prior to surgery, then the nursing team should aim to administer 33% of the MER on day one, 66% of the MER on day two and 100% of the MER on day three after the surgery.

Depending to some degree on the type and grade of the disease, the prognosis for intestinal tumours is generally considered to be better than that for tumours of the stomach due to the relative ease with which complete excision can be achieved with minimal morbidity for the patient. In patients where no metastatic disease can be found and complete excision is achieved the prognosis is reasonable; for example, studies have shown that for intestinal adenocarcinomas the mean survival time is approximately 15 months with 1- and 2-year survival rates being approximately 40% and 33%, respectively. For mesenchymal tumours/GISTs the figures regarding outcome in cases without evidence of metastatic disease are more encouraging still, with 1- and 2-year survival rates of 80% and 67% being seen for small intestinal disease and 83% and 62% for caecal tumours. The prognosis, however, is considerably worse for patients in whom metastatic disease is detected, with survival times of approximately 3 months described for patients with intestinal adenocarcinomas. Part of the reason for this poor outcome is that there are no clear recommendations regarding the use of chemotherapy in dogs or cats in non-lymphoid neoplasia of the intestine. There is a report of improved survival times in cats with intestinal adenocarcinomas given doxorubicin but this finding has not been reported elsewhere. Therefore, at this stage it is difficult to recommend routine adjuvant chemotherapy following surgical excision of any tumour except lymphoma.

Alimentary lymphoma can present quite differently in dogs and cats; cats often have a single solid mass that is frequently palpable, with diffuse disease being less common. However, dogs much more commonly have multifocal, diffuse disease infiltrating the submucosa and lamina propria, sometimes affecting several areas of the intestinal tract. Chemotherapy is the first-line treatment of choice for an alimentary lymphoma but the degree of success seen with chemotherapy can vary widely. The substage of the patient before treatment starts appears to be especially important; animals that appear significantly poorly with alimentary lymphoma frequently do not respond well to treatment. Once the staging process has been completed and a diagnosis of lymphoma has been reached, the choice of protocol to use comes down to one of personal preference based on experience, cytotoxic drug-handling facilities and available finance from the client. In the UK, COP is still most often used in primary practice, although many specialists will recommend using a doxorubicin-containing protocol such as the Madison-Wisconsin protocol.

There have also been two reports of successful treatment for feline alimentary lymphoma with just chlorambucil and prednisolone with good success rates (average survival time of 704 days in one study) and it is important to remember that cats usually tolerate chemotherapy very well. Remission rates of between 56% and 80% have been reported with average first remission times of approximately 7 months, although 2-year survival rates of up to 34% are reported in one study. The prognosis for alimentary lymphoma patients also appears to be dependent on whether or not a complete remission can be achieved, as patients who only achieve a partial remission generally have significantly shorter survival times. In summary therefore, chemotherapy is always worth attempting in cases of feline alimentary lymphoma unless the cat is significantly unwell, but it is difficult to be very accurate regarding the probable outcome. However, in general many cats will enjoy a good quality of life with chemotherapy, so its use should not be discounted.

Tumours of the gastrointestinal tract of the rabbit include mandibular osteosarcoma, which presents as a hard swelling of the mandible and could be easily confused with dental disorders. This is considered to be rare. The diagnosis is made by radiography and computed tomography. These can show disruption of bone density. Metastasis to the lungs, pleural cavities, and abdominal organs can be found. Surgical removal is possible and hemimandibulectomies have been reported. Adenocarcinoma and leiomyosarcoma of the stomach and intestine can be seen. These may metastasize locally to adjacent organs. Other tumours reported include bile duct adenoma or carcinoma and hepatocellular carcinoma.

If there is no evidence of haemorrhage found, identifying patients with haemolysis can sometimes be simple if many spherocytes can be identified on the blood smear, as these are the product of incomplete immune-mediated erythrocyte damage but it is important to remember that immune-mediated haemolytic anaemia (IMHA) can be either a primary (idiopathic) condition, or secondary to another underlying disease including neoplasia. The most common tumours that have been associated with IMHA are haemolymphatic malignancies such as lymphoma, myeloma and leukaemia but IMHA can also occur secondarily to the presence of solid tumours such as splenic haemangiosarcoma or histiocytic sarcoma. Patients that are identified as having IMHA therefore require a thorough clinical examination and careful diagnostic imaging (thoracic radiographs and a full abdominal ultrasound scan) to see if a neoplastic focus can be identified. A complete blood count and a blood smear examination are also required to investigate the possibility of there being an underlying leukaemia, along with detailed serum biochemistry to look for evidence to support a diagnosis of myeloma such as a hyperglobulinaemia. If a blood smear reveals the presence of cells that may be neoplastic, then obtaining a bone marrow aspirate and/or core biopsy is likely to be required to reach a diagnosis. An alternative approach would be to analyse any abnormal cells seen with flow cytometry, as this is likely to confirm whether or not the cells in question are indeed neoplastic. It may also reveal what their cell lineage is, thereby enabling a definite diagnosis to be reached. Currently the only centre in the UK where flow cytometry is available is the University of Cambridge Veterinary School (see Appendix 6) but it is an extremely useful technique frequently utilized at the authors' clinics.

If a diagnosis of a secondary IMHA due to a cancer is made, then although the patient may be stabilized initially with treatment for the anaemia, the

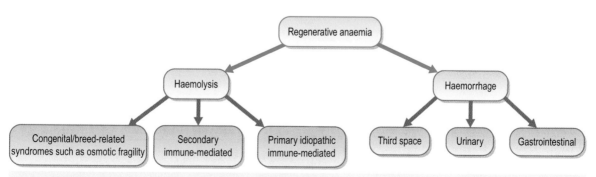

Figure 11.11 The general differential diagnoses for a patient with a regenerative anaemia

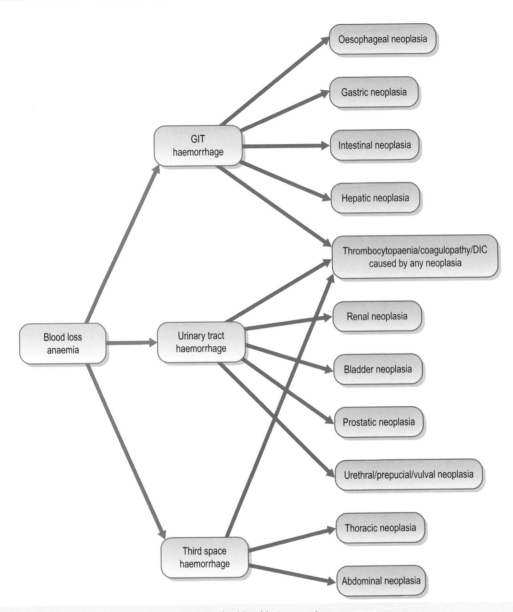

Figure 11.12 The neoplasia differential diagnosis list for blood loss anaemia

immune-mediated component is unlikely to stop unless the underlying cause is treated so all efforts must be made to identify and treat the primary source if possible. The IMHA usually requires concurrent treatment, so these cases require prompt, accurate diagnoses and careful, accurate treatment.

CLINICAL CASE EXAMPLE 11.3 – NON-REGENERATIVE ANAEMIA IN A LABRADOR WITH GRADE V LYMPHOMA

Signalment

12-year-old neutered female Labrador dog.

Presenting signs

Dull and lethargic with a reduced appetite.

Case history

The relevant history in this case was:

- The dog was fully vaccinated, wormed and had no travel history
- The dog had been 'slowing up' in the owner's opinion for the past 3 months but this had accelerated in the 2 weeks prior to referral in that the dog had become very dull, lethargic and had become progressively inappetant
- The dog had had two lipomas removed by the referring vet 6 months previously without any problems having been noted.

Clinical examination

- On examination the dog's mucous membranes were noted to be significantly pale but her heart rate was only 88 bpm, indicating that the anaemia was chronic in nature and that her body had undergone a compensatory response
- Her peripheral pulses were strong
- She appeared to have lost weight but otherwise examination was unremarkable.

Diagnostic evaluation

- A complete blood count confirmed a significant anaemia (PCV 16%) that was non-regenerative in nature (absolute reticulocyte count 45×10^9/L)
- Serum biochemistry revealed mild elevations in ALT and ALP, consistent with an anaemic animal but was otherwise unremarkable
- Survey thoracic and abdominal radiographs were unremarkable
- Abdominal ultrasound revealed a heterogeneous, diffusely hyperechoic appearance to her hepatic parenchyma so fine needle aspirates were obtained. These diagnosed extramedullary haematopoiesis to be present but no pathological cause for this was identified at this stage
- A bone marrow aspirate was obtained which interestingly revealed up-regulation of the erythroid series to the point of reticulocyte formation but very few reticulocytes were visible. What was visible was the presence of macrophages engulfing erythroid cells, a process known as erythrophagocytosis. Furthermore, a significant number of atypical lymphoid cells were

identified in the bone marrow. As samples of the bone marrow had not been obtained for flow cytometry, these abnormal cells were assessed by PCR for antigen rearrangement ('PARR' analysis) and this returned to indicate that the lymphoid cell population identified on the cytology was a clonally expanded population of T-lymphocytes

- PCR analysis for *Borrelia* and *Bartonella* were negative
- Serum thymidine kinase was strongly positive for lymphoma (22.3 U/L).

Diagnosis

- Intramedullary haemolytic anaemia secondary to an intramedullary lymphoid neoplasia, almost certainly lymphoma.

Treatment

- The dog was initially treated with a packed red cell transfusion whilst the results of the PARR analysis were awaited. Once these results were available the dog was started on a CHOP chemotherapy protocol.

Outcome

- Sadly the dog developed significant steroid side effects, so the owners requested that all treatment be withdrawn and she was euthanized 4 weeks later.

Theory refresher

A non-regenerative anaemia usually indicates that the bone marrow has become unable to respond to the hypoxic drive caused by a low red cell count but like regenerative anaemia cases, it is not possible to concentrate solely on one body area in the initial clinical evaluation (Fig. 11.20). Once an anaemia has been classified as non-regenerative, then the major two possible causes from a cancerous disease point of view are whether there is intramedullary disease present (myelophthisis), or whether the bone marrow is being depressed by an extramedullary neoplasm, such as a renal tumour. Intramedullary neoplasia that causes anaemia will often cause a bi- or pancytopaenia; indeed the presence of a bi- or pancytopaenia warrants a bone marrow aspirate to enable further investigation. Intramedullary neoplasia can be one of four different types:

1. Leukaemia
2. Grade V lymphoma
3. Myeloma
4. Metastatic neoplasia.

In this particular case, the cause of the anaemia was not overcrowding in the bone marrow with large numbers of neoplastic cells as may have been expected; rather it was the presence of the neoplastic lymphoblasts that had triggered an immune-mediated reaction against the reticulocyte stage of erythroid maturation, thereby generating an apparently non-regenerative anaemia picture in the peripheral blood despite there being a regenerative process taking place within the marrow. The PARR analysis proved to be extremely useful, so although it is currently only available from Colorado State University, USA, it certainly should be considered in appropriate cases. PARR analysis has been shown to have >90% specificity for the diagnosis of lymphoid neoplasia, because it assesses whether a population of lymphoid cells are a monoclonal or polyclonal expansion. Other than for neoplasia, monoclonal expansion can be seen in ehrlichiosis, Rocky Mountain spotted fever, Lyme's disease and *Bartonella* infection. The dog in this case had not travelled outside of the UK and was shown to be negative on PCR assessment for *Borrelia* and *Bartonella*, so the positive PARR analysis was taken to be very highly supportive for the fact that the abnormal lymphoblasts visualized were neoplastic, although a definitive diagnosis was never reached as the owner declined a bone marrow core biopsy. Nevertheless, the use of thymidine kinase analysis was strongly supportive of a diagnosis of lymphoma. Thymidine kinase (TK) is an intracellular enzyme which is involved in a 'salvage pathway' of DNA synthesis. It is activated in the G1/S phase of the cell cycle, and its activity has been shown to correlate with the proliferative activity of tumour cells and in particular, canine lymphoma. A study of dogs with lymphoma, compared to dogs without lymphoma showed that a level of TK of greater than 7 U/L was diagnostic of lymphoma. Furthermore, the degree of elevation of TK had important prognostic information too, as dogs with lymphoma that initially had TK >30 U/L had significantly shorter survival times (P < 0.0001). Measuring TK therefore can be a powerful objective tumour marker for prognosis and for predicting relapse before recurrence of clinically detectable disease in dogs with lymphoma undergoing chemotherapy.

Normal bone marrow

In order to understand what happens in bone marrow neoplasia, it is important to review the functions of normal bone marrow. Bone marrow acts as the major production site for all of the cellular components of blood. In young animals this occurs both in flat bones

and throughout the length of the long bones, but in adulthood the production in long bones becomes restricted to their extremities only. All the various components in blood, the erythroid (red cells), the myeloid (neutrophils, monocytes, basophils, eosinophils and platelets) and the lymphoid (B and T lymphocytes and plasma cells) cell series all originate from one common pluripotent stem cell. This stem cell undergoes various differentiation divisions to commit the resulting cells into one lineage or another and once committed, the cells proceed down their appropriate maturation pathway.

In order to assess bone marrow, samples can be obtained in the form of either a bone marrow aspirate or a core biopsy. Indications to take a marrow sample include:

1. Abnormalities in the numbers of more than one cell lineage on a complete blood count (CBC) or a blood smear
2. The abnormal appearance microscopically of one or more cells lines on a blood smear
3. Excessively high or unexplainably low numbers of one or more cell types
4. In the search for a neoplastic process that you cannot locate using more basic diagnostic tests.

Bone marrow aspirates (BMA) and core biopsies can be obtained from many sites, including the wing of the ileum, the neck of the femur, the greater trochanter of the humerus, the sternum and the tibial crest (Figs 11.13–11.19). BMA can be carried out with the animal sedated (if there is help on hand to provide physical restraint if required) and is a relatively safe procedure to

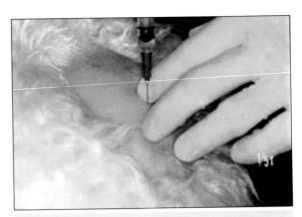

Figure 11.13 The site for bone marrow aspiration is clipped, prepared and then local anaesthetic is instilled in the subcutaneous tissues, the muscle and into the periosteum

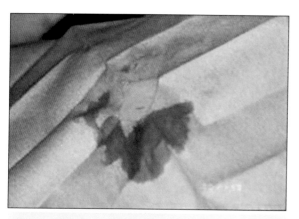

Figure 11.14 The site is cleaned again, draped and then a small stab incision is made

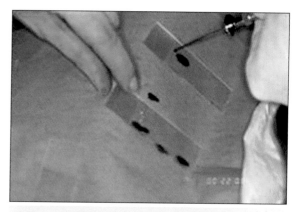

Figure 11.17 The samples are then squirted onto the waiting microscope slides

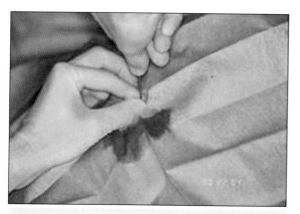

Figure 11.15 The aspiration needle is inserted down into the marrow cavity in a sterile manner

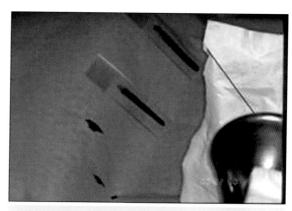

Figure 11.18 Any excess blood is allowed to drain down the slide

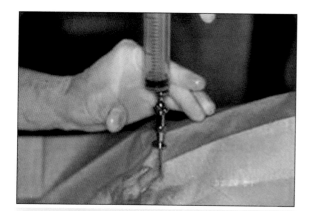

Figure 11.16 Once placed correctly, suction is applied to the needle after the stylette has been removed using a 20 ml syringe until a small volume of blood can be seen entering the hub of the syringe

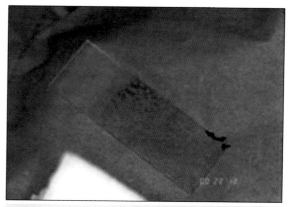

Figure 11.19 Smears of the aspirate are then made from the top portion of the slide

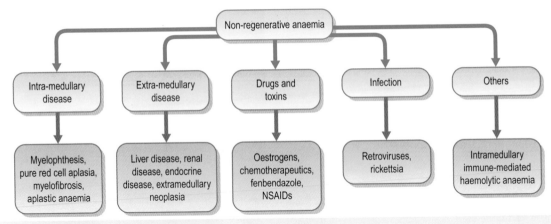

Figure 11.20 The differential diagnoses for a patient with a non-regenerative anaemia

perform in thrombocytopenic animals, whilst a bone marrow core biopsy really requires a brief anaesthesia to undertake. The site is clipped and prepared in a sterile manner before local anaesthetic is infiltrated into the skin, subcuticular tissues, muscle and periosteum. Make a stab incision through the skin and carefully place the Klima or Jamshidi needle into the bone. This requires effort. Once into the marrow cavity, the needle feels embedded into the bone and you have the impression that you could lift the dog on the needle. Remove the stylette and place a 20 ml syringe on the needle. Apply suction (this is the only bit that can hurt, so make sure the animal is restrained well) and once you see a bloody fluid bubbling into the syringe, collect 1–2 ml and then QUICKLY remove the needle and syringe together and start placing drops onto microscope slides that are already prepared at an angle. You need to have 20–30 slides ready and do not discard the marrow in the needle as this is often the best bit. Bone marrow clots extremely rapidly (within 10 seconds), so you need to arrange for one or two assistants to start making smear preparations quickly and allowing them to air-dry. Send the samples to a pathologist or cytologist that you know, trust and can speak to easily on the phone. Most will like it if you can also send a fresh blood smear and a sample of EDTA blood simultaneously.

> ### NURSING TIP
>
> Patients who undergo bone marrow aspiration often appear a little uncomfortable after the procedure, so ensuring they have good analgesia with an opioid such as buprenorphine is very important.

CLINICAL CASE EXAMPLE 11.4 – NON-REGENERATIVE ANAEMIA IN A SPITZ DUE TO ACUTE MYELOID LEUKAEMIA

Signalment

Male Spitz dog.

Presenting signs

The dog presented due to the owner's concern about a marked weight loss in the preceding 2 weeks and the referring vet's finding of a marked non-regenerative anaemia.

Case history

The relevant history in this case was:
- The dog was fully vaccinated, wormed regularly and had not travelled outside of the UK
- The owner had noticed the dog starting to lose weight despite a normal appetite 2 weeks prior to presentation. He was also drinking more than usual
- In the week before presentation he had started to become dull and lethargic
- The owner also thought that the dog had been intermittently lame over this period.

Clinical examination

- On examination the dog was quiet and dull (Fig. 11.21). Examination of his mucous membranes revealed significant pallor but no evidence of petechiation or ecchymoses were noted
- His rectal temperature was elevated at 39.8°C
- His resting HR was 92 bpm, suggesting that a degree of compensatory response had occurred and therefore the anaemia was unlikely to be acute in nature

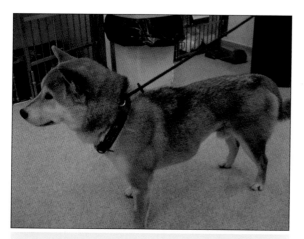

Figure 11.21 *Case 11.4* The dog shows poor body condition

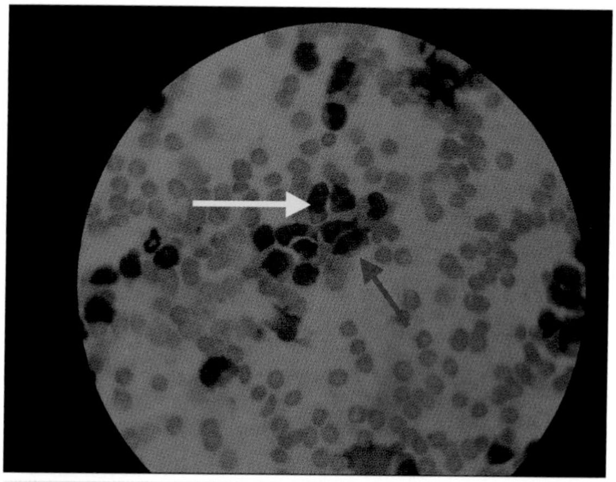

Figure 11.22 *Case 11.4* The appearance of the abnormal cells on the blood smear, as shown by the cluster adjacent to the red arrow. The cells are generally large and abnormal in appearance, with anisocytosis, anisokaryosis, nuclear moulding and variable numbers of nucleoli (as shown in the cell highlighted by the yellow arrow)

- Abdominal palpation revealed him to be significantly underweight, with a mild hepatomegaly palpable. No other abnormalities were noted.

Diagnostic evaluation

- Serum biochemistry revealed mild elevations in ALP and ALT and a moderate elevation in CK
- Survey thoracic and abdominal radiographs revealed no significant abnormalities
- Abdominal ultrasound revealed his liver to be subjectively larger than normal with a heterogeneous appearance, potentially consistent with an infiltrative disease process
- His complete blood count revealed a moderate, non-regenerative anaemia (PCV 28%, absolute reticulocyte count 11×10^9/L) but also a leucocytosis of 65×10^9/L. Blood smear examination revealed that almost all of the white cells present were markedly abnormal in appearance (Fig. 11.22)
- Flow-cyometric analysis of the abnormal leucocytes confirmed them to be of immature myeloid origin.

Diagnosis

- Acute myeloid leukaemia.

Treatment

- In the light of the poor outcome associated with this diagnosis, the owners elected not to treat the condition and the dog was euthanized 7 days later.

Theory refresher

Leukaemia is defined as the proliferation of neoplastic haemopoietic cells from one or more different cell lineages within the bone marrow. This may or may not lead to the presence of these neoplastic cells within the circulation. The more common clinical presentation is to have a marked increase in the numbers of cells from the neoplastic cell line within the circulation, but it is possible to have a situation where although the bone marrow is heavily overpopulated with the abnormal cells, none leak into the circulation. This is termed 'aleukaemic leukaemia'. A slight variation on this situation is where only a low number of abnormal cells are found in the circulation despite the heavy infiltration within the marrow, so-called 'subleukaemic leukaemia'.

Unfortunately there are several different ways to classify leukaemias. The simplest way is to consider the main cell lineages and then consider the clinical course of the disease. From this, leukaemias can be divided into several different types:

- Acute myeloid leukaemia (AML)
- Chronic myeloid leukaemia (CML)
- Myelodysplasia
- Acute lymphoid leukaemia (ALL)
- Chronic lymphoid leukaemia (CLL)
- Plasma cell tumours (multiple myeloma).

Acute leukaemias are generally conditions characterized by large numbers of immature blasts within the circulation and bone marrow that clinically have a rapid rate of onset and often short disease duration. Chronic leukaemias are usually much slower to develop and are characterized by high numbers of mature cells within the circulation and bone marrow. Chronic conditions carry a better prognosis as a general rule.

Myeloid leukaemias

Acute myeloid leukaemia

This is a condition where there is a rapid proliferation of myeloblasts (of any of the myeloid cell series, thereby resulting in ten different subtypes) within the bone marrow that then leak out into the circulation, causing a leukocytosis comprising mainly of these abnormal immature myeloblasts. Their expansion in the bone marrow is rapid, so the other cell lines are often literally squeezed out, resulting in thrombocytopaenia and a non-regenerative anaemia, as was the case reported here.

The duration of clinical signs is usually short (1–2 weeks). Signs include pyrexia, hepatosplenomegaly, mild lymphadenopathy, haemorrhages and various ocular signs. Diagnosis is made by examination of a peripheral blood smear, bone marrow aspirates/biopsies and immunohistochemistry or flow cytometry. Flow cytometry can be extremely useful as it can be carried out on a blood sample alone, as was proven in this case where the use of flow cytometry negated the need to undertake a more invasive bone marrow core biopsy.

The response to treatment for AML is universally poor in dogs, with most papers reporting a mean survival post-diagnosis of only 3 weeks, hence the decision of the owner in the case reported here to take the dog home again once the diagnosis had been reached. Treatment has been attempted using combination therapy with vinblastine, prednisolone, cyclophosphamide and cytosine arabinoside and there is one case report of a dog surviving 240 days with a different protocol of cytosine arabinoside, 6-thioguanine and prednisolone, but two other dogs treated this way were euthanized 10 days into treatment.

Chronic myeloid leukaemia

This is actually quite rare in dogs and is usually seen as an inappropriate overproduction of mature neutrophils. It too, causes quite non-specific clinical signs. There will be markedly elevated neutrophil counts with no (or very few) abnormal blast cells in the circulation.

The diagnosis is made by identifying the neutrophilia, ruling out all possible infectious and inflammatory causes and obtaining a bone marrow sample. The reason an accurate diagnosis is important is that the prognosis for CML is much better than for AML. Treatment with hydroxyurea is reported as being quite effective in restoring normal blood counts, although no large-scale studies have been performed into its effectiveness. Survival times of just under 2 years have been reported.

Myelodysplastic syndrome

This is an unusual condition, the true incidence of which is unclear because many are probably not diagnosed. The bone marrow becomes hyperplastic as in other leukaemic conditions, but less than 30% of the marrow population are blasts and the affected cell line usually does not mature completely ('maturation arrest'). No treatments have been repeatedly reported as being successful. In humans, treatment is focused on causing the affected cell line to complete maturation and there are a small number of case reports on the use of a drug called aclarubicin in dogs, which appears to be able to cause this terminal differentiation but this treatment is not available in the UK.

Lymphoid leukaemias

Acute lymphoblastic leukaemia

Similar to AML, this is defined as a proliferation of neoplastic blasts to over 30% in the bone marrow, but obviously this time the blasts are lymphoblasts rather than myeloblasts. These lymphoblasts escape into the circulation and cause a leucocytosis.

The clinical history is usually slightly longer than in AML (usually 2–4 weeks) but the clinical signs are similar, namely lethargy, anorexia, vomiting and diarrhoea, lameness and PU/PD. Affected dogs usually are quite ill and are in poor condition, thereby differentiating it from stage V lymphoma, in which the dogs can initially seem quite well. In addition, dogs with ALL often only have a mild lymphadenopathy whereas dogs with stage V lymphoma often have a marked generalized lymphadenopathy. Middle-aged dogs are most commonly affected and one study has suggested that German shepherd dogs are possibly predisposed to the disease. The WBC count can be extremely high in these patients, usually > 100 × 10^9/L, and there have been reports of WBC counts up to 600 × 10^9/L. Definitive diagnosis again needs careful examination of a blood smear with or without flow cytometry and bone marrow assessment with or without immunohistochemistry or flow cytometry.

The prognosis for ALL is different from AML, but it is still guarded. If the animal is significantly thrombocytopenic or anaemic, then agents such as vincristine or L-asparaginase, that alone are not usually myelosuppressive, should be used. However, aggressive chemotherapy is probably more appropriate if the animal can tolerate it, so a protocol such as the Madison-Wisconsin protocol should be considered (see Appendix 2). The prognosis is still guarded, however, with a mean survival time of 120 days being reported (with just prednisolone and vincristine).

Chronic lymphocytic leukaemia

As with CML, in CLL there is a hypercellular bone marrow and a leucocytosis, but this is comprised of mature lymphocytes rather than lymphoblasts. It is an interesting condition as dogs can present asymptomatically, although many are lethargic. It is generally seen in older dogs and many clinicians elect not to treat it, but to monitor for progression into a blast crisis and only treat at that point. Treatment if required is usually best done with chlorambucil and prednisolone.

Multiple myeloma

This is a neoplastic proliferation of B-lymphocytes that have already undergone differentiation into plasma cells, thereby explaining why a very common feature of the condition is a monoclonal gammaglobulinaemia, due to the excessive production of one immunoglobulin clone. The problem with myeloma is that it is associated with many different paraneoplastic syndromes, such as hyperviscosity, hypercalcaemia, bleeding diathesis, renal dysfunction, immunodeficiencies, cytopaenias and cardiac failure. It is generally seen in dogs 8–9 years old with a vague history (up to 1 month) of lethargy, weakness, lameness, epistaxis, PU/PD and possibly CNS deficits. Careful ocular examination may reveal retinal haemorrhage, venous dilatation and vessel tortuosity, retinal detachment and possibly even blindness. Severe bony infiltration can result in fractures, which may present as an acute spinal emergency.

Diagnosis is based on finding two or more of the following four diagnostic criteria:
- Excessive globulin concentrations within the serum, which on plasma electrophoresis is shown to be monoclonal
- Plasmacytosis within the bone marrow
- Osteolytic bone lesions
- The presence of globulin fractions within the urine (Bence-Jones proteinuria).

The prognosis for multiple myeloma is generally reasonably good because the majority of dogs will respond to the alkylating agent, melphalan, and response rates can be increased by combining melphalan with prednisolone. Careful blood monitoring is required as melphalan is myelosuppressive, especially to the megakaryocytes. Average survival times of 18 months are common.

12 The polydipsic cancer patient

INTRODUCTION

Polydipsia is defined as when an animal drinks in excess of 100 ml/kg/day, although a high degree of suspicion for polydipsia can be reached when daily water intake exceeds 80 ml/kg. Interestingly, many owners are much more aware of the polyuric aspect of polydipsic patients, which is probably not surprising, especially if the patient is incontinent. Because investigation of polydipsic patients encompasses many possible different medical and oncological conditions, it is vital that a logical and step-wise approach is taken with such patients. Very broadly, polydipsic patients can be grouped in many different ways but the flow diagram in Figure 12.1 gives one possible framework to investigate polydipsic patients along with the major differential diagnoses for each group.

From this it will become apparent that neoplasia is a major cause of polydipsia and polyuria. This can be due to a direct effect of the tumour via the production of non-constitutive hormones such as parathyroid-hormone-related peptide, as can be seen in anal sac carcinoma, or by production of excessive amounts of a constitutive hormone such as cortisol, as seen in adrenal-dependent hyperadrenocorticism. Neoplasia can affect plasma osmolality and viscosity (such as in multiple myeloma), cause renal damage (such as in tumour-associated glomerulonephritis), affect hepatic function (as seen in diffuse hepatocellular carcinomas) and also possibly via mechanisms that are, as yet, not fully understood.

CLINICAL CASE EXAMPLE 12.1 – MEDIASTINAL LYMPHOMA IN A DOG

Signalment

6-year-old neutered male boxer dog.

Presenting signs

Excessive drinking (approximately 120 ml/kg/day), dullness, lethargy and inappetance.

Case history

The relevant history in this case was:
- The dog was fully vaccinated with no travel history and was regularly wormed
- He had become progressively polydipsic and polyuric over the preceding 3 weeks to the point where he was displaying nocturia
- He did not appear dysuric or stranguric and his urine had become very pale in appearance
- The lethargy and inappetance were also progressive, becoming especially marked in the 3–5 days prior to presentation. The owner commented that the dog was very reluctant to eat and that he was unable to walk very far without appearing very out of breath and tired
- He had lost approximately 1.5 kg (from 28 kg down to 26.5 kg) in this period.

Clinical examination

- The dog appeared dull, weak and not particularly interested in his surroundings
- Thoracic auscultation revealed caudal displacement of his apex heart beat and an absence of breath sounds in the cranioventral thorax
- Thoracic percussion revealed dull sounds in the cranioventral lung fields
- Thoracic compressibility was substantially reduced
- Abdominal palpation was unremarkable
- The remainder of the examination was unremarkable.

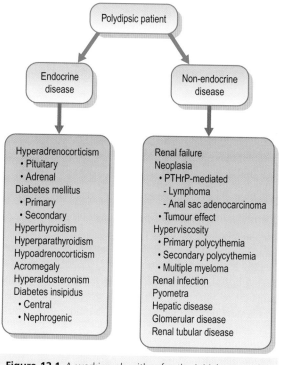

Figure 12.1 A working algorithm for the initial approach to a polydipsic patient

Diagnostic evaluation

- Urinalysis revealed significantly dilute urine (urine specific gravity [USG] 1.009) but with no active sediment and no excessive protein loss (urine protein: creatinine ratio 0.24)
- Serum biochemistry revealed hypercalcaemia (total calcium 3.6 mmol/L, ionized calcium 1.9 mmol/L) with a low-normal phosphate (0.85 mmol/L). Renal parameters were within normal limits
- Digital rectal examination was unremarkable
- Lateral thoracic radiographs revealed the presence of a cranial mediastinal mass occupying a large area within the cranial thorax
- Abdominal radiographs and abdominal ultrasound were unremarkable other than for the ultrasound revealing pyelectasia (as expected in a polydipsic animal)
- Fine needle aspirates were taken from the mediastinal mass under ultrasound guidance. The cytological appearance was highly suggestive of lymphoma. This was confirmed by undertaking flow cytometry which confirmed the mass to be a T-cell lymphoma
- PTHrP was shown to be significantly elevated, whilst PTH was sub-normal thereby confirming the

hypercalcaemia to be a hypercalcaemia of malignancy caused by the mediastinal lymphoma.

Treatment

Whilst waiting for the laboratory results, the dog was hospitalized and received intravenous fluid therapy at four times maintenance (i.e. 8 ml/kg/hour) in an attempt to help reduce his hypercalcaemia. Once the diagnosis was confirmed, the owner agreed to commence chemotherapy, as the optimal treatment for mediastinal lymphoma remains systemic chemotherapy in most cases. A Madison-Wisconsin protocol was used for this dog, as detailed in Appendix 2.

Outcome

The total and ionized calcium normalized within 72 hours of commencing treatment, the dog's demeanour improved significantly during this time and his appetite returned. The intravenous fluids were stopped as soon as the serum calcium normalized and the dog was discharged back to the owner. The dog continued to improve clinically, although the owner noted that the polydipsia did not completely resolve until the prednisolone was stopped at week 5 of the protocol. Thoracic radiographs were repeated at the first doxorubicin administration (week 4) and were found to be completely normal with total resolution of the lymphoma.

The dog remained well after the chemotherapy stopped and he remained well for 11 months, but then he became dull and inappetant again and this time he was also tachypoeic. Thoracic radiographs confirmed relapse of the mediastinal mass with an accompanying pleural effusion. Rescue treatment was instituted with single-agent Lomustine, which was successful in producing a second remission (clear thoracic radiographs again) but this remission only lasted for just under 3 months before he relapsed again and he was euthanized.

Theory refresher

Lymphoma is one of the more common tumours seen in dogs, estimated to account for between 7 and 24% of all reported canine tumours. It is most commonly seen in middle-aged to older dogs and there appears to be no gender predisposition for the disease. Lymphoma and lymphosarcoma are interchangeable terms, although as lymphatic tissue is technically mesenchymal in origin, the term lymphosarcoma is technically more correct. The neoplastic cells develop from a clonal expansion of lymphocytes located in any of the sites within which lymphoid cells may be found. As a result, there are many different forms of the disease and currently several different classification systems, which can make interpretation of pathology reports difficult! However, in practical terms, the classification systems do not really change the initial clinical approach to the disease, which is to:

- Diagnose the condition on either cytology or histopathology
- Establish the location(s) in which the disease exists
  - Multi-centric
  - Alimentary
  - Mediastinal/thymic
  - Hepatic
  - Splenic
  - Central nervous system
  - Cutaneous
  - Other
- Establish whether or not there are any paraneoplastic syndromes present that require concurrent treatment, or that will affect the lymphoma treatment adversely
- Decide on the best treatment option and commence therapy.

Diagnosis can frequently be made simply by cytology on aspirates obtained, either from peripheral lymph nodes, or by ultrasound-guided aspiration of internal organs. It is highly recommended to attempt this in all cases before considering obtaining surgical samples for histopathological diagnosis, as cytology is simpler, cheaper and the results are available more quickly. If ever there is a question over the accuracy of a cytological result then it should be confirmed by histopathology, but cytology is usually the method by which lymphoma is diagnosed in the authors' clinics. The major drawback with cytological evaluation is that it does not allow an accurate assessment of the tumour grade to be undertaken but as illustrated above, the grade rarely impacts significantly on the treatment.

The clinical usefulness of cytology can be enhanced by having flow cytometry undertaken at the same time. Flow cytometry is a technique in which cells are sorted according to their size and then investigated to see what external molecular markers they carry by using monoclonal antibodies that bind to cell surface molecules. Flow cytometry can be extremely useful in the diagnosis of lymphoproliferative diseases, as there are some markers such as CD45, that clearly label a cell as being a leucocyte. There are markers that are unique to B lymphocytes (e.g. CB21 and CD79a) or T lymphocytes (e.g. CD3, CD4, CD8) and markers that are only found on immature cells (e.g. CD34), thereby identifying the cell as

being a blast. By using this specific identification technique, cells can be accurately identified; both by their specific family subtype but also by their stage of maturity and therefore are determined as neoplastic or normal. Flow cytometry has been shown to be especially helpful in the differentiation between thymoma and lymphoma, which cytologically can be a challenge as the thymus contains lymphoid cells in various stages of maturation as a natural physiological feature (see Fig. 8.8). Thymomas can also cause a dog to become hypercalcaemic in a minority of cases (up to 30% in one series), so the identification of hypercalcaemia in a patient with a mediastinal mass does not rule out a diagnosis of thymoma. It has been shown that thymomas in dogs can be identified by undertaking flow cytometry on cells obtained by ultrasound-guided aspirates of mediastinal masses and identifying more than 10% of the cells as having both CD4 and CD8 staining, whereas lymphoma cases stained for these markers on less than 2% of cells. This is why this technique was performed in this clinical case example.

Surgery rarely has a role in the management of lymphoma, because (a) the disease generally shows a good response to chemotherapy and (b) because frequently a single lymphoma lesion will be part of a systemic multicentric disease even if gross evidence of the disease cannot be easily identified. Surgery can obviously be useful in solitary, stage I disease and also in obtaining lymph node tissue for biopsy if cytological evaluation does not elucidate the diagnosis. The question of whether chemotherapy should be administered to a patient following the diagnosis of a splenic lymphoma excised at laparotomy to investigate splenomegaly is a slightly difficult one, but the opinion of the authors is that splenic lymphoma should probably be considered a manifestation of multicentric disease. Therefore, should this scenario develop, a full investigation should be undertaken postsurgery to try to establish the exact clinical stage of the disease but frequently the use of systemic chemotherapy will be warranted.

If histopathology is undertaken, the classification system in Box 12.1 is the one most frequently referred to in the UK.

What the various classification systems have been useful to show is that:

- In general, B-cell lymphomas will respond better to treatment and have longer remission durations than T-cell lymphomas
- High-histological grade tumours often respond more completely to chemotherapy than low-grade tumours

Box 12.1 World Health Organization Clinical Staging System for Lymphosarcoma in Domestic Animals

Anatomic site
A. Generalized
B. Alimentary
C. Thymic
D. Skin
E. Leukemia (true)*
F. Others (including solitary renal tumour)

Stage
I   Involvement limited to a single node or lymphoid tissue in a single organ†
Ia   Stage I without systemic signs
Ib   Stage I with systemic signs
II   Involvement of many lymph nodes in a regional area (with or without the tonsils)
IIa Stage II without systemic signs
IIb Stage II with systemic signs
III Generalized lymph node involvement
IIIa Stage III without systemic signs
IIIb Stage III with systemic signs
IV   Liver and/or spleen involvement (with or without stage III disease)
IVa Stage IV without systemic signs
V   Manifestation in the blood and involvement of bone marrow and/or other organ systems (with or without stages I to IV disease)
Va   Stage V without systemic signs
Vb   Stage V with systemic signs

*Only blood and bone marrow involved.
†Excluding bone marrow.

Box 12.2 The main differential diagnoses for hypercalcaemia in the dog and cat

Common neoplastic causes for hypercalcaemia	Non-neoplastic causes of hypercalcaemia
Primary hyperparathyroidism – parathyroid adenoma or carcinoma producing PTH	Hypoadrenocorticism
	Renal failure (chronic or acute)
Lymphoma – producing PTHrP	Vitamin D toxicity
Anal sac adenocarcinoma – producing PTHrP	Granulomatous inflammation (e.g.: histoplasmosis, blastomycosis, granulomatous lymphadenitis)
Multiple myeloma – producing PTHrP	
Other tumours (rare, but has been reported with many different carcinomas)	Idiopathic
	Spurious

- Low-grade tumours will frequently have longer lifespans without chemotherapy when compared to patients with higher-grade disease
- High-grade tumours are more frequently B-cell in origin whilst low-grade tumours are more frequently T-cell in origin.

B-cell lymphoma is the more common variant over T-cell lymphoma but it is also possible to have mixed B- and T-cell tumours and also occasionally lymphoma which shows no clear B- or T-cell immunophenotyping, so-called 'null cell' lymphoma. From a clinical point of view, dogs that appear not to have significant signs of illness (substage 'a') will frequently respond better to treatment than dogs with obvious signs of clinical illness (substage 'b'), both in terms of remission rates and remission times.

Hypercalcaemia is more commonly associated with T-cell lymphoma (although it does develop in B-cell patients) and the identification of hypercalcaemia used to be thought of as a negative prognostic indicator. However, it is now clear that it is the B- or T-cell delineation that has the negative prognostic indications rather than the hypercalcaemia per se. The hypercalcaemia is induced by the production of parathyroid-hormone-related peptide (PTHrP) by the neoplastic cells, as documented in the case presented. PTHrP is elevated in many tumours (with the subsequent development of hypercalcaemia) but it is most commonly associated with lymphoma, anal sac adenocarcinoma and multiple myeloma. The other main differential diagnoses for hypercalcaemia in the dog and cat are given in Box 12.2.

Prognosis

The prognosis for lymphoma patients is variable and depends upon many factors, so it is often difficult to be precise when giving such information to an owner. The tumour cell type (B or T) is important as explained previously, as is the clinical subtype staging ('a' or 'b'). The clinical staging of the multicentric form of the disease also has some bearing, in that dogs with stage V disease often have a poorer outcome, but in general, dogs with stage I–IV disease will respond in a similar way to treatment. For animals with non-multicentric lymphoma, there are few good studies that provide consistent data with regard to prognosis with the exception of cutaneous lymphoma. However, animals with primary CNS lymphoma have been reported to respond to external beam radiotherapy.

The choice of treatment protocol for the multicentric form of lymphoma may also affect the prognosis in some cases. It has been shown that dogs treated with a doxorubicin-containing protocol in general have a reduced risk of relapse and death when compared to dogs treated with a non-doxorubicin-containing protocol. Furthermore, multidrug protocols generally result in longer remission times and greater survival figures when compared to single-agent treatments. Pretreatment with steroids should be avoided if at all possible, as steroids appear to increase the risk of multidrug resistance gene expression, leading to reduced success rates with other chemotherapeutic agents. However, many factors need to be considered when choosing the correct protocol for each case, such as treatment cost, treatment frequency and duration, the suitability of the patient for injectable treatments and the risk of toxic side effects, to name but a few. Therefore, a summary of the most commonly used treatment choices is given below:

1. Single-agent prednisolone
   - Cheap and easy
   - Produces a short-term (1–2 months) remission in approximately 60% of dogs
2. COP (cyclophosphamide, vincristine and prednisolone)
   - Simple, easy to give and relatively low cost
   - Produces a complete remission in approximately 70% of patients
   - Median survival times of approximately 6–7 months
3. Single-agent doxorubicin treatment
   - Treatment once every 3 weeks for five treatments only
   - Moderately expensive
   - Produces a complete remission in approximately 70% of patients
   - Median survival times of approximately 6–8 months
4. CHOP-based protocol
   - More involved treatments
   - More expensive
   - Produces a complete remission in approximately 85–90% of patients
   - Median survival times of approximately 12 months
   - 2-year survival rates of approximately 20–25% reported.

All of these protocols are given in detail in Appendix 2.

It is therefore clear that, if at all possible, a doxorubicin-containing multidrug protocol is the optimal choice for dogs with multicentric or visceral lymphoma and ideally should be given as part of the first remission protocol.

Rescue treatment

As illustrated in the clinical example, it is possible in many cases to achieve a second (and sometimes a third) remission in lymphoma cases, so having a plan for this situation is always recommended. The majority of lymphoma cases will suffer a disease relapse at some point in their lives, but as long as they are still in substage 'a' and also that the duration of their first remission has been satisfactory, it is usually worth attempting rescue treatment. Owners must be aware that the chances of success are approximately half what they were for the first round of treatment at best and that long second remission durations are sadly not usual, but if the dog is well, then it is certainly worth considering. As with the protocols published for first-line therapy, there are many different rescue protocols described but if the relapse occurs after the initial treatment course has been completed, it is usually best to consider attempting a second induction using the same protocol as was used initially. However, if this is not successful, or if clinically this is not indicated (i.e. the relapse occurs whilst still receiving the first-line treatment or the relapse occurs soon after finishing the first-line treatment), then an alternative rescue protocol can be considered, as listed below:

1. Single-agent doxorubicin (to be considered only if not given in first-line treatment; use at 30 mg/m^2 once every 3 weeks for five cycles)
   - Approximately a 40% response rate (30% complete remission reported) with a median remission duration of approximately 5 months
2. Single-agent Lomustine (CCNU)
   - Easy to give (90 mg/m^2 by mouth once every 3 weeks)
   - Approximately 30% response rate (10% complete remission) with a median remission duration of approximately 3 months
3. Single-agent Mitoxantrone
   - Easy to give (5 mg/m^2 by slow intravenous infusion once every 3 weeks)
   - Approximately a 40% response rate (30% complete remission) with a remission duration of approximately 3 months
4. MOPP (Mechlorethamine, vincristine, procarbazine and prednisolone)

- Involved, but not a complicated protocol with both home and hospital administration of medication required
- Approximately a 65% response rate (with 30% complete remission reported) with a remission duration of approximately 3 months
- Moderate expense

5. D-MAC (Dexamethasone, melphalan, actinomycin D and cytosine arabinoside)
   - Involved, but not a complicated protocol with both home and hospital administration of medication required
   - 72% remission rate, (44% complete remission and 28% partial remission) with a median remission duration of 61 days (range, 2–467+ days)

6. LAP (Lomustine, L-asparaginase and prednisolone)
   - Involved, but not complicated protocol with both home and hospital administration of medication required
   - 87% response rate with 52% complete remission reported, with a remission duration of approximately 2–3 months
   - Moderate expense.

From this list, it becomes apparent that there is not one protocol that stands out as being substantially more efficacious than another, so again it becomes a matter of choosing the most appropriate protocol for individual cases depending on the circumstances of each patient. The authors' general preference is to use single-agent Lomustine first, with MOPP as a second choice and D-MAC as a third choice but as the data above show, any of the treatments listed above (and this is not an exhaustive list) could be considered.

CLINICAL CASE EXAMPLE 12.2 – ANAL SAC ADENOCARCINOMA IN A DOG

Signalment
10-year-old neutered male golden retriever dog.

Presenting signs
A 2-week history of being polydipsic and having a markedly reduced appetite.

Case history
The relevant history in this case was:
- The dog was fully vaccinated with no travel history and was regularly wormed

- He had become progressively polydipsic and polyuric over the proceding 2 weeks to the point where he had two episodes of urinary incontinence on his bed
- He did not appear dysuric or stranguric and his urine had become very pale in appearance
- His appetite had become quite rapidly poor, in that initially he was reluctant to finish his food but that in the 3 days prior to presentation he appeared almost totally disinterested in food. However, he had not exhibited any vomiting, diarrhoea or dyschezia in this period.

Clinical examination
- The dog appeared quite bright and nervous but his owners commented that he was not as lively as usual
- Thoracic auscultation revealed normal lung and heart sounds and thoracic percussion was unremarkable
- Thoracic compressibility was normal
- Abdominal palpation was unremarkable
- Digital rectal examination revealed an irregular, hard mass in the right anal sac, measuring approximately 4 cm in diameter
- No further abnormalities were identified.

Diagnostic evaluation
- Urinalysis revealed isosthenuric urine (USG 1.011) but with no active sediment and no excessive protein loss
- Serum biochemistry revealed hypercalcaemia (total calcium 3.3 mmol/L, ionized calcium 2.1 mmol/L). Renal parameters were within normal limits. ALP was mildly elevated
- Fine needle aspirates were obtained from the anal sac mass and the cytological appearance was highly suggestive of a carcinoma
- Lateral thoracic radiographs revealed no abnormalities
- Abdominal radiographs were unremarkable but abdominal ultrasound revealed mild enlargement of the medial iliac lymph node (1 cm in diameter). No visceral metastases were identified
- PTHrP was shown to be significantly elevated, whilst PTH was subnormal, thereby confirming the hypercalcaemia to be a hypercalcaemia of malignancy caused by anal sac adenocarcinoma.

Diagnosis
- Stage 3a metastatic anal sac adenocarcinoma.

Treatment

Because of the finding of an enlarged medial iliac lymph node, the clinical team were concerned this could represent nodal metastasis. However, the size of the node and its proximity to the aorta precluded fine needle aspiration. Therefore, the dog was managed surgically by undergoing an anal saculectomy using the closed technique and then a laparotomy to remove the enlarged medial iliac lymph node. The dog was anaesthetized and placed in sternal recumbency with his legs positioned over the back of the table, the tail elevated and a pad placed underneath his groin to elevate the caudal pelvis. Gauze swabs were placed into the rectum to prevent wound contamination during surgery. Following routine preoperative skin preparation, a probe was inserted into the anal sac and held in place by an assistant whilst a vertical incision was made over the sac and the surrounding tissue (in particular the external anal sphincter). Fibres from the external anal sphincter muscle were carefully freed from the anal sac using a combination of blunt (using fine haemostatic forceps) and sharp (using metzenbaum scissors) dissection. A single absorbable suture was used to ligate the anal sac duct before transection and then the surgical site was carefully and thoroughly lavaged with sterile saline. The wound was closed in a routine manner. A caudal abdominal laparotomy was then performed. The medial iliac lymph node was identified, the blood supply ligated and the node removed. Careful exploration of the abdomen revealed no evidence of further disease, so the abdomen was closed routinely. Postoperatively the dog received NSAID (carprofen for 5 days) and opioid analgesia (methadone for 24 hours followed by buprenorphine for 24 hours) along with oral clavulate-potentiated amoxicillin for 5 days.

CLINICAL TIP

The anal sac is generally adhered tightly to the external anal sphincter muscle, so great care must be taken to avoid excessive trauma to this muscle, and also to the caudal rectal nerve, during dissection. Curved mosquito forceps can be extremely useful to tease muscle fibres of the external anal sphincter from the anal sac.

Follow-up

Immediately postoperatively the dog appeared well and defecated normally within 12 hours. Histopathological analysis of the excised tissue confirmed it to be an adenocarcinoma of the anal sac with metastasis to the medial iliac lymph node. The dog was then treated with carboplatin, administered as a slow intravenous infusion at 300 mg/m^2 once every 3 weeks for four treatments. The dog tolerated this treatment well with no adverse side effects.

Outcome

The dog remained well for 18 months and then represented as the owner was concerned he was losing weight, drinking more again and had a reduced appetite. On examination he was quiet and slightly tachypnoeic, although pulmonary auscultation and percussion were unremarkable. Serum calcium assessment revealed a recurrence of the hypercalcaemia and thoracic radiographs revealed the presence of multiple pulmonary metastases, so the dog was euthanized.

Theory refresher

Anal sac carcinomas are not considered to be common tumours of the dog and they are rare tumours in the cat. However, up to 53% of cases in dogs are associated with PHTrP-induced hypercalcaemia, so many cases will present with signs associated with excessive serum calcium (i.e. polydipsia, polyuria, inappetance and lethargy), as in this case. It is important to note that a significant number of cases of anal sac adenocarcinoma will not be hypercalcaemic, but the tumour still has malignant potential, so finding a dog with an anal sac mass and normocalcaemia does not rule out a malignant tumour. Anal sac adenocarcinomas arise from the apocrine gland cells that line the anal sacs and are generally seen in older dogs (mean age of 9–11 years old). Although some studies have suggested that the disease is more common in female dogs, the most recent publication in the UK found an even male : female occurrence rate. Some breeds appear to be more predisposed than others, with cocker spaniels, golden retrievers and German shepherd dogs seemly over-represented.

Anal sac tumours require surgical excision but it is vital to carefully stage the patients first, as the clinical staging appears to have significant impact on the treatment choices that should be made and also to the prognosis and outcome. A recent case series describing 130

Table 12.1 An adapted TNM staging system for use in dogs with anal sac adenocarcinomas (as suggested by Poulton and Brearley, JVIM (2007) 21(2): 274–280)

Clinical stage	Primary tumour	Nodal disease (regional draining nodes)	Metastasis (distant)
Stage 1	<2.5 cm max diameter	Negative	Negative
Stage 2	>2.5 cm max diameter	Negative	Negative
Stage 3a	Any tumour	<4.5 cm max diameter	Negative
Stage 3b	Any tumour	>4.5 cm max diameter	Negative
Stage 4	Any tumour	Any nodal disease	Present

Table 12.2 The mean survival times for dogs with anal sac adenocarcinomas and the variability found dependant on the clinical staging as found in one large study (adapted from Poulton and Brearley, JVIM (2007) 21(2): 274–280)

Clinical stage	Mean survival time (MST) (days)	MST range
Stage 1	1205	690–1720
Stage 2	722	191–1253
Stage 3a	492	127–856
Stage 3b	335	253–417
Stage 4	71	6–136

dogs with anal sac adenocarcinomas adapted the existing TNM staging system for use in anal sac carcinoma (Table 12.1).

It is from this table that the case described here received its stage 3a designation.

The reasons that the clinical staging is so important are, firstly, because the findings have a significant impact on the treatment that should be recommended and, secondly, because the prognosis is also different depending on the stage of disease identified, as shown in Table 12.2.

The role of surgery in the management of anal sac adenocarcinomas is therefore of paramount importance and this has to be considered the first-line therapy for both the primary disease and also for lymphatic secondaries. Several studies clearly show that surgical removal of nodal metastases significantly improves the life expectancy for these patients, and dogs with this complication should be considered as candidates for referral to a soft-tissue surgery specialist unless the practitioner is experienced and has the suitable hospital facilities to manage these patients postoperatively. Metastasis to visceral organs, however, usually dictates that no further treatment is possible. The question therefore is whether or not there is clearly a role for adjunctive treatment to aid the surgical management of these patients. With regard to chemotherapy, it has been shown that carboplatin can reduce the size of primary tumours by up to 50% in some cases, thereby enabling less radical surgery to be performed to try to reduce the risk of external anal sphincter damage, but this response is variable. More recent work has also suggested a role for carboplatin in dogs with stage 3b disease in an attempt to shrink the nodal metastasis preoperatively. However, whether or not chemotherapy should be utilized postoperatively to treat undetectable microscopic disease is not actually clear and further work is required to clarify the role of chemotherapy in this situation.

Electrochemotherapy has also recently been described as possibly beneficial in an incompletely excised anal sac adenocarcinoma. Two doses of cisplatin were administered 14 days apart in combination with biphasic electrical pulses and the dog was still in complete remission 18 months later. Newer treatments such as electrochemotherapy certainly merit further evaluation in these cases and may represent a further viable treatment option in the near future.

The role of radiotherapy is also unclear, although it is thought that external beam radiation directed at the site of the primary tumour may improve the outcome for these patients, especially if incomplete excision of the mass occurs. Both hypo- and hyperfractionated protocols have been reported to be useful following surgery, although care has to be taken to reduce exposure of the rectum to the beam. One study has described the use of radiotherapy with concurrent mitoxantrone administration with excellent survival times (mean survival time 956 days) but further work is required to establish the role of chemoradiotherapy more clearly. Radiotherapy has also been described following excision of an anal sac carcinoma in a cat with no significant side effects.

CLINICAL CASE EXAMPLE 12.3 – PRIMARY POLYCYTHEMIA IN A DOG

Signalment

5-year-old neutered female Welsh springer spaniel.

Presenting signs

A 4-week history of being polydipsic, polyuric and urinary incontinent.

Case history

The relevant history in this case was:

- The dog was fully vaccinated with no travel history outside of the UK
- No previous history of any medical problems
- The owner had first noted that the dog was unable to get through the night without urinating approximately 4 weeks prior to presentation and had then realized that she was drinking much more than she had used to. When she calculated her daily water intake it averaged at 134 ml/kg/day
- As well as her excessive water intake, the dog had become lethargic at home and reluctant to go for a walk. Her appetite had remained reasonable and not excessive
- She had not lost weight.

Clinical examination

- The dog appeared quiet
- Oral and ocular mucous membranes appeared redder than normal and this was most visible on the buccal mucosa but there were no signs of dehydration
- Thoracic auscultation revealed normal lung and heart sounds and thoracic percussion was unremarkable
- Thoracic compressibility was normal
- Abdominal palpation was unremarkable
- Digital rectal examination was unremarkable
- No further abnormalities were identified.

Diagnostic evaluation

- In the light of the history and presenting signs, polycythemia was considered a significant possibility, so a complete blood count was undertaken first. This revealed a marked elevation in her red cell count (PCV 77%)
- Her serum biochemistry revealed mild elevations in ALT and AST but was otherwise unremarkable

- Urinalysis revealed isosthenuria (USG 1.010) with no active sediment or proteinuria
- Thoracic radiographs were unremarkable
- Abdominal ultrasound revealed no abnormalities
- The serum erythropoietin concentration was in the low-normal range, thereby confirming that the dog had primary polycythemia.

Diagnosis

- Primary polycythemia (polycythemia vera).

Treatment

The dog was hospitalized and initially underwent a phlebotomy. A total of 20 ml/kg blood (340 ml) was removed and the dog commenced intravenous fluid therapy (at 4 ml/kg/hour for 36 hours). This was successful in reducing her PCV to 63%. The dog then started hydroxyurea at a dose of 500 mg once a day (dose equivalent of 30 mg/kg) for 10 days before the dose was reduced to 500 mg every other day. The dog responded well to treatment, with the PCV falling to 53% over a 6-week period and the clinical signs resolved. The dog was lost to follow-up 18 months later but at this time she was still in remission with no clinical signs.

Theory refresher

Primary polycythemia (also known as polycythemia vera and primary erythrocytosis) is the condition in which there is an absolute increase in the number of mature circulating red blood cells. Increased red blood cell numbers can be due to a relative polycythemia in which there is not an absolute increase in the red cell numbers (e.g. severe dehydration, acute splenic contraction or body fluid shifts), a secondary polycythemia in which there is a genuine increase in the number of red cells but as a normal physiological response (e.g. in response to living at altitude, severe chronic pulmonary disease, a left-to-right cardiac shunt), the result of excessive erythropoietin production as a result of underlying pathology such as a renal tumour, or a true primary polycythemia. Primary polycythemia can therefore only be diagnosed once all the other possible conditions have been ruled out.

Primary polycythemia is generally seen in middle-aged dogs and they commonly present with a history of polydipsia and polyuria, lethargy, weakness and sometimes more significant neurological signs (such as ataxia and seizures). Inappetance is frequently described and sometimes patients will present with evidence of a coagulopathy. On examination, the mucous membranes are usually brick red, the scleral vessels appear congested and the PCV will often be markedly elevated (>70%). The best diagnostic approach is to try to rule out all the other possible causes, so a full serum biochemistry profile is to be recommended along with left and right lateral inflated thoracic radiographs, a lateral abdominal radiograph and abdominal ultrasound as an initial diagnostic investigation. Arterial blood gas assessment should be performed if there is clinical or radiographic evidence of pulmonary disease or hypoxia. Serum erythropoietin assessment (undertaken in this instance at Cambridge Specialist Laboratory Services, Cambridge, UK) should always also be undertaken once pulmonary disease has been ruled out or if a renal mass has been identified. In primary polycythemia, serum EPO concentrations are usually low-normal.

Treatment involves initial stabilization of the patient, usually by phlebotomy and fluid therapy. Removing 20 ml blood/kg and replacing this volume with ideally the spun-down plasma, or alternatively crystalloid fluids, usually lowers the PCV by approximately 15%, as illustrated in the case here. The mainstay of medical therapy is hydroxyurea at approximately 30 mg/kg SID for 7 days (although the recommended dose appears to vary between reports from 20–50 mg/kg in the early stages, then reduced to 15 mg/kg SID or EOD as maintenance once the PCV has normalized).

CLINICAL CASE EXAMPLE 12.4 – DIABETES INSIPIDUS DUE TO A PITUITARY TUMOUR

Signalment

9-year-old neutered female boxer dog.

Presenting signs

A 10-day history of sudden-onset marked polyuria and polydipsia with urinary incontinence.

Case history

The relevant history in this case was:
- The dog was fully vaccinated, wormed and had no travel history
- The owner initially thought she had developed urinary incontinence because she had started to urinate indoors. The referring veterinary surgeon had dispensed some phenylpropanolamine but this had not improved the problem. The owner then measured daily water intake and found that the dog was drinking more than 200 ml/kg/day, so she was referred for further evaluation.

Clinical examination

- On examination the dog was bright, alert and in good body condition at 28 kg
- Cardiopulmonary auscultation and percussion were unremarkable
- Abdominal palpation was unremarkable
- Digital rectal examination was normal
- Neurological examination was unremarkable.

Diagnostic evaluation

- In the light of the clinical history, the first evaluation that was undertaken was a free-catch urinalysis, which revealed a USG of 1.004 with no active sediment or proteinuria
- Serum biochemistry (including bile acid stimulation) and a complete blood count were unremarkable
- An ACTH stimulation test was normal
- Thoracic radiographs revealed no underlying pathology
- Abdominal ultrasound revealed no abnormalities other than for pyelectasia, potentially consistent with the dog being polydipsic. A cystocentesis sample was obtained by ultrasound guidance, culture of which was negative
- A water depravation test was undertaken (see Appendix 3), in which the dog lost 5% of her bodyweight within 12 hours of the test starting without showing a significant rise in her USG (which went to 1.008). The dog was then given 2 µg of the antidiuretic hormone analogue, desmopressin (DDAVP; 1-deamino, 9-D-arginine vasopressin) by intramuscular injection and the USG rose to 1.030 within 2 hours and the dog lost no further weight.

Diagnosis

On the basis that all non-endocrine causes of polydipsia and all endocrine causes bar diabetes insipidus and psychogenic polydipsia were ruled out by the diagnostic evaluation, the water depravation test and the response to exogenous DDAVP confirmed the diagnosis to be one of central diabetes insipidus (cDI).

Treatment and initial follow-up

The dog was initially treated with DDAVP drops administered on the conjunctiva (three drops three times a day), which worked well at first with a total resolution of the dog's clinical signs. However, over the following 3 weeks the dog's DDAVP requirement went up by 40% (to five drops three times a day) without generating adequate control of the dog's polyuria so the dog re-presented. On examination, she was still bright and alert but exhibited very slight anisocoria. Neurological evaluation was otherwise still unremarkable. In the light of the history of acquired central diabetes insipidus and the mild anisocoria, it was decided to undertake an MRI scan of the brain to investigate the possibility of there being a tumour within the pituitary and as shown in Figures 12.2 and 12.3 the MRI did indeed reveal the presence of a large pituitary mass.

Outcome

The dog was maintained on ocular DDAVP drops but also underwent external beam radiotherapy to treat the pituitary mass. The radiotherapy was tolerated well with no acute side effects. The diabetes insipidus did not resolve, although the ocular DDAVP dose did stabilize the condition, meaning that the original signs of polyuria and polydipsia were well controlled.

Theory refresher

Diabetes insipidus (DI) is a clinical condition characterized by an often acute onset of marked polyuria and polydipsia and it has two main forms; central (cDI) and nephrogenic (nDI). The condition develops due to either a failure of production of adequate quantities of antidiuretic hormone (ADH), also known as arginine-vasopressin, from the posterior lobe of the pituitary gland (therefore termed cDI), or a failure in the action of ADH at the kidney (therefore termed nDI). The classification of cDI and nDI can be further expanded by determining whether the condition is congenital or acquired. The most common form of the disease is acquired nDI. In this case, however, the condition was an acquired cDI, which should always raise concern in the attending clinician's mind as to the possibility of there being a space-occupying lesion within the pituitary or hypothalamus. ADH is synthesized along with oxytocin in the supraoptic and paraventricular nuclei of the hypothalamus, from which axons extend down into the posterior pituitary. Therefore any lesion that will disrupt or damage this pathway could lead to the development of DI.

In normal animals the stimulus for release of ADH is an increase in plasma osmolality indicating dehydration and this change is detected by specialized hypothalamic osmoreceptors. ADH is released into the circulation to bind to V_2-receptors in the kidney and this binding action stimulates the temporary formation of channels known as 'aquaporins' in the distal convoluted tubules and the

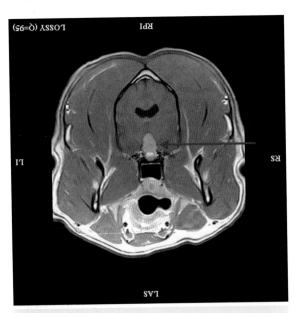

Figure 12.2 *Case 12.4* A transverse T1 plus contrast MRI scan from the dog, revealing the presence of a large, contrast-enhancing mass in the pituitary gland, as shown by the red arrow

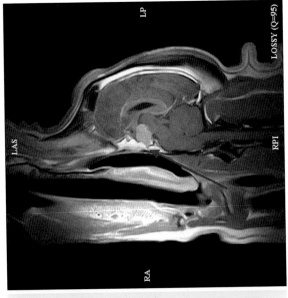

Figure 12.3 *Case 12.4* A sagittal T1 plus contrast MRI, showing the pituitary tumour with a small cord of tissue from it extending ventrally and causing compression of the optic chiasm (shown by the red arrow), thereby explaining the anisocoria seen at the second examination

collecting ducts, thereby allowing the re-absorption of solute-free water along the osmotic gradient established by the solute and urea re-absorption in the more proximal renal tubules. The action of ADH is therefore vital to normal water conservation and balance within the body and without it the kidneys would lose large amounts of water rapidly.

Making a diagnosis of DI therefore firstly involves carefully eliminating all of the more common causes of polyuria and polydipsia, as shown in Figure 12.1, and this can be done quite simply by careful clinical examination, blood testing, urinalysis and appropriate diagnostic imaging. One key point to remember when considering the differential diagnoses is that really the only diseases that will cause the urine specific gravity to fall below 1.006 are DI and primary/psychogenic polydipsia, so if the USG lies between 1.008 and 1.015, a diagnosis of complete DI is unlikely. Therefore, only once all of the other possible differentials have been ruled out should a water depravation test be considered.

CLINICAL TIP

Water depravation tests are potentially dangerous and should never be performed until all of the other possible differential diagnoses have been investigated first.

Another key indicator that a dog has DI is the fact that affected patients often have an insatiable desire to drink water. If this is not reported as a clinical sign it would be sensible to consider other more common differential diagnoses first unless there is a compelling clinical reason not to do so. Such a reason could be a subtle neurological abnormality, as identified on this dog or an extremely low USG (i.e. < 1.006).

NURSING TIP

Dogs or cats who are suspected of having diabetes insipidus must never be left without access to water unless undergoing a controlled water depravation test, as they can become clinically dehydrated quickly.

Brain tumours are not considered to be common, although dogs do appear to be significantly more prone to develop them than cats. They are generally seen in middle-aged to older animals, although they can occasionally be seen in very young animals. Numerous different types of brain tumour have been reported, including many different primary tumours arising from different neurological tissues and metastatic tumours from distant sites (such as mammary carcinoma and haemangiosarcomas) have also been reported. Pituitary tumours are one of the more common intracranial tumours reported in the dog, and occur more frequently in brachycephalic breeds. Considering that the boxer, in particular, is over-represented in the incidence figures for brain tumours, the finding of a pituitary tumour in the case described here was not particularly surprising. However, a pituitary tumour causing diabetes insipidus would not be the form of pituitary neoplasia usually encountered, as the more common form of tumour within this gland is a functional tumour of either the pars distalis or pars intermedia of the anterior pituitary, resulting in the development of pituitary-dependent hyperadrenocorticism.

Treatment for brain neoplasia and of pituitary neoplasia, in particular, can be with surgery or radiotherapy. Surgical excision of a pituitary mass is commonplace in human medicine but is rarely undertaken in veterinary medicine due to the technical difficulties of the procedure. When this approach has been used in dogs with a functional anterior pituitary tumour, the 1- and 2-year survival rates reported were 84% and 80% respectively. A more commonly utilized treatment is radiation therapy and, in particular, external beam radiotherapy in which the use of orthovoltage radiation has been described, but the use of a megavoltage linear accelerator is superior. In a study from 2007 involving 46 dogs with pituitary tumours, 19 of which received radiation treatment and 27 of which did not, the mean survival time for the treated group was 1405 days compared to 551 days in the non-treated group and the 1-, 2- and 3-year estimated survival rates for the treated group were 93%, 87% and 55%, compared to 42%, 32% and 25% for the non-treated group. Several other earlier studies support these findings and indicate that the use of radiotherapy in pituitary neoplasia can significantly improve the longevity of the patient with few treatment-associated side effects being noted and their quality of life being maintained or even improved.

13 The haematuric/stranguric/dysuric cancer patient

Haematuria is defined as the presence of excessive numbers of erythrocytes within the urine and therefore from a cancerous disease viewpoint, haematuria can be caused by neoplasia existing potentially anywhere within the urinary tract. Stranguria usually indicates an obstruction in the lower urinary tract whilst dysuria can be suggestive of either an obstructive lesion or a neurological dysfunction. Cancer causing any of these clinical signs therefore could theoretically be located in a number of different anatomical locations and a logical step-wise approach should be taken to enable an accurate diagnosis to be made as quickly as possible.

CLINICAL CASE EXAMPLE 13.1 – A DOG WITH A UNILATERAL RENAL CARCINOMA

Signalment

6-year-old neutered female doberman dog.

Presenting signs

A 3-week history of passing red-coloured urine intermittently.

Case history

The relevant history in this case was:

- The dog was fully vaccinated including current rabies, having been imported from the USA 3 years previously
- She was being successfully treated for urinary sphincter mechanism incompetence with oral phenylpropanolamine and had remained stable on this medication for the past 2 years
- The owner had noticed abnormal colouration of her urine once or twice last month and then had started to notice that her urine was darker than normal in the majority of her voidings when she urinated on concrete but he couldn't comment on urine colour when she voided on grass. In the 10 days prior to presentation the urine had become more obviously bloody and the owner said that he was now able to see that the urine was blood stained on many surfaces
- The dog was not drinking more than normal and was not exhibiting any stranguria, dysuria or polyuria. However, she had lost a little weight and she was moderately lethargic with reduced exercise tolerance.

Clinical examination

- The dog appeared quiet but alert
- Oral and ocular mucous membranes appeared slightly pale
- Thoracic auscultation revealed normal lung and heart sounds and thoracic percussion was unremarkable
- Abdominal palpation revealed an enlarged mass-like lesion in the region of her left kidney
- No further abnormalities were identified.

Diagnostic evaluation

- Her serum biochemistry revealed mild elevations in ALT and ALP but was otherwise unremarkable
- Her complete blood count revealed a mild anaemia (PCV 33%; normal 37–55%) that appeared to be regenerative based on the presence of marked polychromasia on the blood film
- Her urine did not appear grossly haematuric but urinalysis revealed the presence of many red blood cells per high power field and ++++ blood on a dipstick
- Thoracic radiographs were unremarkable
- Abdominal radiographs confirmed the presence of the enlarged and abnormally shaped left kidney
- Abdominal ultrasound showed the abnormal left kidney to be due to a mass present on the caudal pole measuring approximately 6 × 8 cm. The cranial part of the kidney appeared normal but the mass had

no normal kidney structure identifiable. No enlargement of the draining renal lymph nodes was noted. A small volume of echogenic debris was visible when the urinary bladder was balloted using the ultrasound probe, consistent in appearance with blood cells in the urine.

Diagnosis

- Primary renal tumour with no evidence of metastatic disease.

Treatment

The dog was taken to surgery for unilateral nephrectomy. Once anaesthetized the dog was placed in dorsal recumbency and the skin was routinely prepared. A ventral midline incision was made and the wound held open with a Balfour retractor. The abnormal left kidney was exposed by lifting the descending colon and moving it to the right, thereby using the mesentery attached to this to hold the small intestine towards the right hemi-abdomen. The overlying peritoneum was incised and then manually peeled away from the kidney, using electrocautery to prevent any haemorrhage. The perirenal fat was then reflected to expose the renal vasculature and the ureter. The renal artery and vein were then identified and separated and then individually ligated using 3-0 silk before being transected. The ureter was then isolated and ligated close to the urinary bladder before being transected as well and the kidney removed (Fig. 13.1). The abdomen was then lavaged and closed routinely.

Postoperatively the dog was managed with opioid analgesia (methadone for 12 hours, buprenorphine for 24 hours) along with NSAID medication (carprofen

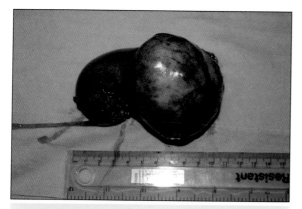

Figure 13.1 *Case 13.1* The appearance of the abnormal left kidney following excision

2 mg/kg BID for 5 days) and she recovered well. No gross haematuria was noted but microscopic haematuria was noted for 3 days.

Diagnosis

- A renal tubular cell carcinoma.

Theory refresher

Cancer of the kidney as a primary disease is actually rather unusual in the dog; indeed renal tumours are more likely to be secondary metastatic tumours than primary disease. This, therefore, leads to the necessity in any patient in whom a renal tumour is suspected for a thorough presurgery evaluation and staging to ensure that there is not a primary tumour elsewhere, as well as trying to establish the extent and severity of the disease. If a primary renal tumour is suspected in a dog, then the majority will be carcinomas (of which there are several different types), but lymphoma can also be seen and this can be bilateral in nature. Bilateral carcinomas were only reported in 4% of cases in a recent multicentre study. More unusually, other tumour types have been reported. In cats, lymphoma is the most common renal tumour type reported.

The clinical signs associated with renal neoplasia can be quite non-specific and haematuria that is noticed by the owner, as in this case, is actually not always reported although microscopic haematuria will frequently be identified. Weight loss, lethargy and inappetance are commonly reported, so a careful clinical examination is required to evaluate the size and shape of both of the kidneys, as identification of a palpable abdominal mass is often the first indication of a serious problem. Animals with renal lymphoma will usually have obviously enlarged kidneys with an irregular outline whereas, as in this case, unilateral renal enlargement due to a tumour may affect only one pole of one kidney.

The clinical pathology findings are also often non-specific. The finding of haematuria in the case reported here is reported in approximately 50% of cases, causing regenerative blood loss anaemia in approximately 33% of patients.

Diagnostic imaging, and in particular ultrasound, therefore, is a very important and useful tool to help establish the diagnosis. Ultrasound-guided aspirates or Tru-cut biopsies can be obtained, although in general the authors will only request an aspirate if lymphoma is suspected. Abdominal ultrasound is also very useful to look for local and visceral metastasis and also to assess whether or not the tumour has broken through the renal capsule to invade the surrounding musculature or vasculature. Whilst local invasion of a primary renal tumour does not prevent surgical excision, it will complicate the surgery, so attempting to establish the extent of the tumour in its locality is a very important function of the ultrasound scan. Radiographs are important to establish whether or not there are pulmonary metastases present and also to look for bony metastases in a patient that may have unexplained discomfort. Renal carcinomas (in common with most carcinomas) certainly have the potential to establish bony secondaries and although not common, will cause significant bone pain which may be difficult to treat. The author (RF), however, has had some success treating bone metastasis with a combination of meloxicam and oral bisphosphonates, in terms of producing good short-term analgesia and restoring quality of life for a limited period. There has been a recent case report of a dog with a transitional cell carcinoma of one renal pelvis causing hypertrophic osteopathy and this dog presented with haematuria and a reluctance to move. Surgical excision of the tumour led to a resolution of all the clinical signs and no further limb pain.

Unless lymphoma is diagnosed, or there are multiple secondary tumours identified, the treatment for renal neoplasia is complete nephrectomy and the diagnosis confirmed by histopathology. The prognosis does vary depending to some degree on the type of tumour identified; in a study of 82 dogs with renal tumours the median survival time for dogs with carcinomas was 16 months (range 0–59 months), for dogs with sarcomas it was 9 months (range 0–70 months), and for dogs with nephroblastomas it was 6 months (range 0–6 months). Interestingly, although not a common diagnosis, renal haemangiosarcoma is associated with relatively longer survival times when compared to other visceral forms of haemangiosarcoma (median survival time of 278 days with a range 0–1005 days in a case series of 14 dogs treated with surgery alone). However, in general, the problem with renal tumours is that they are usually highly malignant, they are frequently diagnosed quite late in their disease course and the tumours usually show very little response to chemotherapy (unless the diagnosis is one of lymphoma), so surgical excision is currently the only realistic treatment for non-lymphoid renal neoplasia.

Outcome

The dog remained well with no evidence of further disease for 19 months, when she re-presented with exercise intolerance and lethargy. On examination she was moderately tachypneoic and sadly thoracic radiographs revealed the presence of multiple pulmonary metastases, so she was euthanized. However, with a disease-free period of 19 months after the diagnosis, she had a longer than average survival and a normal quality of life in this period.

CLINICAL CASE EXAMPLE 13.2 – A DOMESTIC LONG-HAIRED CAT WITH RENAL LYMPHOMA

Signalment

2-year-old neutered male domestic long-haired (DLH) cat.

Presenting signs

Weight loss and inappetance.

Case history

The relevant history in this case was:
- The cat had been in his owner's possession since he was 10 weeks old and other than castration and his routine vaccinations he had had no veterinary treatment
- He had become dull and lethargic 5 days prior to presentation and was taken to the referring vet when he had stopped eating altogether. The owner did, however, report that she thought he had been losing weight for approximately 2–3 weeks before this.

Clinical examination

- Nervous and difficult to examine
- Cardiopulmonary auscultation unremarkable
- Abdominal palpation revealed marked bilateral renomegaly, with the kidneys having a palpably irregular surface, but was otherwise unremarkable
- No other abnormalities were detected.

Diagnostic evaluation

- The cat was referred for further investigations. Abdominal ultrasound confirmed the marked enlargement of both of his kidneys and revealed both kidneys to have a thin irregular outline with some hypoechoiec nodules present within them (Fig. 13.2). The renal cortices had a mottled and stippled appearance and there was a small volume of free fluid in the renal pelvis and a small amount of subcapsular fluid present bilaterally. No other ultrasonographic abnormalities were detected

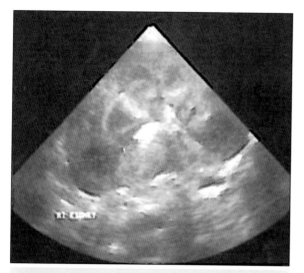

Figure 13.2 *Case 13.2* Ultrasound image of the cat's right kidney, revealing the irregular outline, renomegaly and the presence of hypoechoic nodules and a mottled appearance to the cortex

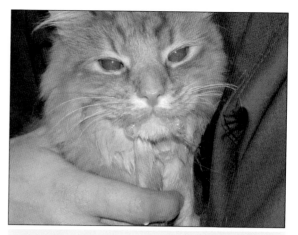

Figure 13.3 *Case 13.2* The cat shows marked salivation and papillary dilation as a result of doxorubicin administration. He was also significantly tachycardic (220 bpm). These clinical changes occurred within 5 minutes of the doxorubicin infusion being started

- Routine biochemistry was unremarkable and the cat was FeLV/FIV negative
- The complete blood count revealed a stress leucogram but no anaemia and a normal platelet count
- Fine needle aspirates of one of the kidneys were obtained. This revealed clusters of large, abnormal lymphoblastic cells exhibiting anisocytosis with variable numbers of variably sized nucleoli, coarse chromatin and nuclear moulding.

Diagnosis
- Renal lymphoma.

Treatment
- The cat was treated initially with a CHOP multidrug protocol but he suffered an acute anaphylaxis to doxorubicin, exhibiting tachycardia, hypotension and profuse salivation (Fig. 13.3). This was managed successfully but further doxorubicin administration was declined so he was maintained simply on a high-dose COP protocol for 12 months and then on an alternating cyclophosphamide/vincritisine once every 2 weeks protocol for a further 12 months before all treatment was withdrawn.

Outcome
- At the time of writing the cat is still alive and well with no evidence of lymphoma at all 4 years after his diagnosis.

Theory refresher

Renal lymphoma is the most common renal tumour found in cats but it is not the most common form of feline lymphoma reported. The disease presents usually in a similar way to that seen in the cat reported here; quite non-specific signs with usually obvious bilateral renomegaly are apparent on abdominal palpation.

> ### CLINICAL TIP
>
> In cats, haematuria could be missed unless the animal uses a litter tray, so renal neoplasia in felines is often detected when the cat presents to investigate other signs such as lethargy or inappetance.

The diagnosis can usually be made using ultrasound-guided fine needle aspiration but it is important to remember that this will cause some degree of renal haemorrhage, so at least an accurate platelet count should be obtained before aspiration is performed. The ultrasonographic appearance of the kidneys can be very suggestive of lymphoma and a study has suggested that there is a significant association between hypo-echoiec subcapsular thickening and renal lymphoma. The positive predictive value of hypoechoeic subcapsular thickening for lymphosarcoma in the study was 80.9%, the negative predictive value was 66.7%. The sensitivity and specificity of hypoechoiec subcapsular thickening for the diagnosis of renal lymphosarcoma were 60.7% and 84.6%, respectively.

The treatment for renal lymphoma for both dogs and cats is not surgery but chemotherapy. By the WHO classification, renal lymphoma is stage V and so variable responses have been reported but this case shows that it is always worth attempting treatment if the cat is relatively well. There are no studies to show a marked difference in efficacy between protocols, but a study from the Netherlands suggests that a COP-based protocol in cats for any form of lymphoma may be more successful than it is in dogs, with a complete remission rate of 75% being reported along with estimated 1- and 2-year disease-free periods (DFPs) in the cats with CR of 51.4 and 37.8%, respectively, and a median duration of remission was 251 days. The overall estimated 1-year survival rate in all cats with lymphoma was 48.7%, and the 2-year survival rate was 39.9%, with a median survival of 266 days. The cat reported in this case far exceeded what the attending clinician had expected in terms of success but the owner was delighted!

CLINICAL CASE EXAMPLE 13.3 – TRANSITIONAL CELL CARCINOMA OF THE URINARY BLADDER

Signalment

7-year-old neutered male Bichon Frise.

Presenting signs

Haematuria and penile haemorrhage.

Case history

The relevant history in this case was:
- The dog was fully vaccinated with no travel history and had received no other veterinary treatment
- Three weeks prior to presentation the owner had started to notice that the dog was licking his prepuce much more than usual. The owner then noticed the presence of fresh blood on the hair around his prepuce but the dog displayed no dysuria
- The dog was treated by the referring veterinary surgeon with antibiotics (oral clavulate-potentiated amoxicillin) but this generated no improvement
- The prepucial haemorrhage became progressively more frequent and then the owner noticed that his urine had become obviously blood-stained so he was referred.

Clinical examination

- On examination the dog was bright and alert with no other clinical signs
- Cardiopulmonary auscultation was unremarkable
- Abdominal palpation was unremarkable
- Examination of the penis and prepuce revealed blood-stained hair in the peri-prepucial region but was otherwise unremarkable
- No other abnormalities were noted.

Diagnostic evaluation

- The dog was admitted for further evaluation
- A coagulation profile was within normal limits
- Serum biochemistry was unremarkable, with the exception of his albumin being slightly subnormal at 24 g/L
- The complete blood count initially appeared normal (PCV 38%) but the blood film revealed moderate polychromasia, suggestive of increased erythroid activity in the bone marrow
- Plain abdominal radiographs were unremarkable
- Abdominal ultrasound revealed a mass lesion to be present within the ventral wall of the body of the urinary bladder. The mass had an irregular surface and measured just under 2 cm in diameter. No local lymph node enlargement was noted and the remainder of the scan was unremarkable
- A retrograde contrast urethrogram revealed no evidence of urethral disease
- Urine cytology revealed many erythrocytes consistent with haematuria but also revealed small clusters of malignant epithelial cell consistent with a diagnosis of a urinary bladder carcinoma (Fig. 13.4).

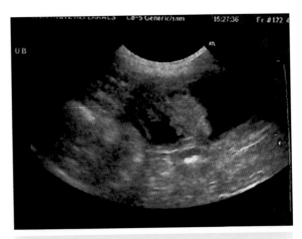

Figure 13.4 Case 13.3 Ultrasound image of the urinary bladder, revealing the presence of the mass on the ventral bladder wall

Diagnosis

- Urinary bladder tumour, probably a transitional cell carcinoma.

Treatment

In the light of the history and clinical findings the dog was taken to surgery and the mass explored. The dog was anaesthetized and positioned in dorsal recumbency and the skin prepared routinely. A ventral midline para prepucial incision was made to allow a midline incision through the linea alba to be performed. The bladder was isolated within the abdomen with moistened laparotomy swabs and the bladder carefully palpated to identify the mass. Stay sutures were then placed in the bladder at the cranial, caudal and lateral aspects of the planned incision (2 cm lateral to the mass) and the bladder drained of urine via cystocentesis using a 23-gauge needle. A stab incision was then made using a scalpel and the incision extended using metzenbaum scissors. The mass was removed with a 2-cm margin (Figs 13.5, 13.6). The surgeons then changed gloves, instruments and drapes to help prevent tumour seeding before examining the remainder of the urinary mucosa and then closing the bladder with a one-layer, approximating suture pattern using absorbable monofilament suture material. The closure was then checked by instilling saline into the bladder via a urinary catheter to cause bladder distension before lavaging the abdomen with warm saline and performing a routine closure.

Postoperatively the dog was managed with a urinary catheter for 24 hours and a combination of opioid (methadone for 12 hours, buprenorphine for 24 hours) and NSAID (carprofen BID for 5 days) analgesia.

Diagnosis

Histopathology confirmed the mass to be a transitional cell carcinoma.

Outcome

The dog made an excellent recovery after the surgery and the haematuria and prepucial haemorrhage stopped. Once the diagnosis was confirmed the dog commenced chemotherapy using oral piroxicam at 0.3 mg/mg SID (2.5 mg) and mitoxantrone at 5 mg/m² by slow intravenous infusion once every 3 weeks for a total of five treatments. He tolerated this treatment well. His progress was assessed by ultrasonographic examination of his bladder every 2 months. At his re-check scan 10 months after the surgery the owner commented that she had seen further haematuria and the scan confirmed regrowth but this time extending caudally towards the trigone. The owner declined further surgery. The dog coped well for a further 9 weeks before the owner described him as starting to display significant stranguria with haematuria, so he was euthanized.

Theory refresher

Cancer of the urinary bladder is not considered to be a common problem in the dog, estimated to account for up to 2% of all canine malignancies and it is even less common in the cat. However, in both species the most common tumour type reported is the transitional cell

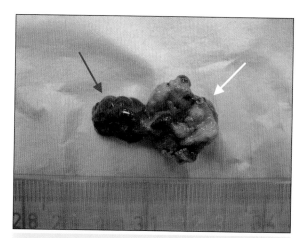

Figure 13.5 *Case 13.3* The appearance of the excised tissue, with the neoplastic tissue highlighted by the red arrow and the normal bladder tissue by the white arrow

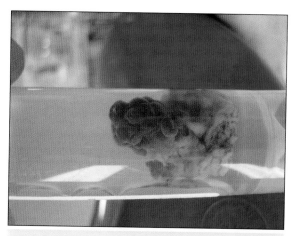

Figure 13.6 *Case 13.3* The excised tissue in formalin, showing how it would have appeared when in situ and illustrating why the ultrasound appearance was as it was

carcinoma (TCC). Other primary bladder tumours, such as squamous cell carcinomas, have been reported but they are not always of epithelial origin and they can be mesenchymal, such as leiomyosarcomas or lymphoma. In addition, the bladder can be affected by extension of prostatic neoplasia in male animals, and also rarely by metastasis from distant tumours such as haemangiosarcoma.

In cats, bladder tumours are usually seen in middle-aged to older male animals, whereas in dogs, females seem more prone to developing the disease. In general, canine bladder tumours are seen in older dogs. There also appears to be significant breed predilections for bladder tumours, with Scottish terriers being by far the most commonly reported breed affected. Shetland sheepdogs, beagles, wirehaired fox terriers and West Highland white terriers also appear to be over-represented in the published case series.

The clinical signs seen with bladder tumours will depend to some degree on the size and location of the tumour, but bladder tumours will cause haematuria in many cases. What was unusual in the case described here was the penile bleeding, as this is not usually a feature of a bladder neoplasm; rather this would usually be associated with a penile, urethral or possibly a prostatic growth. If the tumour is located in the body of the bladder, then haematuria may be the only reported clinical sign. However, the majority of tumours in dogs are located at the trigone, which more commonly results in clinical signs relating to bladder outflow tract obstruction such as stranguria and dysuria. In some cases, urinary incontinence may also be seen. In cats, the tumour is more frequently located at the apex of the bladder which may aid surgical excision, but often means that the tumour will be substantial by the time a definitive diagnosis has been reached as the clinical signs may be less easy for an owner to recognize.

The diagnosis of a bladder tumour is usually initially made on the basis of appropriate clinical signs and then good diagnostic imaging. Plain abdominal radiographs seldom reveal the tumour, but a good contrast radiograph series can be extremely useful, especially if ultrasound is not easily available. Firstly a plain lateral abdominal radiograph is obtained before a urethral catheter (such as a fine Foley or a dog urethral catheter) is placed in the distal urethra. It is sensible not to advance the catheter all the way into the bladder, as a more distal placement will allow for a contrast urethrogram to be performed in addition to a cystogram. A contrast urethrocystogram is then performed followed by a double-contrast film by instilling air through the catheter. This procedure will usually highlight any filling defects and reveal the presence of the tumour and should also indicate whether or not there is any urethral involvement. However, ultrasound is often a more useful diagnostic tool, as this can clearly reveal the presence of a mass. In addition, the local lymph nodes can be assessed for possible metastatic disease. Local metastasis must always be checked for, as a metastatic rate of up to 40% at the time of diagnosis has been reported. Furthermore, in one study 56% of cases had concurrent urethral involvement and 29% of male dogs had prostatic infiltration. Therefore the authors would usually request an abdominal ultrasound first and resort to a double-contrast radiograph series as a second choice, or if urethral involvement was suspected. Radiography of the thorax to check for distant metastasis should always be considered, especially if surgical excision is being planned, as pulmonary metastasis has been reported in up to 17% of canine cases and 15% of feline cases at the time of diagnosis.

Once a mass has been located, obtaining an exact diagnosis can be done in several ways. Ultrasound-guided fine needle aspirates can be considered but they carry a risk of causing tumour seeding, so should be avoided if possible. Careful urinalysis and cytology on a free catch sample can certainly be carried out, but this has poor sensitivity. Therefore, the two main methods used by the authors are firstly to undertake flexible cytoscopy and obtain grab biopsies whilst visualizing the lesion(s), or more simply by the use of a suction biopsy. To perform a suction biopsy, a urinary catheter with side holes is placed into the urethra and advanced to the lesion. Accurate location of the catheter tip can be done by ultrasound guidance. The tip of the catheter can then be pressed downwards into the lesion by digital pressure applied per rectum if required. A 20-ml syringe is then attached to the external portion of the catheter and suction applied. Whilst the suction is still applied, an assistant should pull the catheter out. The tip of the catheter should contain a tumour sample which is suitable for both squash cytology and histopathology. In cases for which cytoscopy is not possible for some reason, this is the preferred method of obtaining a biopsy before surgery for lesions within the urinary bladder, prostate and urethra in the authors' hospitals.

Bladder tumour antigen testing has been described in humans, but the human antigen detection kit has very poor specificity in the dog so its use cannot be recommended. A veterinary version of the bladder tumour antigen (V-BTA) detection kit has been investigated and reasonable results reported, especially when used on centrifuged urine, therefore indicating that this variant of tumour antigen detection may be of use in the clinical veterinary practice, especially in a branch surgery where diagnostic imaging facilities are not available. However, it is not used in the authors' clinics due to the availability of the other modalities discussed.

The most commonly utilized option in the treatment of bladder tumour is excisional surgery as described, but the difficulty in dogs is firstly, that many tumours are located in the trigone region and secondly, that many dogs seem to develop multifocal tumours of the bladder. Surgery is therefore often considered palliative as complete resection is rarely possible. Palliative permanent cystostomy tube placement to relieve urinary obstruction resulted in a median survival of 106 days in a case series of six dogs, which interestingly is approximately the same median survival time as those dogs undergoing partial cystectomy.

The reason that the surgeons changed gloves and instruments in this case is that transitional cell carcinomas exfoliate easily, so it is very easy to contaminate 'clean' tissue with tumour cells once the tumour has been exposed and especially if it is directly handled. A wide margin of excision is also recommended due to the risk of seeding of the tumour along the uroepithelium.

Postoperative chemotherapy has been shown to help improve disease-free periods and such treatment can also be considered in patients with unresectable tumours, either as a sole treatment or as adjunctive therapy in patients in whom a cystostomy tube is placed. The non-steroidal anti-inflammatory COX-antagonist, piroxicam has been shown to generate clinical benefit in TCCs in approximately 20% of cases, with median survival times of approximately 6 months being reported and up to 20% of these patients living for more than 1 year. Combining piroxicam with mitoxantrone (at 5 mg/m^2 by slow intravenous infusion every 3 weeks for four cycles) improves the response rate to 35% with a median survival time of 291 days being reported with a low incidence of toxicity. For this reason, this chemotherapy regimen is the first-line therapy in the authors' clinics, either after surgery or as a palliative treatment. Higher response rates have been described when cisplatin and piroxicam are combined, but this treatment is associated with significant renal toxicity and cannot therefore be recommended as a routine treatment. Carboplatin and piroxicam have also been trialled as a combined therapy and generated remission in 40% of the dogs it

was given to but significant gastrointestinal side effects were reported in 74% of these patients and haematological toxicity seen in 35%. These results indicate that carboplatin combined with piroxicam is also not an optimal treatment for urinary transitional cell carcinoma, despite the response rate. Meloxicam has now been shown to have a protective action against experimental carcinogenesis in rat bladders and there is anecdotal evidence that it may have a clinical effect in veterinary practice but to the authors' knowledge at the time of writing there have been no veterinary clinical trial results published proving clinical efficacy in dogs or cats. However, under the current cascade regulations, as meloxicam is licensed for use in both dogs and cats but piroxicam is not, meloxicam should be used in preference.

Photodynamic therapy has now also been described as a treatment for TCC of the urinary bladder in animal models and this has now also been reported in a small series of dogs with TCC with moderately successful results. PDT may therefore prove to be an effective future treatment but more work is required in this area.

CLINICAL CASE EXAMPLE 13.4 – MULTIFOCAL UTERINE HAEMANGIOMA IN A RABBIT

(Case written by Dr Livia Benato DVM, MRCVS, The R(D) SVS, University of Edinburgh.)

Signalment

2-year-old intact female lion head rabbit.

Presenting signs

Episodes of intermittent mild haematuria.

Case history

The relevant history in this case was:
- The rabbit was fully vaccinated and no signs of previous illness were reported by the owner
- The rabbit was presented with flaky skin, and a few episodes of intermittent mild haematuria and soft faeces
- The owner was reluctant to proceed in the investigation and medical treatment was started. Enrofloxacin oral solution was given once a day for 1 week to treat a possible infection of the urogenital tract, causing the haematuria and a first injection of ivermectin was made subcutaneously to manage the skin problem

- Although, the skin aspect improved, the haematuria started once again at the end of the treatment with enrofloxacin and the owner asked for further evaluation.

Clinical examination

- Upon physical examination the rabbit was alert and responsive
- The cardiopulmonary auscultation was unremarkable
- The rabbit showed mild abdominal pain
- Soft masses were detected upon palpation of the caudal area of the abdomen
- In the perianal area, the fur appeared stained with blood and soft faeces
- The skin appeared flaky and crusty
- No other abnormalities were noted.

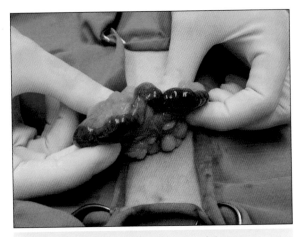

Figure 13.7 *Case 13.4* External aspect of the uterus before performing the ovariohysterectomy. The uterus appears swollen and inflamed

Diagnostic evaluation

- The rabbit was admitted for further investigation
- Haematology and biochemistry were unremarkable
- A urine sample was obtained by cystocentesis and tested negative for blood
- An abdominal radiographic examination was performed and no radiographic abnormalities were found except some soft-tissue density dorsal to the bladder
- Abdominal ultrasonography revealed a swollen and irregular uterus
- On the basis of the history and the physical examination an ovariohysterectomy was recommended
- To investigate the skin problem a deep skin scrape was necessary and a diagnosis of *Cheyletiella* spp., rabbit fur mites, was made.

Treatment

General anaesthesia was induced using a combination of medetomidine, ketamine and butorphanol subcutaneously and, after intubation, the rabbit was maintained on isoflurane and oxygen. An ovariohysterectomy was undertaken. The rabbit was placed in dorsal recumbency and the abdomen was prepared for a midline incision. Upon entering the abdomen, the vagina, the uterine horns and the oviducts were exteriorized. The uterus appeared to be swollen and inflamed (Figs 13.7, 13.8). The ovarian vessels were ligated and transected. The uterine arteries were individually ligated and the double cervix was exteriorized and a single transfixing suture was placed cranial to the vagina. The abdominal wall was closed in two layers with a simple interrupted pattern and the skin was closed with an absorbable

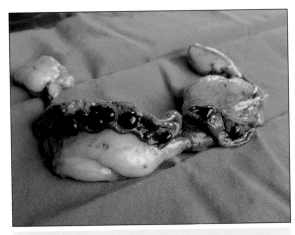

Figure 13.8 *Case 13.4* The protuberant nodules in the uterine lumen were the cause of the haemorrhage and haematuria

continuous subcuticular suture and an 'Aberdeen' knot.

Meloxicam and enrofloxacin were administered postoperatively. The antibiotic treatment was continued for 7 days. The rabbit made an uncomplicated recovery and was discharged the following day.

Diagnosis

- Multifocal uterine haemangioma.

Outcome

Two weeks after the surgery, during the follow-up, the owner reported that she had not seen any further haematuria and that the rabbit had exhibited normal behaviour. Also, she noticed the skin was improving and fewer crusts were present.

After a total of three injections of ivermectin, once a fortnight, the skin healed completely.

Theory refresher

The rabbit, *Oryctolagus cuniculus*, is a mammal belonging to the order of lagomorphs and is the third most popular pet in the UK.

Uterine tumours are commonly found in entire female rabbits older than 5 years of age (up to 80%) but are rare in younger animals such as this case. The most common type of uterine tumour is the uterine adenocarcinoma (Fig. 13.9). It is a malignant tumour which tends to metastasize not only to the lungs but also to the adjacent organs. Other common neoplasms are haemangiomas, haemangiosarcomas and leiomyosarcomas.

The clinical signs seen with uterine tumours are varied but haematuria is the most common symptom of a urogenital problem. Differentiating between these is possible by a urinary dipstick test. In rabbit, the colour of urine can vary from pale yellow to reddish orange due to the presence of porphyrin pigmentation and can be easily confused with blood in urine. Again, if in doubt, a urinary dipstick test can be handy. Other clinical signs can be anorexia, weight loss, decreased activity,

decreased faecal output, swollen mammary glands and anaemia. Also, ascites may be present in advanced cases and dyspnoea in cases of pulmonary metastasis. Haematuria is the most common presenting symptom of urogenital problems in the rabbit. It is important to differentiate between genital and urinary tract disease. Common tumours of the urinary tract are renal neoplasia (renal carcinoma, renal adenocarcinoma and renal lymphosarcoma) associated with nephromegaly and secondary renal failure. Bladder tumours have also been reported and include leiomyomas. Benign embryonal nephroma can also be seen, but normally is considered an incidental finding during post-mortem examination. Single or multiple masses may affect one or both kidneys but do not lead to significant renal impairment. If one kidney is affected then nephrectomy is curative, should this be deemed necessary. Uterine adenocarcinoma is considered the most common tumour of female rabbits. With abdominal palpation it is possible to localize multiple masses affecting both of the uterine horns. This type of tumour can metastasize locally and via the bloodstream to the lungs, brain, bone, skin, mammary glands and liver. Other common neoplasms of the genital tract are uterine haemangioma, uterine haemangiosarcoma, uterine leiomyosarcoma, and squamous cell carcinoma of the vaginal wall. Ovariohysterectomy is recommended as both treatment and prevention. Other clinical signs associated with urogenital neoplasia are urinary scalding and dysuria. This means that cystitis is an important differential.

In this case, the rabbit also presented with skin problems due to ectoparasites. This is a common symptom for an immune-suppressed animal suffering from underlying disease or stress. Although, ectoparasites are normally present in the skin of a healthy rabbit, when skin disease is evident a full evaluation of the rabbit should be taken into consideration.

Uterine tumours can be diagnosed by several methods. Clinical history and physical examination are important to make a differential diagnosis list and rule out any other diseases. Abdominal palpation, in the caudal quadrant, may reveal uterine masses. A radiographic exam will enable a confirmation of what has already been found during the clinical examination and, most of the time, is enough to establish a diagnosis. Chest radiographic examination is useful in cases where pulmonary metastasis is suspected. Ultrasonography and explorative laparotomy provide further information about the nature of the uterine tumour. The first test is not invasive and it can be performed without sedation and allows a

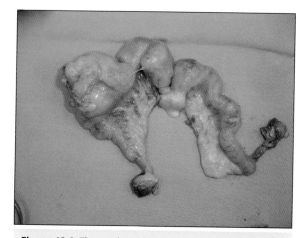

Figure 13.9 The cytological appearance of the neoplastic prostatic epithelial cells, as described above (Giemsa stain, ×100 magnification). Courtesy of Mrs Elizabeth Villiers

guided needle biopsy. Explorative laparotomy should be the last diagnostic test to consider. However, a thorough examination of all the abdominal organs, in search of abnormalities or metastasis, is possible. If indicated the surgeon can proceed immediately with surgical treatment.

The treatment of choice for uterine tumours is surgery. Ovariohysterectomy offers the best option to remove the tumour completely, particularly if benign or at an early stage, and to treat clinical symptoms like, for example in this case, haematuria. Although the general anaesthesia might be considered problematic, an ovariohysterectomy is considered a routine surgery and a very safe procedure with, most of the time, a quick recovery. In this case the skin was closed using an absorbable continuous subcuticular suture to avoid contamination of the surgical wound and to stop the rabbit removing the stitches.

To avoid complications due to the surgery, exact management of the rabbit pre- and postoperatively is essential. Prior to surgery, fluid therapy and treatment with gut stimulants and analgesics are mandatory. In the case of an anorexic rabbit, assisted feeding for 2 or 3 days before surgery would be considered appropriate. Following surgery the patient should be allowed to recover in a warm and calm, stress-free environment. The rabbit can be sent home as soon as she shows appetite and there are no signs of stasis of the gastric enteric tract.

If there is no evidence of metastasis, the prognosis is normally considered good with no recurrence. The preventive treatment for uterine tumours is to spay the rabbit at 4–6 months of age.

The diagnosis can be made by radiography, ultrasonography, laparoscopy and exploratory laparotomy. When possible, the best treatment is surgical resection. Chemotherapy has been advocated in cases of haemangiosarcoma where surgical resection is not possible.

CLINICAL CASE EXAMPLE 13.5 – A GOLDEN RETRIEVER WITH A PROSTATIC CARCINOMA

Signalment

11-year-old neutered male golden retriever.

Case history

The relevant history in this case was:

- The dog was fully vaccinated. He had osteoarthritis of both hips and was on an oral non-steroid anti-inflammatory drug (carprofen) and oral glycosaminoglycans to treat this. Otherwise he had received no other veterinary treatment in his life.
- For approximately 4 weeks prior to referral the owner had noticed that he took longer to urinate than he used to, in that he would stand for several seconds before the urine flow would start. The owner also thought that this was becoming gradually worse but put this down to an old-age change
- Over these 4 weeks the owner also described that he had become 'listless'
- Approximately 2 weeks prior to referral she had noticed he had started to strain to defecate and then that his faeces appeared to be much thinner than normal; she described them as being 'ribbon-like'
- Two days prior to referral the dog had developed blood-stained urine and was straining significantly to urinate.

Clinical examination

- On examination the dog was quiet and in reasonable body condition
- Cardiopulmonary auscultation was unremarkable
- Caudal abdominal palpation was resented by the dog and appeared uncomfortable but revealed a full urinary bladder
- Digital rectal examination revealed substantial enlargement of his prostate, palpation of which appeared to cause the dog discomfort
- No other abnormalities were noted.

Diagnostic evaluation

- The dog was admitted for further evaluation
- Serum biochemistry revealed only a mild elevation in ALP (460 iu/L; normal 10–100) but otherwise no abnormalities
- The complete blood count revealed no abnormalities
- Urinalysis revealed a positive (+++) reading for blood and protein on the dipstick, but there was no active sediment and cytology was unremarkable
- Plain abdominal radiographs revealed significant prostatomegaly and distension of his urinary bladder but no sublumbar lymph node enlargement
- Thoracic radiographs revealed no significant abnormalities
- Abdominal ultrasound revealed the prostate to be irregular and asymmetrically enlarged with a well-defined heterogeneous parenchyma. Cavitary lesions were also noted along with some echogenic foci that caused acoustic shadowing

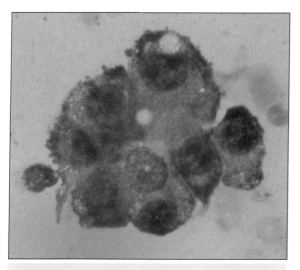

Figure 13.10 *Case 13.5* The cytological appearance of the neoplastic prostatic epithelial cells, as described in the text (Giemsa stain, ×100 magnification). Courtesy of Mrs Elizabeth Villiers, Dick White Referrals

- Fine needle aspirates of the prostate were obtained under ultrasound guidance. These yielded moderate numbers of nucleated cells (Fig. 13.10). There were many rafts of cohesive epithelial cells in a background of red cells with moderate numbers of inflammatory cells. The cohesive epithelial cells were large and pleomorphic. They had large nuclei containing coarsely clumped chromatin, often with two or three nucleoli. There was moderate to marked anisokaryosis. Significant numbers of binucleated and occasional multinucleated cells were seen. The cytoplasm was basophilic and generally devoid of vacuoles, although some cells had foamy cytoplasm. Within the cell clusters there was considerable cell crowding and disorganisation with streaming random cell arrangements. The cells were round to polygonal to elongated (the latter with streaked cytoplasm). There were also small numbers of small uniform prostatic epithelial cells. The nuclei were approximately one quarter the diameter of the large pleomorphic cells.

Diagnosis

Prostatic carcinoma with associated inflammation.

Treatment

In the light of the aggressive nature of prostatic carcinomas, the age of the dog and his concurrent arthritis

problem, it was decided to simply treat the dog with oral meloxicam (swapping from the carprofen) and lactulose as a faecal softener and to assess his progress.

Outcome

The dog became moderately brighter and exhibited less stranguria over the next week. The dyschezia improved considerably on the lactulose. Six weeks later he developed marked stranguria again and appeared very uncomfortable, so he was euthanized by the referring vet.

Theory refresher

Prostatic tumours are actually quite rare in dogs and even less common in cats. It is generally seen in older animals (mean age of 9 years in the dog) and the Bouvier des Flandres appears to be at an increased risk of developing the condition. Although prostatic carcinoma can be seen in both castrated and entire dogs, there are reports indicating that the disease is more common in castrated dogs. Furthermore, although castration does not initiate the development of canine prostatic carcinoma, it does favour tumour progression with an increased risk of metastatic disease. It is important to remember that benign prostatic hyperplasia is associated with entire males, not castrated ones, so an enlarged prostate gland identified on digital examination and diagnostic imaging in an elderly castrated male should raise a suspicion for the possibility of prostatic neoplasia.

Prostatic cancers are usually epithelial in nature (prostatic carcinoma and transitional cell carcinoma are the two most common tumours reported), although a recent report of a prostatic haemangiosarcoma has been published and there are previous reports of lymphomas, squamous cell carcinomas, leiomyomas and leiomyosarcomas being diagnosed. The tumour can be focal or disseminated within the prostate, meaning that any aspirate or biopsy samples must be representative of the tissue that appears to be abnormal to ensure that an accurate diagnosis is made.

The clinical signs associated with prostatic carcinoma can be variable but were quite well summarized by the case described in this section. Dysuria is often reported and this can be accompanied by haematuria, but haematuria is not a consistent finding in all cases. Urinary incontinence may also be seen. Concurrent bacterial infection of the tumour may result in clinical evidence of a urinary tract infection with active urinary sediment observed cytologically on a centrifuged sample. Some patients may occasionally present exhibiting moderate

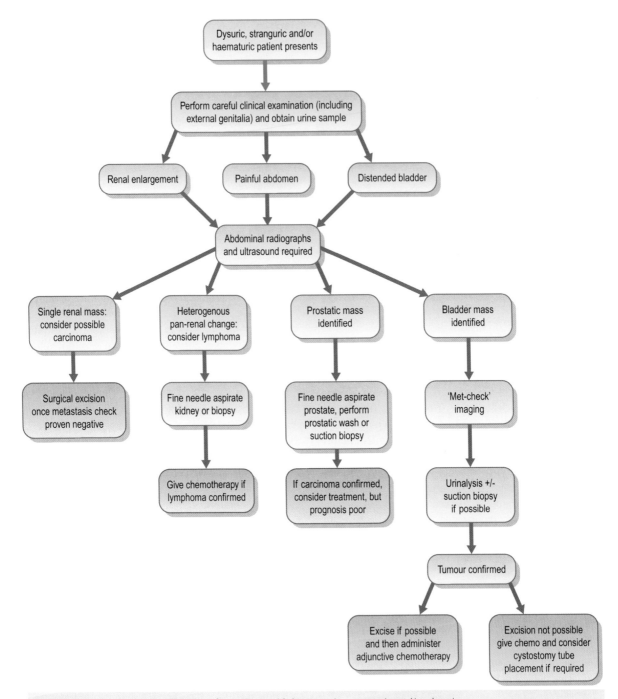

Figure 13.11 Diagnostic plan flowchart for patients with haematuria, stranguria and/or dysuria

to marked pain on urination or defecation, but this is unusual. Changes to the appearance of the faeces, caused by direct compression of the colon by the prostatomegaly can occur, resulting in the reported 'ribbon' faeces in this case.

Prostatic carcinomas are usually aggressive tumours which metastasize readily, initially to the vertebral venous sinuses and the iliac lymph nodes and also potentially to the bladder, rectum or pelvis. In advanced cases there can be metastasis to the lumbar vertebrae or pelvic musculature which can result in lameness, hind-limb weakness or back pain. Distant metastases are unusual but it is important to undertake abdominal and thoracic 'met-check' radiographs in these cases and also undertake a thorough abdominal ultrasound examination to look for lymphatic and visceral metastasis.

Radiographically, some prostatic tumours can be associated with a 'sunburst' reaction on the pelvic bones, but this is not pathognomonic for the disease, as it could result from other metastatic or primary neoplasia or other aggressive lesions such as osteomyelitis. Radiography also cannot easily distinguish between the causes of prostatomegaly unless there is obvious lymph node enlargement suggestive of metastatic disease. However, ultrasound can be extremely useful as a study showed that multifocal, irregularly shaped, parenchymal mineral densities (as described in this case) were observed only in dogs with prostatic carcinoma or prostatitis. It should then be possible to use urinalysis, fine needle aspirates or biopsy to distinguish between these two conditions. Ultrasound is also very useful for investigation of the local lymph nodes for metastatic disease and can also be used to obtain fine needle aspirates for cytological evaluation. There has been concern that fine needle aspiration may lead to seeding of tumour cells along the needle track, but this is an inconsistent finding and in the authors' opinion, relatively less serious than the risk of the disease itself and not reaching a definitive diagnosis.

Treatment for prostatic carcinoma is frequently difficult due to the aggressive nature of the tumour, the propensity to develop bony metastases and also the fact that many cases are diagnosed relatively late in the disease course. Treatment is further complicated by the fact that prostatic carcinoma appears to respond poorly to adjunctive chemotherapy. The prognosis therefore for this disease is generally guarded and giving conservative treatment as described is often the correct decision. Surgical prostatectomy has been reported but is often associated with significant complications such as the development of urinary incontinence and as such is rarely recommended. Surgical placement of a cystostomy tube can certainly be helpful for dogs that develop urethral obstruction as a result of their tumour by improving their quality of life but such a measure will only ever be a short-term palliative option. Photodynamic therapy may hold more promise in the future as several studies have shown that several different photosensitizers can be targeted to the prostate, but this technique is not yet readily available in veterinary medicine.

The use of cyclo-oxygenase 2 (COX-2) antagonists such as meloxicam also holds promise, as it has been shown that normal prostatic tissue does not express COX-2 but up to 75% of prostatic carcinomas do express COX-2, suggesting that COX-2 may have some function in tumorigenesis. However, the exact role and clinical usefulness of COX-antagonists remains unclear. One small trial has also indicated that dogs with prostatic carcinoma have a significantly longer mean life expectancy when given non-steroidal anti-inflammatory drugs compared to dogs given no treatment.

14 The lame cancer patient

The identification of an animal being lame due to a neoplastic disease usually causes owners significant distress as they face the possibility of considering amputation of the affected limb, whilst for the veterinary surgeon some careful diagnostic evaluation will be required for the case to ensure the tumour found is primary as opposed to being secondary, to ensure that there are no detectable secondary tumours present and also to consider all of the treatment options available. It is also important to remember that lameness may indicate spinal or neurological disease, so thorough clinical evaluation is essential to be sure that the clinical extent of the condition has been fully established.

CLINICAL CASE EXAMPLE 14.1 – OSTEOSARCOMA IN A DOG

Signalment
7-year-old neutered female rottweiler.

Presenting signs
A 2-week history of progressively worsening right hindlimb lameness.

Case history
The relevant history in this case was:
- The dog was vaccinated, wormed and had travelled to Europe on regular holidays with his owners
- The dog had started to limp after returning from a walk 10 days prior to presentation and this had not improved despite a course of oral NSAIDs
- The lameness worsened suddenly after she had gone out into the garden, to the point of being practically non-weight-bearing, so she was referred.

Clinical examination
- On examination the dog was non-weight-bearing lame on her right hind leg and the dog resented palpation and manipulation of her right stifle

- Cardiopulmonary auscultation revealed the dog to be tachycardic but she was otherwise unremarkable
- Abdominal palpation was unremarkable.

Diagnostic evaluation
- In the light of the clinical findings, the dog was immediately taken to radiography and radiographs of the right hindlimb obtained. These revealed the presence of an osteolytic lesion within the femur with an accompanying periosteal reaction, as shown in Figure 14.1.

Differential diagnosis
- Primary bone tumour
  - Osteosarcoma
  - Chondrosarcoma
- Metastatic bone tumour.

Treatment
- In the light of the radiographic findings, the diagnosis was made that the dog had a bone tumour, likely to be a primary bone neoplasm
- In the light of the degree of pain she was obviously in for her to be non-weight-bearingly lame, the decision was made not to biopsy the mass because it was felt that knowledge of the tumour type would not affect the initial treatment (i.e. the limb required amputation if any treatment was to be considered), but knowledge of the tumour type would influence whether or not postoperative chemotherapy should be recommended
- The popliteal lymph node was carefully examined but was found not to be palpable
- Left and right lateral inflated thoracic radiographs were obtained which revealed no gross metastatic disease
- The dog therefore underwent a full hindlimb amputation
- Histopathology confirmed the tumour to be an osteosarcoma.

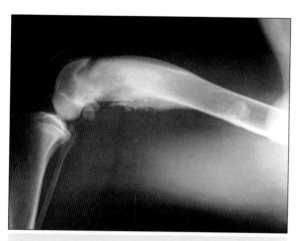

Figure 14.1 *Case 14.1* A lateral radiograph of the femur revealing the presence of a bone tumour characterized by osteolysis and a large periosteal reaction on the caudal border of the femur. Courtesy of Dr Hervé Brissot, Dick White Referrals

Outcome

The dog received chemotherapy in the form of alternating carboplatin and doxorubicin given once every 3 weeks for a total of six treatments. The dog was alive and well with no evidence of pulmonary metastasis at 12 months after the surgery.

Theory refresher

Osteosarcoma (OSA) is a highly malignant mesenchymal tumour originating in primitive bone cells that has been reported to account for up to 85% of all skeletal malignancies in the dog. It is a disease seen most frequently in large/giant-breed dogs in particular. There is a positive correlation with the height of the animal and the development of the disease. It is not surprising therefore to see that the breeds that develop the disease most frequently are Saint Bernards, great Danes, dobermans, Irish setters, rottweilers, German shepherd dogs and golden retrievers. The disease is reported in small-breed dogs but with very low frequency (no more than 5% of all cases). Most cases involving the appendicular skeleton develop in middle- to older-aged dogs with an average age of 7 years (although it can certainly develop in quite young dogs), but OSA of the rib is most commonly seen in younger dogs at approximately 5 years of age. There may be a slight gender predilection for males developing the disease, but the data in some studies suggest there is no gender bias in OSA, so this question is currently unresolved. The tumour, as in this case, most

commonly develops in the metaphyseal region of the long bones and the front limbs appear to be affected more frequently than the hind legs.

The tumour has significant local effects, with new bone development and osteolysis often occurring concurrently. This leads to distortion of the periosteum, microfracture formation and often quite marked pain. It is not possible to definitively diagnose an OSA on radiographs alone (although suspicion can be very high), but it is this mixed pathology that generates the 'classic' peripheral pallisading new bone appearance admixed with (sometimes patchy) cortical lysis and obvious soft tissue swelling on radiographic examinations. In addition to being locally destructive, OSA also usually exhibits aggressive metastatic behaviour, with the lungs being the primary target location for the development of secondary disease. This is why it is mandatory to obtain good-quality left and right lateral inflated thoracic radiographs as a minimum diagnostic imaging evaluation prior to undertaking any surgical treatments. Other potential metastasis sites include other bones or any soft tissues.

Any dog therefore presenting with a non-resolving lameness that has an accompanying soft-tissue swelling should always undergo a radiographic evaluation, with OSA as a major concern if the dog is a large or giant breed. However, it is very important to remember to examine the whole dog, as it is possible that the tumour could be a secondary lesion. Bony metastases often originate from a carcinoma, so the anal sacs need to be evaluated with a digital rectal examination as does the prostate, along with a careful palpation of the mammary glands, as part of a detailed physical examination to try to establish whether there is disease elsewhere or not.

If the presentation of the patient is potentially consistent with a primary bone tumour, a decision has to be made whether or not to biopsy the lesion. Although in most scenarios it is vitally important to obtain a definitive diagnosis before contemplating a treatment such as amputation, if the dog, as in the case reported here, is obviously in substantial pain and the opinion of the attending clinician is that amputation may actually be the best form of analgesia the dog can receive, surgical removal of the problem with postoperative histology may be acceptable. If amputation is a treatment option that is declined by the owners, then it is essential to obtain samples for biopsy. Usually the simplest and safest way to obtain a bone biopsy sample is to use a Jamshidi needle device. These needles can be quite large but it is very important to get as much tissue as it is safely possible to do, as the histological appearance can vary within individual biopsy samples and a superficial or small biopsy may generate a misleading result. A simple closed biopsy procedure under a brief general anaesthesia is usually more than adequate, but the owners must be warned regarding the risk of pathological fracture at the biopsy site due to the pre-existing bone weakness and distortion.

Once the diagnosis has been confirmed, the first-line treatment is to surgically amputate the affected limb and then to give adjunctive chemotherapy, as it is likely that microscopic metastases will be present in virtually all cases. Limb amputation is the most common surgical treatment for canine and feline appendicular OSA. Most animals with OSA will have naturally shifted the majority of their weight bearing onto three legs for some time prior to the surgery so tend to function well after the procedure. There are in fact few contraindications for limb amputation and even dogs with mild to moderate degenerative joint disease in other joints can do extremely well, as do the giant breeds of dogs. However, although the majority of owners are pleased with the outcome the decision to amputate must be discussed carefully and owners' sensitivities towards the operation taken into account.

For forelimbs it is easier to perform a complete forequarter amputation (involving removal of the scapula) rather than shoulder disarticulation. The cosmetic result is very good using this technique as there is no muscle atrophy that occurs over the scapula associated with the latter technique. It also allows for complete removal of local disease. For the hind limbs a coxofemoral amputation is generally recommended for complete disease excision, however, with distal tibial tumours then a midshaft femoral amputation is also acceptable, with some surgeons preferring this as it affords some protection to male genitalia. For any amputation, electrocautery is a useful means of controlling haemorrhage from smaller vessels. However, it should not be used excessively and ligation techniques are necessary for larger arteries and veins. If possible muscles should be separated at their origins or insertions. Arteries and veins are ligated separately (and in this order) with major vessels double ligated before division. Nerves are sharply divided after infiltration with local anaesthetic. When closing the wound the surgeon should focus on eliminating dead space and controlling haemorrhage to help avoid complications such as wound seroma and dehiscence.

> ### CLINICAL TIP
>
> Spending time on haemostasis and eliminating dead space by multilayer closure will allow quicker healing times with fewer complications. The need for drain placement if this is done is negated.

> ### NURSING TIP
>
> Placement of a comfortable bandage postoperatively helps to prevent bleeding from small vessels and also makes the patient feel more comfortable. Particular attention must be given to analgesia.

> ### NURSING TIP
>
> These patients often display the 'wind-up' phenomenon seen in patients with long-term pain, so they require excellent analgesia in their premedication, through surgery and in the immediate 24–48 hours postoperatively. They require regular reassessment to establish their levels of pain control.

Once the limb has been amputated and the dog has recovered, attention must turn to adjunctive chemotherapy. Without follow-up treatment, secondary disease often develops very rapidly (within as short a time as 3 months) and this is thought to be due to the fact that microscopic metastatic disease is likely to be present in most cases by the time they present. Many different drug regimens have been evaluated and it is clear that the platinum drugs definitely generate substantial improvements in life expectancy and outcome. Doxorubicin also shows activity against OSA but with less efficacy as a single agent when compared to the platinum drugs, so currently the authors use an alternating carboplatin/doxorubicin protocol where the drugs are given at 21-day intervals for a total of six treatments. The authors generally use carboplatin in preference to cisplatin due to its relative ease of handling, lower side effect risk and the relatively fewer health and safety concerns regarding carboplatin. This protocol has been reported to generate median survival times of 321 days with a 1-year survival rate of 48% and a 2-year survival rate of

18%. However, many other treatment combinations have been reported in which the drugs used (cisplatin, carboplatin, lobaplatin, doxorubicin), the doses used and interdose intervals are all varied and a general observation would be that most protocols generate median survival times of approximately 1 year and have 1-year survival rates of between 30 and 50%. Two-year survival rates with this approach are low.

To try to improve these figures, alternative treatment possibilities have been reported. 'Limb-sparing' surgery has been extensively investigated and performed at the Colorado State University Animal Cancer Center (CSU ACC) in the USA and also at several other centres around the world and this has proved to be a successful technique in most cases but the procedure requires an experienced and dedicated clinical team and very dedicated owners. It is a technique that can be performed for radial, ulnar, tibial or fibular OSA and in essence the procedure involves surgically excising the tumour and then replacing the bone deficit usually with a cortical allograft, although the use of metal endo-prostheses has been described, as has pasteurizing the excised bone tumour section before re-implanting it. A review of over 200 cases at CSU from the 1990s reported that the 1-year survival rates were 60% with the 1-year local disease-free rate being over 75%. Currently this is not a commonplace procedure in the UK but with more surgeons visiting and training in the USA, it may well become a more routine procedure in this country.

If surgery is not a viable option for any reason, then external beam radiotherapy can help to generate some significant analgesia for OSA patients for up to approximately 3 months when given as a two-fraction treatment, usually administering up to 10 Gy per fraction. The concern regarding radiotherapy is that it may increase bone weakness at the tumour site and therefore lead to an increased risk of the dog developing a pathological fracture, especially if the analgesic action is sufficient for the dog to use the leg almost normally. Analgesia can be augmented with the NSAID meloxicam, as not only is it a highly effective non-steroidal anti-inflammatory analgesic, it is now under investigation as an antineoplastic agent itself. In addition, the author has had some experience of using oral and injectable bisphosphonates in OSA patients. Bisphosphonates are osteoclast inhibitors and it is thought that osteoclast activity is one of the major causes of pain in bone cancer, so antagonizing these cells may help OSA patients (Figs 14.2, 14.3).

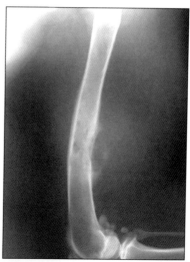

Figure 14.2

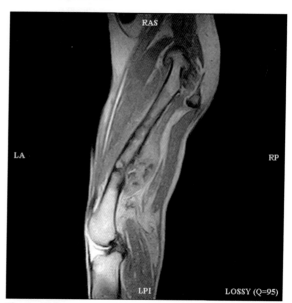

Figure 14.3

Figures 14.2, 14.3 Lateral radiograph and T1 plus contrast sagittal MRI scan of the femur of a Gordon setter with a large osteosarcoma in the mid-section of the bone with a large resultant local soft-tissue involvement. Note the significant extension of the tumour through the medullary cavity that is visible on the MRI but there is no evidence of it on the radiograph. Amputation was declined, so the dog was treated with two cycles of external beam radiotherapy, single-agent carboplatin chemotherapy, oral meloxicam and the bisphosphonate 'alendronate'. The dog became completely sound again and remained non-lame for 6 months. Courtesy of Dr Hervé Brissot, Dick White Referrals

If amputation or limb-sparing surgery are not undertaken, however, the fact that OSA is a painful disease must come first in the clinician's mind and at no time must the dog be allowed to endure discomfort unnecessarily, especially in the face of a disease that is virtually always terminal for the patient.

The importance of obtaining a bone biopsy comes when the differential diagnosis for a bone tumour is considered. Chondrosarcomas (CS) are the second most common primary bone tumour encountered in dogs, accounting for up to 10% of all bone tumour cases. Unlike OSA, CS does not exhibit aggressive metastatic behaviour, although it is a malignant tumour and secondary disease usually does develop, albeit slowly when compared to OSA. One study reported a median survival time following amputation of 540 days (although this was only a small study of five cases) with no adjunctive treatment being given. The reason for this is that a consistently efficacious chemotherapeutic against CS has not been reported in dogs. If CS therefore is diagnosed, the outlook for the patient is considerably better than if an OSA is diagnosed.

Fibrosarcomas (FSA) of bone have been reported rarely, as have haemangiosarcomas (HSA) and the prognosis between these two tumours varies considerably too. Primary bone HSA is a highly malignant tumour that usually leads to secondary disease within 6 months of the diagnosis, so the prognosis for this disease is poor. FSA on the other hand, although a malignant tumour, appears slower to metastasize. There are few good studies into its behaviour and no consistently efficacious chemotherapy but if treated early by complete excision then there may be a long-term disease-free period.

Primary bone cancer in cats is considered to be rare but when it occurs, up to 90% will be potentially malignant in nature and the most frequently reported tumour type is OSA. Interestingly, however, OSA in cats does not appear to be as aggressive as it is in dogs, as median survival times after amputation without adjunctive chemotherapy of between 24 and 44 months have been reported. Currently therefore, the treatment of choice should be surgical excision.

Mandibular OSA has been reported to develop in rabbits. The tumour presents as a hard swelling of the mandible and could therefore be easily confused with dental disorders. Mandibular OSA is considered to be rare but an appropriate investigation should always be undertaken if there is clinical suspicion of a tumour. Radiography is obviously very useful as a diagnostic tool, but computed tomography can also be very useful where available. Both modalities can show disruption of bone density at the site of the primary tumour and also obviously potential metastasis to the lungs, pleural cavities and abdominal organs. If no metastatic lesions are identified then surgical removal is possible and hemimandibulectomies have been reported.

CLINICAL CASE EXAMPLE 14.2 – METASTATIC ANAL SAC CARCINOMA CAUSING LAMENESS IN A DOG

Signalment

9-year-old neutered female cocker spaniel.

Presenting signs

A 3-week history of a progressively worsening lameness affecting her right hind leg. The owner also commented that she had stopped wagging her tail and he felt she was having to strain considerably to pass faeces.

Case history

The relevant history in this case was:

- The dog was fully vaccinated, wormed and had not travelled outside of the UK
- The owner had first seen her limp possibly up to 3 months previously but this had been intermittent and he had put it down to her having arthritis
- Approximately 6 weeks prior to examination, the dog had started to intermittently strain more than normal to pass faeces but this had not been investigated
- The lameness affecting her right hind leg progressed to become constant and the owner described her as also appearing weak on this leg, with it sometimes appearing to 'give way' for no reason
- In the 10 days prior to presentation, the dog had appeared to lose the use of her tail but it was not painful to touch
- The dog had started to lose a little weight and had become dull and lethargic.

Clinical examination

- On examination she was quiet and obviously lame on her right hind, although she was weight bearing
- Cardiopulmonary auscultation was unremarkable
- Abdominal palpation revealed an obvious, consistent pain response in the mid-lumbar region. There was no palpable swelling but she significantly resented digital palpation in this area
- Neurological examination revealed proprioceptive deficits in her right hind along with mild weakness in

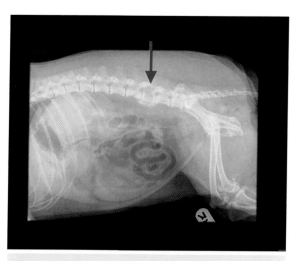

Figure 14.4 *Case 14.2* A right lateral abdominal radiograph revealing the metastatic lesion within L$_5$, as shown by the red arrow

this leg and reduced perianal sensation, but no other defects were noted. No painful focus could be found anywhere in the right hind leg itself
- Digital rectal examination revealed the presence of a mass within the right anal sac measuring approximately 2 cm in diameter.

Diagnostic evaluation
- Fine needle aspirates of the anal sac mass confirmed the mass to be an anal sac carcinoma
- Thoracic radiographs were unremarkable
- Abdominal radiographs revealed an osteolytic lesion in L$_5$ which radiographically appeared to have almost totally destroyed the vertebral bone (Fig. 14.4)
- Abdominal ultrasound revealed mild enlargement of the right colonic and sublumbar lymph nodes
- Ultrasound was used to obtain guided fine needle aspirates of the lesion in L$_5$. These confirmed the presence of a malignant carcinoma.

Diagnosis
- Anal sac carcinoma with bony metastasis to the vertebrae (stage IV disease).

Treatment
- The owners understood that surgical excision of the disease was not possible and that the efficacy of chemotherapy would be poor, so palliative treatment was commenced with oral meloxicam, oral Tramadol and the oral bisphosphonate, Alendronate.

Outcome
- The dog made rapid and good progress for the first 3 months of treatment, with the lameness almost totally resolving and her tail also regained some limited movement. Furthermore, the discomfort noted on her previous lumbar palpation appeared to be markedly reduced. However, 5 months after treatment had commenced the owners requested a repeat examination because they were concerned that she was uncomfortable again and the dog certainly had palpable lumbar pain. Repeat radiographs were obtained which showed progression of the vertebral metastasis, so the decision was made to have the dog euthanized.

Theory refresher
A review of anal sac carcinomas has been given in Chapter 10 so this will not be repeated here. Rather, the rationale for presenting this case was to illustrate how multimodal analgesia can work very well in some cases as short-term palliative care and generate an almost normal quality of life for the patient. The dog in this case was terminally ill and in pain, so it would not have been wrong to advise for her to be euthanized. However, it was decided that initially a 7-day course of medication should be administered to see how she was and, after the first week, it was obvious that there had been a clinical improvement, so the course was extended under very close supervision. The treatment restored her quality of life, albeit for a relatively short period of time.

Meloxicam is a COX-2 selective NSAID that has both human and veterinary licences as an anti-inflammatory analgesic and it is being investigated for possible anti-neoplastic actions, mainly against carcinomas. These were the reasons it was chosen in this case and it was very well tolerated. However, the use of meloxicam alone would probably not have been sufficient to control the discomfort in the initial stages of the disease, hence the rationale for prescribing Tramadol. Tramadol is a synthetic opioid μ-receptor agonist that also antagonizes monoamine and serotonin uptake and it is thought that it is the synergy of these actions that generates the potent analgesic action of this drug, because its efficacy at the μ-receptor is weak. It is not licensed for use in the dog but as there is no other licensed alternative, its use was justified under the cascade system. In human medicine it is used to treat moderate to severe pain and in particular, neuralgia, and as it was felt that there was a significant neurogenic component to the pain seen in this case, it appeared to be a logical choice. Doses of between 0.5–2.0 mg/kg twice a day have been recommended and it appears to be very well tolerated by dogs. In this particular case it was used for the first 4 weeks and then discontinued because the dog appeared so comfortable.

The potential usefulness of bisphosphonates in veterinary oncology was alluded to in Chapter 12. Bisphosphonates act by inhibiting osteoclasts and this inhibition allows the osteoblasts an opportunity to function without interference, thereby strengthening the existing bone and potentially allowing the creation of new bone. Increasing the strength of the existing bone is thought to help to decrease the risk of fractures, and stronger bone is less painful. In laboratory studies, bisphosphonates have also been shown to have a directly toxic effect on bone cancer cells which contributes to their death and that this action may mean that bisphosphonates have a future role in the inhibition of metastasis. There is also evidence that they can help to antagonize cancer growth by inhibiting angiogenesis within the tumour. Lastly, there is a small but growing body of evidence to suggest that there can be significant improvement in pain control when bisphosphonates are used. Further, large-scale veterinary studies are therefore required to try to establish firstly whether or not these results are reproducible and secondly, which form of bisphosphonate (oral or injectable) is most efficacious, but this class of drug holds promise as an adjunctive treatment in many different neoplastic conditions in the future.

CLINICAL CASE EXAMPLE 14.3 – SQUAMOUS CELL CARCINOMA OF THE DIGIT IN A COLLIE-CROSS

Signalment

7-year-old neutered female collie-cross.

Presenting signs

Two-week history of mild–moderate, progressive lameness affecting her left fore leg. The owner had also noticed that she was licking her left fore paw more than normal.

Case history

The relevant history in this case was:
- The dog did not have up-to-date vaccination status but had been recently wormed and had no travel history

- The dog was walked off-lead for approximately 1 hour every day and had no history of previous orthopaedic difficulties
- The dog had started to exhibit mild lameness in her left foreleg during her walks 2 weeks prior to presentation and she seemed less keen to run as far as normal
- The owner had also noticed that the dog had started to lick her left forepaw excessively. The owner thought she had a foreign body in the pad but on examination found an ulcerated area on one of the toes, so presented the dog for veterinary attention.

Clinical examination

- On examination the dog was bright, alert and in good body condition at 22 kg
- Cardiopulmonary auscultation and percussion were unremarkable as was abdominal palpation
- Orthopaedic examination confirmed the dog to be mild–moderately lame on the left fore leg but able to consistently bear weight. Saliva staining was also noticed on the hair from the carpus distally
- Digital examination revealed the presence of an ulcerated lesion on the ventro-medial aspect of digit five, which when clipped appeared erosive in nature (Figs 14.5, 14.6).

Diagnostic evaluation

- Due to the erosive and ulcerated appearance of the lesion, the presence of a tumour was strongly

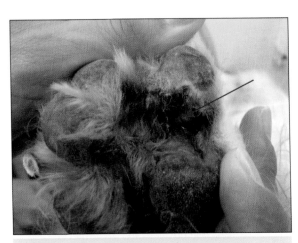

Figure 14.5 *Case 14.3* The initial appearance of the lesion, illustrating the ulcerated appearance and the matting of the hair with an exudate

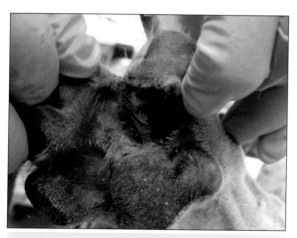

Figure 14.6 *Case 14.3* The appearance of the lesion once the hair was clipped, revealing the erosive appearance

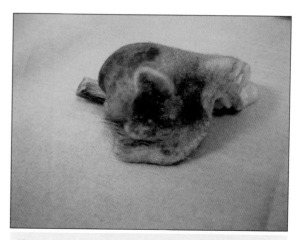

Figure 14.7 *Case 14.3* The digit was amputated by disarticulation at the carpometacarpal level

suspected. Impression smears were obtained but these were non-diagnostic

- The prescapular lymph node was carefully palpated and found not to be enlarged
- A dorsopalmar radiograph of the foot was obtained which showed no bony involvement or changes in P_5
- Left and right lateral inflated thoracic radiographs were unremarkable
- The dog was taken to surgery and the digit was amputated by disarticulation at the carpometacarpal level and the wound then closed routinely (Fig. 14.7).

Diagnosis

- The whole toe was sent for histopathological analysis which confirmed the tumour to be a squamous cell carcinoma.

Theory refresher

Digit tumours can develop on any part of the skin of the toe, but, unlike in this case, frequently arise from the nail bed epithelium, giving rise to subungual tumours. They are more commonly seen in older, larger-breed dogs but primary tumours in this location are considered to be rare in cats. In one study evaluating 124 different digital masses in dogs, 61% were malignant neoplasms, 20% were benign lesions and 19% were pyogranulomatous inflammation, so any mass or ulcerative lesion identified on a toe, especially if it appears to arise from the nail bed should be considered as a potential neoplastic growth and most likely a primary tumour. However, in cats, a tumour in this location is most likely to represent a metastatic lesion from tumours such as

bronchial adenocarcinoma (as illustrated by the case on page 68). Affected patients can present because a mass is visible, or with lameness, pedal discharge or haemorrhage or simply because they are licking the affected foot more frequently, meaning that a foreign body is a significant differential diagnosis to consider at initial presentation. Indeed, many digit tumours have secondary bacterial infection, therefore explaining why some cases are initially misdiagnosed as pedal dermatitis or paronychia, depending on the location of the lesion.

The most common tumour found on the digit of a dog is squamous cell carcinoma (SCC), followed by malignant melanoma, soft-tissue sarcoma and mast cell tumour. The concern regarding SCCs is that again, especially if they arise from the subungual epithelium, up to 80% will have invaded the underlying bone potentially causing bone lysis. This was not identified in the case illustrated here but good-quality dorsopalmar and lateral radiographs should always be obtained of a foot if a potentially neoplastic lesion is found on examination. As explained, SCC is frequently locally invasive but is generally considered to have a low metastatic potential at this site, especially if the tumour is a subungual one. The location of the tumour does appear to be important with regard to the behaviour of an SCC, as tumours that are not subungual in origin (as in the case illustrated here) appear to have higher rates of metastatic disease and lower survival times than when compared to dogs with subungual SCC. Careful examination of the draining lymph nodes must therefore always be undertaken and if they are found to be enlarged they should be aspirated. Unfortunately, melanoma of the digit is frequently malignant, so the clinician must always be alert to this risk at the initial examination and especially if such a diagnosis is confirmed.

The treatment of choice for digit tumours is amputation of the affected digit including disarticulation of the proximal digit joint and submission of all the tissue for histopathological assessment. Inflated left and right lateral radiographs must be obtained prior to any surgery because only 13% of dogs with SCC have pulmonary metastases but up to 32% of dogs with malignant melanoma will have developed metastatic disease at the time of diagnosis. At the time of writing no consistently efficacious adjunctive chemotherapy has been recommended but if a diagnosis of malignant melanoma is reached, then xenogenic DNA vaccine therapy is certainly worth undertaking, as discussed in Case 6.2, page 56.

The prognosis therefore can be very variable but the 1- and 2-year survival rates quoted in an American study showed that for subungual SCCs, 95% of dogs were alive after 1 year and up to 75% were alive at 2 years. This figure interestingly drops for digital SCC that is not subungal in nature, with figures of 60% and 44% for the 1- and 2-year survival times respectively. The prognosis for malignant melanoma is less favourable than SCC, as melanoma of the digit is reported to have a median survival time of 12 months, with the 1- and 2-year survival rates being reported as 42% and 13% respectively, when treated with surgery alone. Mast cell tumours (MCT) that are subungual in nature are usually high-grade tumours that behave aggressively but soft-tissue sarcomas (STS) of the digit have a much less aggressive nature compared to MCT and often good surgery for STS will generate potentially long-term survival times.

Outcome

The dog in this case made excellent progress and showed no signs of further disease before it was lost to follow up 18 months after the diagnosis.

15 The cancer patient with general lumps and bumps

A large number (if not the majority) of veterinary cancer patients present in general practice either because the owner has noticed a mass growing or because a mass is palpated by the veterinary surgeon during an examination. The variety of tumour types that are encountered in this way is significant, so it is very important that a logical and step-wise approach is taken in every case to ensure that a diagnosis is reached, if possible, before definitive surgery is attempted. If this is not undertaken for whatever reasons, making a definitive diagnosis post-surgery is essential. The general rule is that 'if a mass warrants removal, it warrants knowing what it is!' If the cost of histopathology really is a concern to the owner, at the very least the attending clinician should obtain representative tissue samples and store them in formalin for 2 years, so that if a mass recurs at or near the initial surgical site in the future, a diagnosis can hopefully still be reached before a second surgery is undertaken that may not be the most appropriate treatment when an adjunctive treatment may be better.

CLINICAL CASE EXAMPLE 15.1 – CUTANEOUS HISTIOCYTOMA IN A DOG

Signalment

6-month-old entire male boxer dog.

Presenting signs

A rapidly enlarging mass on the skin of his left cheek.

Case history

The relevant history in this case was:
- The dog had been fully vaccinated and wormed
- His owners reported him to be very well with no apparent abnormalities
- They had first noticed a small mass located on the skin on the surface of his left cheek. The mass was raised and reddened but did not seem to bother him

- The mass had doubled in size in 5 days, so he was brought to the vet.

Clinical examination

On examination he was very bright and alert. Dermatological examination revealed a firm, raised, reddened, dome-like lesion on the left cheek measuring 1.5 cm in diameter. The mass did not appear to be painful or to be causing him to be pruritic and there was no enlargement of the sub-mandibular lymph node (Fig. 15.1).

Diagnostic evaluation

A fine needle aspirate of the mass was obtained and this revealed clusters of medium-sized round cells (slightly larger than neutrophils) with an obvious pale blue cytoplasm and a low nuclear : cytoplasmic ratio, round to oval nuclei with a finely stippled chromatin pattern. Some nuclei contained nucleoli but this was not a consistent feature in all cells.

Diagnosis
- Cutaneous histiocytoma.

Treatment

In the light of the diagnosis and the potential for natural resolution, no further treatment was undertaken, but the dog was examined at 7-day intervals to ensure that there was not continual tumour growth. Although the tumour did grow a little more to approximately 2.0 cm in diameter, after 5 weeks the tumour appeared to be shrinking and within 2 further weeks the tumour had resolved completely.

Outcome

No further tumours were seen on the dog.

Theory refresher

Histiocytomas are benign tumours that are almost always seen on the skin of young dogs, especially between 1

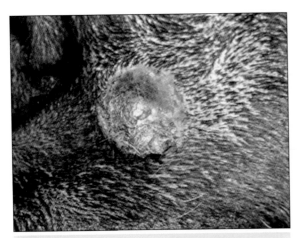

Figure 15.1 *Case 15.1* The appearance of the mass at initial presentation. Courtesy of Professor Dick White, Dick White Referrals

and 2 years of age, although they can develop at any point in a dog's life. In a recent UK survey of insured animals, canine cutaneous histiocytoma was the most common single tumour type reported, with a standardized incidence rate of 337 per 100 000 dogs per year. In other publications, histiocytomas account for approximately 12% of all skin tumours in the dog and are therefore considered to be common throughout the world but they are rarely seen in the cat. There appears to be no gender predisposition but Scottish terriers, boxers, dobermans, Labradors and cocker spaniels have been reported to have a higher incidence than other breeds. They usually present as solitary lesions, more commonly on the head and neck, but they can also very occasionally occur in multiple locations. They appear as raised, often erythematous, initially smooth, dome-like mass lesions that grow rapidly and they can become ulcerated. They are histologically fascinating, as under a microscope they often appear to a non-veterinary pathologist to be a high-grade, malignant neoplasm and yet they are benign and many, as in this case, will spontaneously regress. Fine needle aspiration therefore is always a sensible recommendation, as this is an easy cytological diagnosis and although many histiocytomas do require surgical excision, a large number can be treated conservatively without concern. If the mass is not ulcerated then recommending regular re-examination and no further treatment is usually best. However, if the mass becomes ulcerated, if the dog is troubled by the tumour, or if the cytology is uncertain then surgical excision is to be recommended. Surgical removal, when undertaken, is by simple cutaneous excision and routine closure. Cryosurgery has also been reported to give good results. The prognosis therefore for cutaneous histiocytomas is usually excellent.

Cutaneous histiocytosis is similar in some ways to histiocytoma, in that this condition is caused by collections of proliferating histiocytes resulting in the development of multiple nodules and plaques affecting the head and face, trunk and limbs and also possibly erythema, swelling and depigmentation of the nasal planum or nares. It too is seen in young dogs but a recent study suggested that the mean age of occurrence was 4 years of age (i.e. slightly older than the peak age of occurrence for cutaneous histiocytomas). Cutaneous histiocytosis is also a benign condition but it naturally regresses less commonly than cutaneous histiocytoma and so many cases require treatment in the form of immunosuppression, with prednisolone being the most commonly used first-line treatment and drugs such as azathioprine or cyclosporine being reserved for persistent cases. There is also evidence to suggest that a combination of tetracycline and niacinamide may be effective in some cases, along with vitamin E and essential fatty acid supplementation. Some dogs do require long-term treatment, and recurrence appears to be significantly more likely in dogs with nasal planum or nares lesions than dogs without lesions in these locations.

Systemic histiocytosis is a variant on cutaneous histiocytosis, in which aggregations of benign proliferating histiocytes occur resulting in dermatological lesions as previously described but in systemic histiocytosis there is systemic involvement with nodular lesions developing in internal organs. It is therefore considered that systemic histiocytosis and cutaneous histiocytosis represent two different clinical manifestations of similar reactive proliferative dermal dendritic cells with different predilection sites and as such they are often grouped together as 'reactive histiocytosis'. The reported target sites for systemic histiocytosis include the liver, the spleen, the lungs, lymph nodes, bone marrow and ocular tissues. Clinically the patients with this form of the disease are usually middle-aged and present with nodular or plaque-like skin lesions but with accompanying non-specific signs such as lethargy and inappetence. The clinical examination findings will vary depending on the organs affected. The diagnosis is made by histopathology. The clinical lesions can wax and wane but spontaneous recovery is not common, hence treatment with immuno suppressives is usually required. Interestingly, some studies suggest that the response of systemic histiocytosis to corticosteroids alone is variable but the response is more consistent using drugs such a cyclosporine and luflenomide.

Disseminated histiocytic sarcoma (previously known as malignant histiocytosis), is a serious malignant neoplasm which, despite the similarity in the name to the three conditions described above, has a significantly different presentation and prognosis. The disease was first reported in Bernese mountain dogs but there also appears to be breed predispositions in the flat-coated retriever and the rottweiler and it has been reported to occur in other breeds. The initial clinical presentation varies depending upon whether the disease is localized to one organ (solitary histiocytic sarcoma) or whether it has disseminated widely through the body (disseminated histiocytic sarcoma, or malignant histiocytosis), but in general the signs can be quite non-specific (e.g. lethargy, inappetance, weight loss, vomiting, diarrhoea or coughing). Clinical examination can reveal lymphadenopathy and organomegaly whilst clinical pathological testing can reveal anaemia (often regenerative in nature), thrombocytopaenia, elevations in hepatobiliary markers and hypoalbuminaemia. Diagnosis is based on histopathology (including on bone marrow biopsies). In the disseminated form of the disease, the condition can progress extremely rapidly and is invariably fatal, with mean survival times of approximately 3 months being reported. The response to chemotherapy is generally not good, although one report describes the use of Lomustine with some limited success. Solitary histiocytic sarcomas require surgical excision but the time to recurrence is often short and the prognosis guarded.

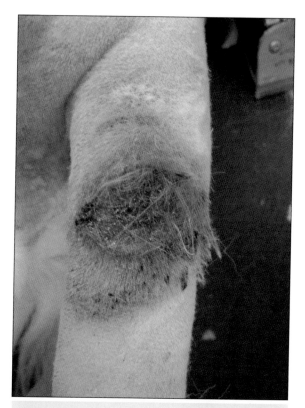

Figure 15.2 *Case 15.2* The appearance of the lesion at the base of the tail after it had been clipped

CLINICAL CASE EXAMPLE 15.2 – MAST CELL TUMOUR IN A DOG

Signalment

10-year-old neutered female golden retriever.

Presenting signs

A non-healing ulcer at the base of her tail.

Case history

The relevant history in this case was:
- Dog fully vaccinated
- She had had two grade II mast cell tumours removed from the lateral aspect of both her left and right thighs 3 years previously

- Otherwise she was a healthy dog with no other previous medical problems.

Clinical examination

The tail was clipped and cleaned to reveal a large, raised ulcerated lesion as shown in Figure 15.2. No other masses were palpable and no other abnormalities were noted.

Diagnostic evaluation

Fine needle aspirates and impression smears were obtained from the mass. These revealed large numbers of medium to large round cells with an obvious granular cytoplasm, the granules staining purple-red under Giemsa staining. The cells had large nuclei with obvious nucleoli. Some of the cells had fractured in the preparation and there were many granules obvious extracellularly.

Diagnosis

- Mast cell tumour.

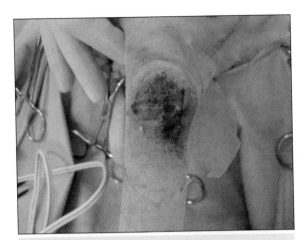

Figure 15.3 *Case 15.2* The use of a surgical marker pen to draw where the incisions will be to achieve a 2-cm lateral margin

Treatment

In the light of the location of the tumour, surgical excision was thought to be the most appropriate first-line treatment with a view to submitting the mass for histopathology for grading. The mass was excised with lateral margins of 2 cm and a deep margin of one fascial plane, as shown in Figures 15.3 and 15.4.

The deficit then required closure, which was achieved with a rotation flap, as shown in Figures 15.5–15.7. The reason a rotation flap was used is that this avoids tension at the surgical repair site which is especially important in an area of skin that is hard to immobilize. Attempting simple appositional closure at this site would have inevitably led to postoperative dehiscence and the need for more complicated reconstructive surgery.

Outcome

The histopathology returned to confirm the tumour to be a grade II mast cell tumour with complete surgical margins in all planes, so no further treatment was recommended.

Theory refresher

Mast cells are inflammatory leucocytes located within the dermis and subcutis that play an important role in allergic responses, wound healing and in acute and chronic inflammatory responses. As such, mast cells contain a number of different inflammatory mediators including histamine, heparin and the proteases tryptase and chymase which explains why some mast cell tumours

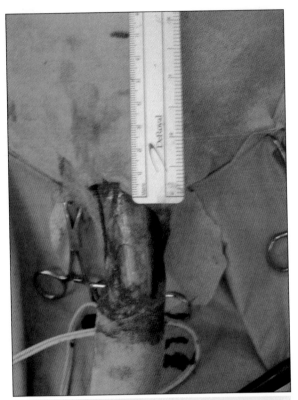

Figure 15.4 *Case 15.2* The tail after the mass has been excised as described and the surgeon is now measuring the size of the flap required to repair the deficit

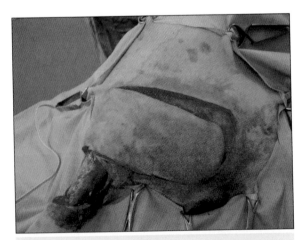

Figure 15.5 *Case 15.2* A skin flap the width of the deficit that requires closure is made utilizing skin from the lateral aspect of the right thigh

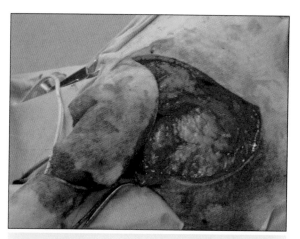

Figure 15.6 *Case 15.2* The skin flap is rotated into place to repair the tail wound and stapled routinely

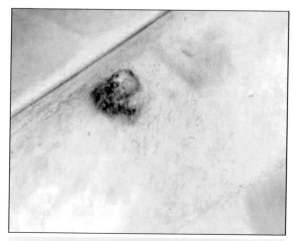

Figure 15.8 *Case 15.2* A small, well-demarcated skin lesion that was firm to touch. Fine needle aspiration revealed the mass to be mast cell tumour

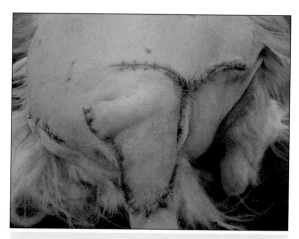

Figure 15.7 *Case 15.2* The deficit over the right thigh is then closed, making every effort to avoid wound tension

cause a local inflammatory reaction around themselves and also why there is the potential for mast cell tumours to cause paraneoplastic problems such as gastric ulceration via parietal cell stimulation. Mast cell tumours (MCT) are common, being cited as the most frequently diagnosed cutaneous tumour of the dog and the second most frequently diagnosed cutaneous tumour in cats. In dogs, MCTs account for approximately 20% of all cutaneous tumours and there is a predilection for the disease in some breeds, such as boxers, bulldogs, Staffordshire bull terriers, Boston terriers, Rhodesian ridgebacks, pugs, weimaraners, Labrador retrievers, beagles and golden retrievers, thereby implying a

genetic component to the aetiology of the disease. In cats, the Siamese seems over-represented in the incidence reports.

MCTs are a heterogeneous group of lesions, in that they have a variety of different presentations and that their behaviour can vary markedly from animal to animal and also from tumour to tumour. They can look like a well-circumscribed nodule that may or may not be erythematous or alopecic (Fig. 15.8). They can also arise from lesions that have been present for significantly long periods of time, initially appearing like a mass which should cause no concern for many months or even years. In addition, as well as solid cutaneous masses, MCTs can also present as soft, fluctuant subcutaneous lesions that may be initially misdiagnosed on palpation as a lipoma (Fig. 15.9). More aggressive MCTs, however, can develop rapidly into large, ulcerated, exudative lesions which may cause considerable morbidity for the patient.

It is primarily because of this variation in appearance and the propensity of MCTs to mimic the appearance of other different cutaneous tumours that the authors have to recommend that all cutaneous masses undergo fine needle aspiration prior to any surgical excision being attempted. This argument is made stronger by the fact that mast cells are usually easily identified by cytology; MCTs often exfoliate large numbers of individual round cells that have round nuclei which often seem pale in appearance compared to the cytoplasm. The cytoplasm itself usually contains large numbers of granules that stain purple-red when using a Wright-Giemsa

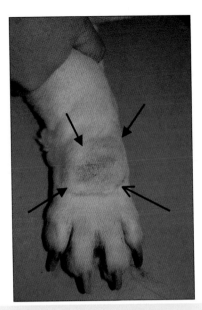

Figure 15.9 A soft, fluctuant swelling on the carpus of a 2-year-old English bull terrier, fine needle aspiration of which revealed the mass to be a mast cell tumour. The dog was treated with 7 days of prednisolone to reduce the size of the mass and then taken to surgery for excision. However, at surgery it was not possible to remove the entire tumour despite the cytoreductive steroidal therapy. Histopathology was suggestive of an intermediate grade tumour so postoperatively he was treated with hypofractionated external beam radiotherapy

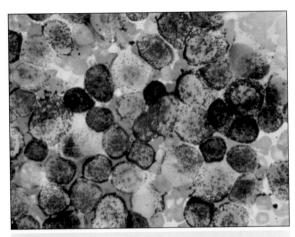

Figure 15.10 A fine needle aspirate from a high-grade mast cell tumour, illustrating the individual round cells and their highly granular cytoplasm with the magenta coloured granules characteristic of mast cells. Preparation stained with Wright-Giemsa stain and viewed at ×100 magnification. Courtesy of Mrs Elizabeth Villiers, Dick White Referrals

preparation and frequently the cells will have granules scattered in the space around them from other mast cells that were shattered in the process of obtaining the aspirate and forming the smears (see Fig. 15.10). Diff-Quick can be used and will also usually show the presence of the granules but sometimes Diff-Quick will not reveal the presence of the granules as well as a Giemsa stain, so it is recommended that Romanowski stains are used for this cytology whenever possible.

The one drawback of cytology is that it cannot accurately determine the grade of the tumour, so this is a useful technique simply to identify the tumour preoperatively. Tumour grading can only be done by histopathology and generates three possible outcomes; grade I (well differentiated), grade II (intermediately differentiated) and grade III (poorly differentiated). Tumour grading is important, as it is the strongest indicator yet available as to the tumour's behaviour; the median survival times of dogs with grades I and II tumours were reported to be in excess of 1300 days in one study in comparison with 278 days for dogs with grade III tumours.

Once a MCT has been identified, all thoughts turn to treatment but it is important to remember that all MCTs have a metastatic potential and that whilst some will be essentially benign, some will be highly malignant and most fall somewhere between these two extremes. There is also some variation in behaviour between breeds; although boxers, bulldogs and pugs are very prone to developing MCTs they frequently behave less aggressively in these breeds. Overall, however, there have been many studies assessing the behaviour of MCTs and their response to treatment to establish the optimal way to approach this disease. One clear principle emerges: the best first-line treatment for MCTs is surgical excision if at all possible. Although there are difficulties and inconsistencies, both with the histological grading systems that are generally utilized and between different pathologists, it appears that well-differentiated tumours (grade I) are best managed by local excision alone and intermediately differentiated tumours (grade II) should be managed by local excision with 2-cm lateral margins and a deep margin of one facial plane. Whilst poorly differentiated, grade III tumours still require surgery as a first-line treatment, adjunctive therapy should usually be considered postoperatively but which adjunctive treatment to use is also subject to debate. The concern with grade III MCTs is that they have a higher metastasis rate and lower survival times after surgery alone when compared to dogs with grade I or II tumours so further treatment is sensible to help remove any metastasizing cells or secondary tumours. The problem comes in that no large scale studies have been published to indicate which is the most effective chemotherapeutic approach to take in these cases. However, there are three approaches the medical author (RF) usually uses in cases that require chemotherapy:

1. Combined prednisolone and vinblastine treatment (see Appendix 2). This has been reported to generate a clinical response rate of 47%, with 33% seeing a complete remission when used in dogs with gross disease. The median response duration has been quoted as 154 days (range 24–645). However, this study was only on 15 dogs so it is difficult to take these figures too literally. When used postoperatively, the reported success rates in a study containing 61 dogs are higher, with an overall survival time of 1374 days being reported.
2. Combined chlorambucil and prednisolone treatment (see Appendix 2). This is a very recently published approach and it appeals because both of the medications used are given per os and therefore require no hospital treatment. The combination is also usually very well tolerated. In a study of 21 dogs with inoperable MCTs there was a 38% overall response rate (complete remission in 14%), a median progression free interval for the responders of 533 days and median survival time for all dogs in the study of 140 days. No toxicities were detected in any of the dogs in the study
3. Lomustine (CCNU). This has been reported to have been effective in a study of 19 dogs with MCT, eight of which (42%) showed a measurable response for a mean duration of 109 days (range 21–254 days).

A fourth, new approach lies in the recent development of the tyrosine kinase inhibitor, masitinib, for veterinary medicine. Tyrosine kinase is known to play a critical role in the development of canine MCT and masitinib blocks the KIT receptor on this enzyme and has now been shown to be safe and effective in delaying tumour progression in dogs with non-resectable grade II or III tumours.

In general therefore, the authors will recommend chemotherapy for all cases with grade III tumours or possibly as palliative treatment for cases with non-resectable grade II tumours and would utilize masitinib first, then either prednisolone and vinblastine, or chlorambucil and prednisolone, depending on the individual animal's situation, and reserve Lomustine for cases that do not respond to either of the first three options.

Radiotherapy has also been cited as a useful treatment in canine MCT and has generally been reported as adjunctive therapy to incompletely excised grade II tumours, with up to 97% 1-year survival rates being reported. It can also be useful as a cytoreductive treatment to be used before surgery in very large tumours or those that may prove to be difficult to resect, using the radiation to shrink the tumour mass to facilitate easier or more complete excision. However, there is a concern that irradiating the large number of mast cells present in a gross tumour mass may precipitate substantial histamine release resulting in paraneoplastic problems such as gastro-duodenal ulceration and more concerningly, a hypotensive crisis. Therefore it is usual for up to 14 days of prednisolone +/- vinblastine to be given before the radiotherapy to help prevent these difficulties.

The use of deionized water to treat incompletely excised tumours has been reported in the literature, based on the rationale that mast cells are highly sensitive to hypotonic shock. Its usefulness is still unclear, as although after the initial reports of the technique were encouraging, one study showed it generated no benefits at all. However, a more recent study in The Netherlands suggested it may be an efficacious technique, so further work is required to clarify whether this technique has any merit. However, at this time the authors do not recommend its use.

The clinical approach to MCT cases, therefore, must be to firstly make an accurate diagnosis using cytology whenever possible and the authors highly recommend undertaking fine needle aspirates of any cutaneous mass before considering surgical excision in an attempt to establish the diagnosis. Once this has been done, the draining lymph nodes must be carefully palpated and if enlarged, they must be aspirated too. Abdominal ultrasound should be undertaken, as if there is a malignant potential for the tumour then secondary disease in the abdominal lymph nodes, liver or spleen is possible and this should be assessed before the primary tumour is excised. Pulmonary metastasis with MCTs is very unusual but thoracic radiographs should be considered as well. If there are considerable cost restrictions, as the majority of cases will be grade I and II with a lower metastatic potential than a grade III tumour, it is not unreasonable to simply undertake a good surgical excision once the aspirates have confirmed the mass to be an MCT (2-cm lateral margins and one fascial plane deep if possible) and submit the tissue for histopathology. The exceptions to this are MCTs found on the subungual area (the nail bed) and on mucocutaneous junctions, as tumours in these regions frequently behave aggressively and full staging before surgery is necessary. If after the histopathology the tumour is shown to be grade III, then postoperative staging is also essential.

Examination of the buffy coat is not considered necessary by the authors in canine cases, as systemic mastocytosis is rare in the dog and therefore this test is rarely of diagnostic use unless a complete blood count indicates bone marrow pathology. Likewise, MCT metastasis to the lungs is unusual, so thoracic radiographs should only be considered if there is evidence suggestive of pulmonary disease on the clinical examination (i.e. tachypnoea, dyspnoea, cyanosis despite normal lung sounds, coughing, dull areas on thoracic percussion, etc.).

Although currently the histological grade is the strongest predictor of MCT behaviour, there are some newer tests that are likely to become more commonplace to help assess how aggressive an MCT may be. Ki-67 is an antigen expressed during the cell cycle and appears to be strongly associated with the prognosis of MCTs in a manner that is independent of the histological grade. The immunohistochemical quantification of Ki-67 is an important tool in our assessment of MCTs and is worth requesting to be assessed in cases where either the pathologist is unable to be certain as to the grading, or if there is a clinical suspicion that the tumour may be behaving aggressively (e.g. rapid development of lesion, location on a mucocutaneous junction). Likewise, KIT is a stem cell factor receptor that activates tyrosine kinase usually located on the cell membrane but many MCTs express the receptor within the cytoplasm, indicating a mutation in the proto-oncogene *c-kit* which encodes for KIT. Assessment for aberrant cytoplasmic KIT may also be a helpful marker to predict MCT behaviour.

A common problem following MCT excision is to find that the tumour was a grade II but that the margins are dirty. In this situation there are three main options:

1. Surgical excision of the original scar if possible, again attempting to obtain 2 cm margins laterally and one fascial plane deep
2. External beam radiotherapy. This is a highly effective treatment against MCTs as mentioned earlier and postoperative irradiation of the surgical site (once healed) is probably very useful in cases with dirty margins, especially on distal limbs where there may be inadequate soft tissue and skin present to facilitate a good reconstruction following a second surgery

3. Careful monitoring with no further treatment. Many cases of grade II tumours with dirty margins do not recur despite the apparently non-curative surgery. This option is not ideal and probably should only be reserved for cases for which referral for radiotherapy and an oncology specialist's opinion is not an option. However, this is an option that is frequently utilized without a problem and in such cases, the patient should be carefully examined at least once every 4 weeks for 1 year. Any recurrence of a mass lesion should be aspirated as soon as possible to assess for the presence of mast cells.

Multiple MCTs produce a unique challenge, as traditionally, dogs with multiple MCTs are classified as having advanced disease because, by the WHO assessment, they have stage III disease (as if they had gross metastases). However, this does not appear to be clinically accurate, as each tumour needs to be assessed individually and in this situation the WHO grading system is not useful. Dogs with multiple MCTs do justify careful clinical staging with lymph node palpation and aspiration if appropriate, abdominal ultrasound and thoracic radiography before surgical excision and submission of all the tumours for grading. The treatment that needs to be undertaken is surgical excision of all the lesions individually if at all possible. If all the tumours are grade I or II and the surgery was carried out well, then the authors would not routinely recommend adjunctive therapy in these cases.

FELINE MAST CELL TUMOURS

Feline mast cell tumours are not common tumours in cats in the UK, although interestingly they are recognized as the second most common cutaneous tumour of cats in the USA. In the cutaneous form they are most commonly found on the head or neck and usually present as papular or nodular lesions that may be hairy, alopecic or have an ulcerated surface. The key issue in cats is that there are two main types of MCT in this species, namely cutaneous MCTs and visceral MCTs.

Cutaneous MCT is the more common presentation, and in cats two different sub-types of this tumour are reported:

1. Mastocytic MCTs, which have a histological appearance similar to that of canine MCTs
2. Histiocytic MCTs, which have an appearance more consistent with a histiocytic mast cell.

The majority of cats with cutaneous MCT develop the mastocytic variety and in particular, a subtype known as 'compact mastocytic MCT'. These tumours generally behave in a relatively benign manner, growing locally but showing little metastatic potential. There is a second subtype of mastocytic MCTs called a 'diffuse mastocytic MCT' and these tumours do show relatively more aggressive behaviour with an increased likelihood of local recurrence following excision and an increased risk of causing metastatic disease. However, pleasingly, they are not as common as the compact mastocytic form (accounting for up to only approximately 15% of cases of mastocytic MCTs). Histiocytic cutaneous MCTs are generally considered to exhibit benign behaviour with many being reported to spontaneously regress, although this can take up to 2 years. Histiocytic MCTs occur most frequently in young cats (less than 4 years old). Siamese cats may be pre-disposed to this form, whilst the more common mastocytic form is most commonly seen in middle-aged animals (average age of 9 years old) with no breed or gender predilection. The mastocytic MCTs usually present as solitary, firm, round, well-circumscribed, variably sized masses (0.5–3.0 cm in diameter) that are dermoepidermal or subcutaneous in origin, whereas the histiocytic MCTs usually present as multiple, raised, firm, round, well-demarcated papules and nodules that are generally small (0.2–1.0 cm in diameter). It is important to note that it is also possible to see multiple mastocytic MCTs, so the presence of multiple lesions does not necessarily imply a diagnosis of the histiocytic form of the disease.

The second main form of MCT in cats is the visceral form, in which the MCT affects the spleen or the intestines as the primary tumour site with secondary metastases developing from this. This form is much more common in cats than it is in dogs, with approximately 20% of all feline MCTs being splenic in origin. Visceral MCT has a much higher metastatic potential than the cutaneous form and of these, the intestinal form of feline MCT is the most aggressive, with metastasis to the local lymph nodes and liver often occurring with metastasis to the spleen and less commonly the lungs, also recorded. Patients with the visceral form usually present for investigation of non-specific signs of illness, such as weight loss and lethargy. Cats with the splenic form often present with vomiting and anorexia, due to the development of gastroduodenal ulceration as a result of the release of histamine into the circulation causing hypergastrinaemia. Cats with intestinal MCT vomit much less frequently than cats with the splenic form and this is thought to be due to a lack of histamine granules in the cells in this form of the disease.

The diagnostic approach to a cutaneous mass that may be an MCT in a cat, therefore, is similar to that described previously for the dog, namely firstly to undertake a detailed clinical examination to establish whether or not there is any evidence of local lymph node enlargement or other systemic disease. The primary mass then should be aspirated for cytological evaluation, as should any enlarged local lymph node. If a solitary mass is confirmed as an MCT, then the treatment recommendation is to excise the mass if possible but as the tumours are frequently relatively benign, it does not seem to be as important to achieve large margins in cats as compared to dogs. The excised tissue must be sent for histopathology to confirm the diagnosis and also if possible identify the subtype of the tumour as detailed earlier, as this will have a significant prognostic significance. If the tumour is confirmed as a histiocytic MCT, then usually no further action is required, as such a lesion may have spontaneously regressed anyway. If a compact mastocytic tumour is diagnosed, as these tumours are also frequently benign no further treatment is required but a note of caution must be sounded, as some of these cases will recur and it is not possible to view these as tumours without any metastatic potential at all, as a small number will develop distant disease. Further evaluation in terms of a staging evaluation and regular re-examinations, whilst not essential, could be considered as good practice. If a diffuse mastocytic tumour is diagnosed, then there is a risk of recurrence and/or distant metastasis in approximately 20–30% of cases. If full diagnostic staging was not undertaken in the preoperative assessment with abdominal ultrasound and thoracic radiographs, this should be completed once the diagnosis has been made. Regular repeat examinations for at least 12 months following the surgery are also to be recommended in this situation. Recurrence should be treated with further surgical excision if the recurrence is simply cutaneous but tumour recurrence is usually associated with a poorer prognosis due to the increased risk of metastatic disease developing.

When a patient presents with a suspected visceral MCT, the diagnosis is still relatively easy to obtain. A detailed abdominal ultrasound will be required, but aspiration of an intestinal or splenic mass is possible and advisable. A middle-aged to older, vomiting or inappetant cat presenting with obvious splenomegaly that appears heterogeneous on ultrasound is highly suspicious for a splenic tumour, so aspiration may not be necessary as splenectomy is indicated anyway. If surgery is planned, it is highly advisable to undertake a detailed abdominal ultrasound pre-operatively to assess for metastatic disease within the draining lymphatics (the mesenteric nodes, or the gastrosplenic nodes depending on the site of the primary tumour) and the liver and also to undertake left and right lateral inflated thoracic radiographs. It has been estimated that up to 30% of cats with splenic MCT will have either peritoneal or pleural effusions, so if identified these need to be aspirated and assessed for malignancy before surgery is performed. Cats with intestinal MCT can usually be considered to have a poor prognosis, due to the high incidence of metastatic disease but if there are no metastatic lesions found then undertaking excision is still recommended. Surgery must aim to remove at least 5 cm of intestine either side of the tumour, as it has been shown that the tumour frequently extends beyond the visible margins.

Cats with a splenic MCT should undergo splenectomy as there are reports of extended survivals following surgery of up to 18 months even when there is bone marrow involvement. However, these cases obviously warrant a cautious to guarded prognosis to be given and compared to the cutaneous form of MCT the survival times are reduced. Between 30 and 50% of cats with visceral MCT have been shown to have bone marrow involvement resulting in a circulating mastocytosis, so unlike in dogs, it is worth considering buffy coat assessment in cats with this form of the disease. This does not always resolve after excision of the primary mass and the presence of mast cells in the buffy coat does not necessarily change the treatment required, but it would help to make the decision as to whether adjunctive treatment should be considered or not and for some owners, whether the initial surgery should actually be performed. However, the authors would generally still recommend surgery for these cases unless the animal is obviously unwell.

CLINICAL TIP

If a cat presents with vomiting and is suspected to have a splenic MCT, an H_2 antagonist such as cimetidine or ranitidine should be given before surgery to help reduce the effect of any histamine release as a result of the splenic manipulation at surgery. Continuing this treatment postoperatively is also sensible, especially if the patient continues to vomit or has poor appetite, to help reduce the risk of gastroduodenal ulceration developing.

Table 15.1 Staging system for feline mast cell tumours

Tumour stage	Criteria for tumour stage
1	One dermal tumour with no spread to regional lymph nodes
2	One dermal tumour with spread to regional lymph node
3	Multiple dermal tumours or large infiltrating tumours with regional lymph node involvement
4	Any tumour with distant metastasis or recurrence with metastasis
Substage a	Stage x with no evidence of systemic disease
Substage b	Stage x with evidence of systemic disease

In the largest study of feline MCTs, the following staging system was used and this is clinically useful as it helps give prognostic information (Table 15.1).

In this study, no figures were available for survival times with stage 1 or 2 disease because more than half the cats were alive at the time of the study being written. However, for cats with stage 3 disease the median survival time was 582 days (range 3–994) and for stage 4 it was 283 days (range 1–375). These figures confirm the broad theory that cats with MCT have a variable prognosis but that solitary cutaneous feline MCTs without spread to the local lymphatics usually manifest as benign disease with a relatively protracted course. However, multiple cutaneous tumours, recurrent tumours and primary splenic or lymph node disease should receive a guarded prognosis due to the relatively short median survival times associated with these forms of the disease.

The role of chemotherapy in feline MCT has not been completely clarified. There is anecdotal evidence that some cases will respond to prednisolone but clear consensus as to whether or not there is a consistent response to this has not been established. However, a recent report has shown that Lomustine (CCNU) given at approximately 50 mg/m² in a variety of different stages of feline MCT produced complete remission in 18% of cases and partial remission in 31% of cases with a median response duration of 168 days (with a range of 25–727 days). The authors therefore certainly would consider adjunctive therapy using Lomustine at the above dosage at 4–6-weekly intervals, and/or prednisolone for cases in which local excision is not possible, or in patients in whom there is metastatic disease that cannot be treated surgically. If this treatment is used, either as a sole treatment or as adjunctive therapy following surgery, clear explanation to the owners that the prognosis is uncertain is very important. The main dose limiting toxicities of Lomustine in cats are neutropaenia and thrombocytopaenia, so careful haematological monitoring is required and a complete blood count must be undertaken prior to each dose.

CLINICAL CASE EXAMPLE 15.3 – MAMMARY CARCINOMA IN A FEMALE DOG

Signalment

10-year-old entire female Bassett hound.

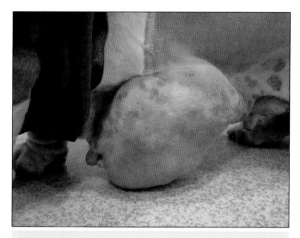

Figure 15.11 *Case 15.3* The appearance of the mass at initial presentation

Presenting signs

A rapidly growing mass affecting her second mammary gland on the left-hand side.

Case history

The relevant case history in this case was:
- The dog was fully vaccinated, wormed and had not travelled outside the UK
- History of recurrent otitis externa, thought to be due to atopy but no full investigation had been undertaken in this regard
- The owner noticed a mass during regular examination at home. Initially the mass was felt to be approximately 2 cm in diameter, firm but movable and located underneath the skin
- Over the following 12 weeks the mass grew such that it was starting to touch the floor and cause the dog ambulatory inconvenience, so referral advice was sought.

Clinical examination

- On examination the dog was quiet and not particularly co-operative. However, she allowed palpation of the mass without any apparent signs of discomfort. The mass now measured 15 cm in diameter (Fig. 15.11). The mass was firm to touch and somewhat irregular in outline. There were no skin abrasions and there was no discharge from the associated nipple
- Cardiopulmonary auscultation was unremarkable
- Abdominal palpation was unremarkable
- Careful palpation of the axillary lymph node failed to reveal any enlargement of this structure.

Diagnostic evaluation

- In the light of the size of the mass and the rapidity of its development, it was felt this was very highly likely to be a mammary tumour. Left and right lateral inflated thoracic radiographs were obtained which revealed no evidence of metastatic disease
- Abdominal ultrasound was undertaken to assess in particular the inguinal lymph nodes, the liver and the spleen; these were all normal.

Diagnosis

- These findings are highly suggestive of the mass being a mammary carcinoma, stage III.

Treatment

- In the light of the negative findings on the staging investigation, the dog was taken to surgery and underwent a regional mastectomy, during which glands 1, 2 and 3 on the left-hand side were all excised 'en-bloc'
- Active suction drains were used to reduce the risk of fluid accumulation following the excision of such a large mass. However, the postoperative recovery of the dog was good and she was discharged 3 days later.

Outcome

- The histopathology confirmed the mass to be a high-grade complex carcinoma. The owners declined any adjunctive treatment and the dog remained well for 8 months and at the time of writing is still well.

Theory refresher

Mammary tumours are one of the most common tumour types encountered in clinical practice and the most common tumour that develops in female dogs. A survey of insured dogs in the UK reported a standardized incidence of 205 cases per 100 000 dogs whilst a survey from Sweden (where routine ovariohysterectomy is less commonplace compared to the UK) revealed a much higher incidence at 111 cases per 10 000 dogs. This Swedish study is interesting, as it is now accepted that the hormone environment in the bitch plays a significant role in the initial development of mammary tumours and progesterone is known to induce tumour development in dogs (by several mechanisms, including up regulating growth hormone concentrations in the mammary gland tissue). Mammary tumours in male dogs are rare (and usually benign when they do develop) and there is a significant reduction in the occurrence of mammary tumours in neutered bitches compared to the incidence in dogs left entire. A study in the late 1960s showed that compared to entire bitches, the risk of a bitch developing malignant mammary neoplasia if she was spayed before her first oestrous, was 0.05%. Spaying before the second oestrous was associated with a risk of 8% and the risk rises to 26% if they are spayed after their second season. Spaying a bitch in later life does not seem to affect the incidence of malignant mammary tumours developing but it probably does result in a reduction in the risk of benign tumours developing. Mammary tumours also show increased incidence with increasing age; the average age of mammary tumour development is 10 years old, it is a rare disease in dogs less than 4 years old and the incidence rises with increasing age. Spaying bitches before their first or second season therefore definitely confers significant protection for the future development of mammary neoplasia in later life but there are obviously other factors that need to be considered when discussing whether or not to neuter a dog and the possible benefits with regard to mammary cancer cannot be used on its own in this regard.

Other factors that have been shown to influence the development of mammary neoplasia include obesity in the first year of life and also somewhat unexpectedly, the feeding of a home-cooked diet as opposed to a commercially available one. Both of these increase the risk of developing the disease.

Approximately half of all canine mammary masses will be malignant and of these, approximately 50% will have metastasized at the time of diagnosis. The most frequently diagnosed tumours are of epithelial origin (i.e.: carcinomas). Histologically, these tumours can then be subdivided into several different subtypes and there is a World Health Organization classification system which groups the tumours by descriptive morphology. The carcinomas are divided into non-infiltrating carcinomas, complex carcinomas and simple carcinomas (of which there are three types; tubulopapillary carcinoma, solid carcinoma and anaplastic carcinoma) and this reflects increasing malignant potential respectively. The only flaw in this classification system is that it does not describe 'ductular carcinoma', a term frequently used by many pathologists. There is also a separate classification for so-called 'inflammatory carcinomas', which are poorly differentiated tumours that grow rapidly and present with obvious cutaneous inflammation and oedema. Inflammatory carcinomas have a high metastatic rate and a poor prognosis (Fig. 15.12).

Mammary tumours generally develop in older dogs as already outlined. They can be single or multiple in nature and approximately two-thirds of tumours will develop in the two most caudal mammary glands (i.e. glands 4 and 5), but tumours in these glands do not have any different behavioural characteristics compared to tumours in glands 1, 2 or 3. This anatomical propensity of mammary tumours to develop in glands 4 and 5 is thought to be due simply to the larger volume of mammary tissue in these two glands. Tumours can be associated with the nipple but are more commonly located within the mammary tissue itself. Benign tumours are generally

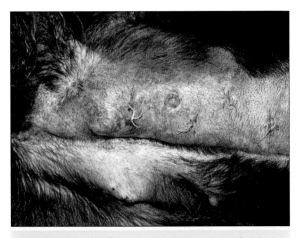

Figure 15.12 An inflammatory carcinoma in a Labrador bitch, showing breakdown at the biopsy site and the cutaneous inflammation characteristic of this tumour type. Courtesy of Professor Dick White, Dick White Referrals

Table 15.2 TNM classification for mammary tumours

T1	Tumour up to 3 cm in diameter
T2	Tumour between 3–5 cm in diameter
T3	Tumour greater than 5 cm in diameter
N0	No lymph node metastasis detected either by cytology or histology
N1	Lymph node metastasis detected either by cytology or histology
M0	No distant metastasis detected
M1	Distant metastasis detected

Table 15.3 Five different stages of disease, identified from the TNM classification for mammary tumours

Stage I	T1N0M0
Stage II	T2N0M0
Stage III	T3N0M0
Stage IV	AnyTN1M0
Stage V	AnyTN1M1

small and appear to be well circumscribed but all mammary masses should be viewed with suspicion as possible malignancies and therefore investigated as soon as possible. Once a mass has been palpated, the initial diagnosis of mammary neoplasia may be made with fine needle aspirates and a recent Brazilian study indicated that cytology is accurate in this regard in up to 92% of cases. However, cytology will not be able to accurately subtype the tumour so histopathology will still be required and surgical excision is the first-line treatment for canine mammary neoplasia. It is therefore reasonable to omit fine needle aspiration in the diagnostic evaluation procedure, as knowledge of the tumour type is realistically not going to change the clinical approach, which is to surgically remove the mass. Before surgery is undertaken, however, clinical staging to establish the extent of the disease is essential and use of the TNM system provides both a logical framework to base the staging investigation on and also important prognostic information. The TNM classification for mammary tumours comes from the World Health Organization publication of 1980 and gives the divisions shown in Table 15.2.

From this, five different stages of disease can then be established (Table 15.3).

To establish the clinical stage therefore, any dogs with mammary lumps or bumps should undergo a thorough and detailed clinical examination, taking care to palpate all of the mammary tissue and also the draining lymph nodes if possible. It is also important to assess the dog for any evidence of respiratory compromise which could indicate pulmonary metastasis or hind limb oedema, which may indicate lymphatic enlargement due to tumour spread. Although there is lymphatic communication between all the glands, thereby making the drainage complicated, in general, glands 1 and 2 drain cranially into the axillary lymph node whilst glands 4 and 5 drain caudally into the superficial inguinal lymph node. Gland 3 can drain both cranially and caudally. The axillary lymph nodes are usually easily palpable when enlarged but in overweight dogs the superficial inguinal node may not be easily apparent, so sometimes ultrasound can be useful or required to assess this structure and also to facilitate fine needle aspiration. Abdominal ultrasound will be required to assess the inguinal and sub-lumbar lymph nodes along with the mesenteric nodes, liver and spleen for the presence of metastatic disease. Good-quality, inflated thoracic radiographs (left and right laterals as a minimum) are also to be recommended before undertaking surgical excision of any mass to ensure that there are no gross pulmonary metastases.

Once the clinical stage of the disease has been established the decision can be made whether or not the dog should/can undergo surgical excision of the primary tumour with or without the draining lymph nodes if found to be enlarged but unless there is obvious metastatic disease, surgical removal of the tumour is the treatment of choice. If distant metastases are diagnosed, then in the light of the poor survival times it is often appropriate to decline excision of the primary tumour(s). However, if no distant metastases are found, which surgical procedure to undertake to remove the primary tumour is a matter of debate. Despite its popularity in general practice, studies have shown that undertaking a complete mastectomy (a so-called 'mammary strip') for single lesions does not generate any improvement in outcome when compared to simple, local mastectomy. It is therefore most reasonable to suggest the following approaches:

1. If the mass is less than 1 cm in diameter, firm and not adherent to the underlying structures (i.e. most likely to be benign), then a simple local 'lumpectomy' should be performed using blunt dissection to remove the abnormal tissue through a simple skin incision. If the histopathology reveals the mass to be malignant, then further more extensive surgery can be performed as detailed below.

2. If the mass is larger than 1 cm but located relatively centrally within one gland and/or feels fixed, then that gland should be removed entirely. This is known as 'mammectomy'. The surgeon should make an eliptical incision around the gland leaving at least 2 cm margins around the mass, before removing all of the skin, subcutis, glandular tissue and any adherent subcutis.

3. Another approach to masses larger than 1 cm or for those that feel fixed is to undertake a 'regional mastectomy'. In this procedure the glands are grouped together and removed according to their lymphatic drainage, so that glands 1, 2 and 3 are removed together and glands 4 and 5 are removed together, should a mass be present in any of them individually. If adjacent glands develop tumours at the same time, regional mastectomy is the treatment of choice. The surgical procedure is as for a mammectomy except that the incisions extend over the whole length of the tissue to be excised. If gland 5 is to be removed, then it is recommended that the superficial inguinal lymph node be removed at the same time due to its close association with the mammary tissue.

4. If multiple masses are present, then removing all of the mammary tissue on one side may be indicated in a regional mastectomy (often termed a 'mammary strip'). To do this, the superficial caudal epigastric artery and vein must be identified and ligated, but otherwise the procedure is as described above. In the light of the length of the incision, care should be taken to minimize blood loss using electrocautery and closure must be tension free to help reduce the risk of dehiscence. Although unilateral or bilateral mastectomies are frequently performed in practice, as previously explained there have not been any studies that have shown that this radical surgery offers any increase in survival times compared to regional mastectomy, hence the reason for recommending this procedure only when it is truly necessary.

The question of whether or not to neuter an entire female dog at the time of removing a mammary tumour remains somewhat unanswered. There are a few studies that suggest that ovariohysterectomy does improve recurrence rates and survival times but there are more studies that suggest that ovariohysterectomy at the time of mammary tumour removal does not improve the outcome for the dogs at all in terms of disease-free periods, recurrence rates or survival times. Therefore on balance, currently the literature suggests that neutering does not appear to significantly improve the prognosis for the dogs with regard to their cancer. It is, however, clear that ovariohysterectomy at an early age does have a protective effect, as discussed previously. If it is decided by the surgeon that neutering the dog at the same time as removing a mammary tumour would be beneficial for other reasons (e.g. to remove the risk of the dog developing pyometra), then the ovariohysterectomy should be performed before the mammectomy/mastectomy procedure and the skin and abdominal incisions made for the neutering procedure must be positioned and performed carefully so as to avoid contaminating the laparotomy with tumour cells from the mammary glands.

If malignant mammary cancer is confirmed by the histopathology, thoughts turn to adjunctive treatments, especially when there are now several well publicized medical treatments available in human medicine. The problem in veterinary medicine is that no clearly efficaceous treatments have been described. A small case series of 16 dogs in Greece with stage III or stage IV disease has been published, in which eight of the dogs were treated with regional mastectomy surgery alone and eight were given cyclophosphamide (100 mg/m^2) and 5-fluorouracil (150 mg/m^2) once a week for 4 consecutive weeks following the same surgical procedure. The dogs in the surgery group had a disease-free period of 2 months and a median survival time of 6 months compared to the chemotherapy-treated group who were all alive at 2 years postsurgery. Although a small study, these results are encouraging and suggest that there may be a role for adjunctive chemotherapy but much more work is required to establish if such results are consistent. Likewise, electrochemotherapy using cisplatin has produced encouraging results in a study of seven dogs with a variety of different neoplasms including mammary carcinoma, so this may prove to be a useful tool in the future but more studies are required to prove consistent efficacy in canine mammary neoplasia.

Hormonal therapy with anti-oestrogens such as tamoxifen have become standard therapy for many human mammary cancer patients with good success rates, but unfortunately this success has not been seen in canine patients. A study of the usefulness of tamoxifen in canine mammary cancer concluded that use of this agent could not be recommended in dogs due to the high incidence of oestrogenic side effects, such as significant vulval swelling, vulval discharge, oestrous-like signs and urinary incontinence and due to these side effects it was not possible to establish whether or not tamoxifen did generate any survival benefit. Therefore, at the time of writing there appears to be no role for adjunctive hormonal therapy for canine mammary neoplasia. Likewise, postoperative radiotherapy is a mainstay of treatment in human mammary neoplasia but its role in canine mammary neoplasia remains to be clarified and therefore it is not currently recommended routinely.

The prognosis for dogs with malignant mammary neoplasia, therefore, is variable and is dependent on many factors. Studies have shown that the main clinical factors that indicate prognosis are:

1. Primary tumour size. Tumours of less than 3 cm have a better prognosis than dogs with tumours greater than 3 cm diameter. One study reported a mean survival time of 22 months for dogs with malignant tumours of less than 3 cm diameter compared to a mean 14 month survival if the primary tumour was greater than 3 cm in diameter. A different study reported that dogs with carcinomas greater than 5 cm in diameter had median survival times of 10 months compared to 26 months if the primary tumour was less than 5 cm at the time of excision.
2. Histological tumour type. Different subtypes of mammary carcinoma carry different prognoses, with simple carcinomas having a poorer prognosis when compared to non-invasive carcinomas. Inflammatory carcinoma is associated with a very poor prognosis, with mean survival time as low as 25 days being reported with simple conservative treatment. Likewise, mammary sarcomas have a guarded prognosis with the majority of dogs dying from the disease within 1 year of diagnosis.
3. Histological tumour grade. Low-grade tumours are associated with longer disease-free periods and lower recurrence rates when compared to high grade tumours. Studies report that low-grade tumours have a recurrence/development of metastatic disease rate of 19–24% within the first 2 years post-excision, but that the recurrence/metastasis rate rises to 90–97% in the same 2-year period with high histological grade tumours.
4. Lymph node involvement. The presence of metastatic cells within the draining lymph nodes has been shown to be associated with significantly shorter survival times, with recurrence rates of up to 80% within 6 months of diagnosis being reported along with death rates of 86% within 2 years in patients with positive nodal disease.
5. Presence of distant metastases. Metastatic lesions beyond the draining lymph nodes are associated with poor survival. One study reported that dogs with mammary carcinomas in whom distant metastasis were diagnosed had a median survival time following excision of the primary tumour of only 5 months compared to a median survival time of 28 months for dogs in whom no metastatic disease was identified.

It is therefore difficult to accurately predict the outcome for individual patients but their owners can be counselled using some of the data given above to indicate the severity of their dog's condition. These data also show the importance of undertaking accurate clinical staging before surgery is contemplated and the value of sending all the samples to a specialist pathologist for analysis so that an accurate diagnosis can be reached in every case.

CLINICAL CASE EXAMPLE 15.4 – FELINE MAMMARY CARCINOMA

Signalment
13-year-old female neutered domestic long-haired (DLH) cat.

Presenting signs
An ulcerated mass in the cranial ventral thoracic region.

Case history
The relevant case history in this case was:
- The cat was an outdoor cat, fully vaccinated and wormed
- The owner had once previously noticed some blood on the cat's fur in the left cranial ventral thoracic region. On further examination the blood was associated with a mass
- The bleeding was intermittent and the cat presented to the hospital for further investigation.

Clinical examination
- The cat was bright and alert with no other clinical signs
- Thoracic auscultation and abdominal palpation were unremarkable

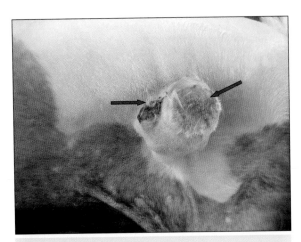

Figure 15.13 *Case 15.4* The appearance of the mammary mass at presentation and preoperatively. Areas of ulceration are present and indicated by the red arrows

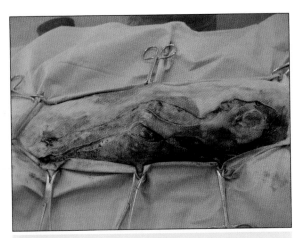

Figure 15.14 *Case 15.4* A unilateral chain mastectomy was performed to treat an isolated mammary mass in the cat

- Examination of the ventral thorax revealed a mass measuring approximately 3 × 2 cm associated with the left cranial thoracic mammary gland. The mass was ulcerated in areas and fixed to the overlying skin (Fig. 15.13).
- No further masses were palpable in any of the remaining glands on either side.
- Local axillary lymph nodes were not palpable.

Diagnostic evaluation

- Careful palpation of the axillary and inguinal lymph nodes was performed, however, no enlargement was found
- Thoracic radiographs (right and left lateral and ventrodorsal views) were undertaken, however, no evidence of detectable metastasis was documented
- Fine needle aspiration of the mass was performed revealing the presence of malignant epithelial cells.

Diagnosis

- Mammary gland neoplasia, probably an adenocarcinoma.

Treatment

As the tumour was likely to be malignant a unilateral chain mastectomy was performed which included all four mammary glands on the left side (Fig. 15.14). The cat was positioned in dorsal recumbency and the mass was excised with 2-cm margins. The incision was also extended caudally to include the remaining mammary tissue on the same side. Closure was achieved using simple continuous sutures of polyglecaprone for the subcutaneous layer and nylon skin sutures after gloves and instruments were changed. The entire chain was submitted for histopathology.

Outcome

The cat recovered well after surgery and was discharged 48 hours later after frequent wound checks and the administration of systemic opioid and non-steroidal anti-inflammatory analgesics. The sutures were removed 10 days after surgery when the wound had healed without complication. The histological diagnosis of the mass was a tubulopapillary carcinoma. The mass appeared to have been completely removed. However, a high level of mitosis and a moderate level of necrosis were observed although no apparent lymphatic invasion was present in the sections examined.

Theory refresher

Mammary tumours are relatively common in the cat, accounting for approximately 17% of all cancer found in this species. Unlike the dog, however, most mammary tumours in the cat (85–90%) are malignant and as a breed the Siamese cat is commonly over-represented. Notable features with this disease in the cat are lymphatic invasion and a high rate of metastasis to other organs such as lungs, liver and kidneys. Lymph node metastasis occurs in almost half of patients with malignant disease. Most mammary tumours in cats are adenocarcinomas with subdivisions of tubular, papillary, solid and cribriform carcinomas. Other types of carcinomas and sarcomas are not as common, however, an important differential diagnosis is a condition called fibroepithelial hyperplasia which is associated with oestrus in entire cats. The clinical appearance of this condition is one of enlarged mammary glands which may become ulcerated and necrotic. Treatment involves ovariohysterectomy and with this the clinical signs normally resolve over a period of a few weeks. Spontaneous resolution is also possible.

Treatment of mammary cancer in cats is surgical if there is no evidence of distant metastasis, so it is important to undertake a thorough clinical staging procedure pre-operatively as described for the dog. Using surgery in combination with chemotherapy (doxorubicin) may be useful and provide better outcomes although more studies need to be performed to definitively prove the efficacy of this combination. For surgical management radical mastectomies are recommended to reduce the chance of local recurrence in the light of the fact that the vast majority of mammary masses are malignant, which is a different situation from that described in the dog. If the mammary mass or masses are located on one side only then a unilateral mastectomy is indicated. If masses are present on both sides then bilateral chain mastectomies are advised which can be staged a few weeks apart to reduce tension at the surgical site. If the axillary lymph node is enlarged then this should also be excised, although there does not appear to be any benefit in removing this node prophylactically. The inguinal lymph node is easily and often removed with the caudal mammary gland. Ovariohysterectomy does not seem to improve survival or prevent recurrence of malignant lesions, however, it may be beneficial in some benign conditions such as fibroepithelial hyperplasia.

The prognosis for cats with mammary neoplasia is almost always guarded due to the high level of malignancy encountered in this species and the average survival time for cats with malignant mammary cancer is 15 months, even with aggressive surgery. The age at time of diagnosis and the breed have been shown to have no prognostic significance at all. However, two main clinical prognostic factors have been identified and these are:

1. Tumour size. As found in dogs, the size of the primary tumour at diagnosis has been shown to help predict the outcome. Cats with tumours less than 2 cm diameter at the time of surgery have had median survival times reported in excess of 3 years, compared to tumours measuring less than 3 cm

in diameter having median survival times of just under 2 years (21 months), whilst cats with tumours measuring more than 3 cm have median survival times of between 4 and 12 months. Large tumours are therefore definitely associated with a poorer prognosis, supporting the fact that early diagnosis and treatment is of paramount importance.

2. Histological tumour grade. As intuitively expected, tumours with a lower histological grading are associated with longer survival times. The tumour type is also important. As in dogs, cats with complex mammary carcinomas (i.e. tumours comprised from both mammary luminal epithelial cells and myoepithelial cells) have significantly better survival times compared to simple mammary carcinomas, with mean overall survival times of 32 months and 15 months respectively being reported in a recent study.

The extent of surgery undertaken probably also has a prognostic implication, with one study showing that more extensive surgery does improve survival time whilst others have suggested that radical surgery only improves the disease-free period but not the overall survival period. However, until this has been clarified the recommendation to undertake a full mastectomy remains in the light of the high rate of malignant tumours encountered in the cat.

CLINICAL CASE EXAMPLE 15.5 – AN INTRASCAPULAR FIBROSARCOMA IN A CAT

Signalment
6-year-old neutered female domestic short-haired (DSH) cat.

Presenting signs
A rapidly growing mass located between her scapulae, just to the left of the midline.

Case history
The relevant history in this case was:
- The cat was fully vaccinated (FHV, FCV, FPV, FeLV) and had received her last booster vaccination 4 months previously. However, the cat had not travelled outside of the UK and was not vaccinated against rabies
- The cat had no other previous medical history
- The owners had noticed the mass as the size of approximately 'a garden pea' 4 weeks prior to presentation and had then found it had grown rapidly

- The cat was otherwise bright and appeared well
- The referring veterinary surgeon had performed an incisional biopsy which had returned to confirm a high-grade soft-tissue sarcoma with features consistent with a vaccine-associated sarcoma.

Clinical examination

- General clinical examination was unremarkable but on palpation in the intrascapular area there was a solid mass palpable that measured approximately 2 cm in diameter
- No other abnormalities were detected.

Diagnostic evaluation

- Unfortunately, at the time of presentation there were no available MRI or CT scanners to enable an accurate assessment of the tumour's borders

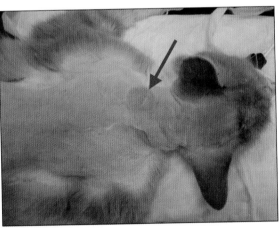

Figure 15.15

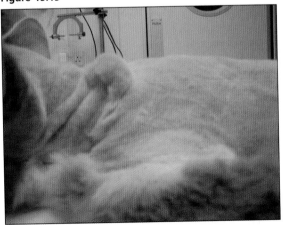

Figure 15.16

Figures 15.15, 15.16 *Case 15.5* The dorsoventral and lateral appearance of the mass immediately before surgery

- Inflated left and right lateral and DV thoracic radiographs were within normal limits with no evidence of metastatic disease or obvious tumour involvement with the dorsal spinous processes.

Treatment

- In the light of the fact that the diagnosis was one of a high-grade soft-tissue sarcoma with features consistent with a vaccine-associated sarcoma, the cat was taken to surgery and underwent an aggressive resection (Figs 15.15–15.19).

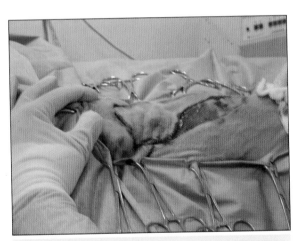

Figure 15.17 *Case 15.5* The aim was to remove the mass en bloc with 3-cm lateral margins plus removal of the dorsal spinous processes

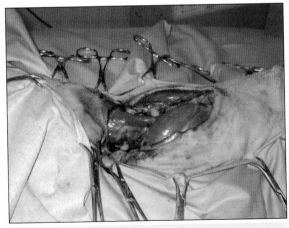

Figure 15.18 *Case 15.5* The mass was dissected out leaving a significant deficit

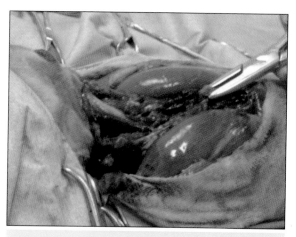

Figure 15.19 *Case 15.5* Finally before closure, the dorsal spinous processes were removed to try and ensure that all potentially contaminated tissue was removed

Outcome

- The cat made a full and rapid recovery from surgery, requiring hospitalization for analgesia for only 72 hours
- The cat remained well for 8 months before the owner found another mass just lateral in location to the first mass. The referring veterinary surgeon biopsied it again and found the tumour to have recurred. The owners had declined any further work-up or surgery, so the cat was put to sleep 6 weeks later.

Theory refresher

Vaccine-associated sarcomas are a specific subtype of soft-tissue sarcoma (STS) recognized only in the cat. They were first reported in the USA in the early 1990s and the resulting epidemiological studies showed a strong correlation between the administration of inactivated vaccines, in particular the FeLV vaccine and rabies vaccine, and the subsequent development of an aggressive form of STS at the vaccinal site. However, the fact that cases are seen regularly in the UK, where rabies vaccination is not commonplace, indicates that it may be the act of vaccination per se that triggers the development of the tumour in susceptible individuals. To support this, a feature of a vaccine-associated sarcoma (VAS) is the presence of an inflammatory cell infiltrate around the periphery of the tumour, leading to the theory that the act of vaccination leads to uncontrolled fibroblast and myofibroblast proliferation, which then eventually leads to neoplastic transformation and tumour genesis. Histologically, VASs are also similar to the STS that arise within eyes of cats that have been traumatized, which again supports a significant role for inflammation in the genesis of the tumour. Furthermore, a study from UC Davis in California found that there was evidence to suggest that certain long-acting injectable medications may also be associated with sarcoma formation, so it may be more appropriate to call these tumours 'injection-site sarcomas'. However, at the time of writing, the exact aetiology of this tumour remains unclear.

The problem with this condition in the USA was such that a Vaccine-Associated Feline Sarcoma Task Force was established and this group has made many recommendations regarding the prevention and optimum treatment for this disease. The main difficulties with VAS are: their high grade, meaning they grow quickly; the fact that they are poorly encapsulated and are highly invasive into the surrounding tissues; and their ability to extend along fascial planes for some distance, therefore making complete excision very difficult. Because of this, and particularly in relation to the last point, whenever possible, pre-surgical MRI or CT scanning is to be recommended in order to be able to do everything possible to establish the size and location of the tumour. VASs are almost always larger than they seem merely from palpation and the attending clinician should always assume the palpable mass is the proverbial 'tip of the iceberg'. Thoracic 'met-check' radiographs (fully inflated left and right lateral views and a fully inflated DV view) are also recommended, as VAS exhibit pulmonary metastasis in up to 20% of cases.

Any mass in the intra-scapular region of a cat should be viewed with suspicion as being a possible VAS, as it has been shown that the tumour can develop up to 10 years after a vaccination was last given. Excisional biopsy should not be attempted, as this has been shown to reduce the likelihood of complete excision at a later date. Rather, an incisional biopsy or a Tru-cut biopsy should be considered and then the biopsy tract should be excised with the tumour at surgery. However, as a study in 2000 clearly showed that the best option for these cases was referral to a specialist surgeon experienced in aggressive resection and reconstruction at the earliest stage possible, it is advisable that specialist advice is taken as soon as a possible VAS has been examined.

Aggressive surgery, aiming to excise a minimum of 2 cm lateral and deep to the tumour margin has been recommended by the task force. However, even with this approach, the 1-year disease-free period has been published to be only 35% with a median survival time of 19 months. The role of adjunctive therapies is therefore theoretically very important, but the role of chemotherapy is a little unclear. Doxorubicin has been shown to be beneficial by substantially increasing the disease-free interval following surgery in one study, but this finding was not reproduced in another study. Radiotherapy has been studied in a number of projects and has been shown to increase the disease-free periods and survival times, but local disease control is still a problem even with aggressive treatment combinations and there is a risk of radiation-induced spinal cord injury, so it is vital to talk to a radiation oncology specialist to see if a particular case would benefit from this treatment in their opinion or not.

The prognosis for VAS therefore is poor, as is shown by this case example, even with the best possible surgery, VASs are aggressive tumours that are likely to prove to be terminal within 2 years of initially developing.

VASs, although mesenchymal in origin, behave significantly differently from most other soft tissue sarcomas (STSs). The term STS encompasses a large number of heterogeneous tumours that share some common characteristics and hence can be considered together as a group. STSs can develop in mesenchymal tissue located in almost any structure, so their subgrouping comes from the tissue of origin, although the STS group generally excludes tumours arising in haemopoietic or lymphoid tissue. Examples of STS include fibrosarcoma, myxosarcoma, leiomyosarcoma, peripheral nerve sheath tumour (also known as haemangiopericytoma), rhabdomyosarcoma and liposarcoma. The characteristics shared by these tumours include:

- They may appear or feel well encapsulated, but they have diffuse margins and grow in a manner which is very invasive locally
- Achieving complete excision can therefore be difficult and local recurrence rates are high
- They generally have a low metastatic potential (this is dependent to some degree on histological grade) but if it occurs, metastasis is usually via the haematogenous route.

It is because of these characteristics that tumours such as histiocytic sarcoma, haemangiosarcoma and lymphosarcoma, which are obviously quite different, are not included in the STS group and are considered as different conditions.

CLINICAL CASE EXAMPLE 15.6 – A SOFT-TISSUE SARCOMA IN A GERMAN SHEPHERD DOG

Signalment

2-year-old neutered female German shepherd dog.

Presenting signs

A rapidly growing mass on the face, situated rostromedially to the medial canthus of the left eye.

Case history

The relevant history in this case was:
- The dog was fully vaccinated and had not travelled outside of the UK
- The owner had first noticed a lump near the dog's eye 6 weeks previously and had elected to monitor it but it grew steadily, although it did not appear to be causing the dog any discomfort
- The dog was taken to the referring vet who initially prescribed clavulanate-potentiated amoxicillin and carprofen but this made no difference and the mass continued to enlarge. Fine needle aspirates were then attempted but they were non-diagnostic so the dog was referred for further evaluation.

Clinical examination

- On examination the dog was very bright and alert. The only abnormality identified was the mass near her left eye (Fig. 15.20). The mass measured 2.5 cm × 1.5 cm × 2 cm and was solid to the touch. It felt attached to the underlying tissues but was not immovable

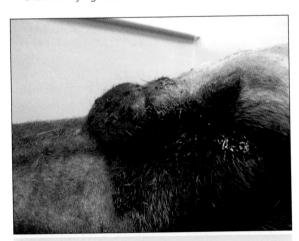

Figure 15.20 *Case 15.6* The appearance of the mass after the area had been clipped, viewed from the left lateral aspect

- The left submandibular lymph node was not palpable
- The dog exhibited epiphora from the left eye but no conjunctivitis or episcleral congestion.

Diagnostic evaluation

- Fine needle aspirates with applied suction using a 5 ml syringe (as described on page 170) were obtained, which revealed the presence of a population of mesenchymal cells. The cells were variable in size with a low–moderate amount of mild blue cytoplasm but obvious nucleoli in variably shaped and sized nuclei were frequently visible. Many of the cells appeared subjectively less spindloid than a normal mesenchymal cell, having a plump and more oval appearance. This appearance was considered consistent with either reactive fibroplasia or a mesenchymal tumour such as a fibrosarcoma
- Left and right lateral thoracic radiographs were unremarkable
- An MRI scan was undertaken, which revealed a solid mass to be present in the subcutaneous tissue but with no apparent invasion into the underlying bone (Fig. 15.21)

- As the appearance of the mass was most consistent with a tumour but the fine needle aspirates were not definitively diagnostic, a Tru-cut biopsy was obtained which confirmed the mass to be a fibrosarcoma.

Diagnosis

- An intermediate grade (grade II) fibrosarcoma.

Treatment

- It was decided to undertake wide surgical excision of the mass, as the proximity of the mass to the eye and the age of the dog meant that conservative surgery in combination with post-operative radiotherapy would not be ideal, had a lower chance of cure and might be associated with radiation-induced ocular damage. However, because of the location and size of the mass there was concern that there would not be adequate skin present in the immediate area for primary closure. Therefore an axial pattern flap based on the cutaneous branch of the superficial temporal artery was planned (Fig. 15.22–15.26). The mass was excised with 2 cm lateral margins and one fascial plane deep. The flap was then created based on the landmarks of the caudal aspect of the zygomatic arch caudally and the lateral orbital rim rostrally for the base of the flap. The length of the flap extended to just beyond the middle of the dorsal orbital rim of the contralateral eye. The flap was then carefully elevated and rotated rostrally through 90^0 to cover the original

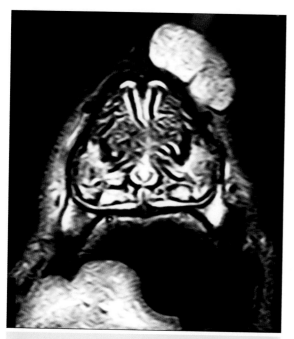

Figure 15.21 *Case 15.6* The transverse appearance of the mass on MRI, revealing the presence of a discrete hyperintense mass on the dorsolateral aspect of the nose without obvious invasion into the underlying bone

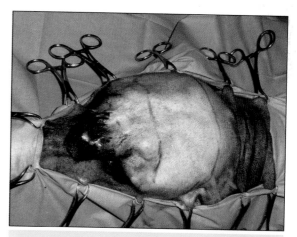

Figure 15.22 *Case 15.6* The dog placed in sternal recumbency and a sterile marker pen indicating the site for the incisions to form the axial pattern flap based on the cutaneous branch of the superficial temporal artery to cover the deficit at the tumour site

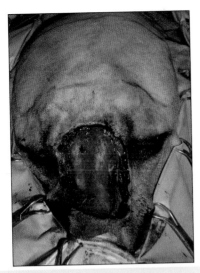

Figure 15.23 *Case 15.6* The intraoperative appearance of the dog following excision of the primary tumour with wide margins

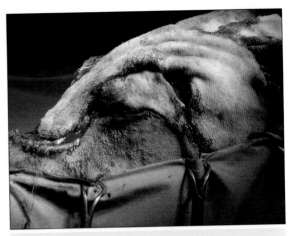

Figure 15.25 *Case 15.6* The advancement flap was rotated rostrally after creating a bridging incision to cover the defect

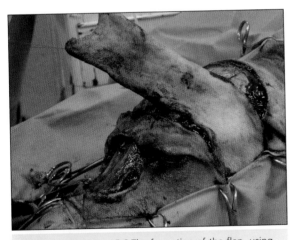

Figure 15.24 *Case 15.6* The formation of the flap, using stay sutures to handle the tissue to reduce trauma and thereby not compromising the viability of the flap

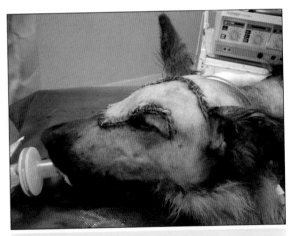

Figure 15.26 *Case 15.6* The immediate postoperative appearance of the dog, showing good tension-free wound closure and no compromise to the aperture of the left eye

skin deficit. The wound was closed after a negative suction drain was placed and the dog recovered uneventfully.

Outcome

- The dog made an uneventful recovery from his surgery. The drain was removed after 72 hours and the staples removed after 14 days. Histopathology revealed complete excision from the sections examined. The dog was then re-examined every 2 months and at 15 months after the operation, he was still free from any signs of tumour disease.

Theory refresher

STSs are considered to be quite common, being quoted to account for 15% of all cutaneous tumours and 7% of all subcutaneous tumours in the dog and cat respectively. They usually present in middle-aged to older animals as a lump that is growing slowly and often may be mentioned by an owner as an almost incidental finding but as in the case described here, STSs can develop in young animals and they can develop rapidly. Any such mass should initially be investigated with fine needle aspiration for cytology but it is important to remember that STSs arise from mesenchymal tissue, which by definition usually comprises cells which are well adhered together and therefore do not exfoliate easily. As a consequence, the authors recommend that a non-suction fine needle aspiration technique is attempted initially but if the sample quality is poor, then the needle should be placed into the mass attached to a 5 ml syringe. Apply suction with the syringe and then rapidly but not forcefully move and re-direct the needle several times. Release the vacuum in the syringe before removing the needle from the mass and then expel the contents of the needle onto a microscope slide before preparing the sample in the standard way (see also fine needle aspiration technique description on pages 1–4). The use of the vacuum generated by the syringe is usually sufficient to produce an adequate sample. However, it is important to note that fine needle aspiration of STSs is not always diagnostic, with false negative results being the main concern. In order to obtain a definitive pre-surgical diagnosis therefore, a solid tissue biopsy may be required in the form of a Tru-cut biopsy (as described in this case), an incisional biopsy or possibly an excisional biopsy, although due to the fact that the surgical margins required at excision are generally 3 cm, attempting an excisional biopsy is not recommended. As explained in Chapter 1, any biopsy procedure must also take into account the fact that the biopsy tract will need to be removed during the definitive surgery, so planning the best approach for the biopsy with the definitive surgery in mind is essential.

Although it is true to say that there is a relatively low metastatic potential with most STSs, diagnostic imaging for pulmonary metastasis is still to be recommended with inflated thoracic radiographs before excisional surgery. More advanced imaging techniques such as MRI or CT can also be extremely useful to help establish the exact size and extent of the tumour before excision is attempted. This can be particularly useful if the tumour is large and a substantial reconstruction procedure is going to be required. Once the full staging procedure has been completed, the first-line treatment for STS is wide surgical excision. Because STSs are locally aggressive typically the tumour cells extend beyond the pseudocapsule. STSs should be removed with 2–3-cm margins of normal tissue laterally and include one fascial plane in the deep margin. Remember that the first surgery is the best surgery to achieve complete resection. All of the

tumour, if possible, should be sent for histopathological assessment, grading and a margin report and if the margins come back as dirty or only just clean, then it is important to assume that it is highly likely that there will be skip metastases present (see page 12) and that further treatment may be necessary. Requesting a histological grading is also important; STSs can occur as low-grade, intermediate-grade or high-grade forms (grades I, II and III respectively):

- **Grade I (low)**: well differentiated, with few mitotic figures per high-powered field and minimal tumour necrosis
- **Grade II (intermediate)**: 10–19 mitotic figures per HPF but < 50% necrosis
- **Grade III (high)**: > 20 mitotic figures per HPF with > 50% tumour necrosis.

The histological grade appears to be predictive of metastases and prognosis in dogs with STS. In one study, 13% of dogs with grade I tumours developed metastases whereas 41% of dogs with grade III tumours developed metastases. Dogs with >19 mitotic figures/hpf had a median survival time of 236 days compared with 1444 days with < 10 mitotic figures/hpf. The percentage of histological necrosis was also prognostic for survival (dogs with > 10% necrosis were approximately three times more likely to die of tumour-related causes than dogs with < 10% necrosis.

Because of the locally invasive nature of these tumours, it is quite common to find that the margins after excision of the primary tumour are dirty. Options for further treatment firstly include surgical excision of the scar from the first surgery but it is not always possible, depending on the location of the scar and the amount of tissue free for reconstruction to be performed. However, a retrospective study in the USA showed that residual tumour was identified in nine of 41 (22%) resected STS scars and the study concluded that if incomplete resection of STS occurs, resection of local tissue should be performed, even if excisable tissue margins appear narrow because following a second surgery undertaken by an oncological surgical specialist, the local recurrence rate was only 15%.

If a second surgery is not easily possible, external beam radiotherapy can alternatively be performed. Although traditionally, STSs have been thought of as relatively radio-resistant tumours and as a single treatment modality, radiotherapy is not particularly effective, two studies at the turn of the century showed that the use of radiotherapy in incompletely excised STS was helpful, with local control rates of between 80% and 95% at one year post-surgery and 72% to 91% at 2 years postsurgery. Referral of cases with incompletely excised STS to a radio-oncologist is therefore certainly an option, especially if surgical excision of the scar is going to be difficult. Chemotherapy for STSs is more difficult to recommend as they are generally poorly responsive to chemotherapy due to their slow growth rate and possibly some inherent chemoresistance. Some studies have shown a response to doxorubicin-based protocols and anecdotally the authors have seen some very good responses to carboplatin in grade III tumours, but in general, a response has only been reported in up to one third of cases. However, an interesting recent report described the use of metronomic administration of cyclophosphamide (given at 10 mg/m^2) and piroxicam (given at 0.3 mg/kg) in dogs with incompletely excised STS. The medication was given on a daily or every other day basis to 55 dogs and the outcomes compared to 30 dogs who received surgery alone. The results showed that the disease-free interval (DFI) was significantly prolonged for STSs of all sites (trunk and extremity) in treated dogs compared with untreated control dogs. The DFI also was significantly longer in treated dogs when tumour site (trunk and extremity) was compared. The authors therefore concluded that further evaluation of this approach is warranted as adjunctive therapy in dogs with incomplete resected STS and also in dogs with highly metastatic tumours such as osteosarcoma and melanoma.

The authors would therefore generally recommend that the best treatment for STS is wide, complete surgical excision, as described in this case. Some cases of STS should be referred to surgical specialists if the primary clinician is uncertain of their ability to totally excise the mass and then close the resulting deficit. If the margins are dirty, then a second surgery should be considered or the patient could be referred for radiotherapy if a second surgery is not possible, with the further option of metronomic chemotherapy also a viable option. If the tumour returns as a grade III histologically, then adjunctive chemotherapy should be considered, either using doxorubicin or carboplatin alone (given once every 3 weeks for five treatments) or with metronomic administration of cyclophosphamide and piroxicam as detailed above.

In general, the prognosis for STS depends on the histological grading and the site of the primary, but most cases will do well with good treatment. The median survival times for dogs with STS ranges from approximately 1400 days for cases managed with surgery alone, up to over 2200 days for cases managed with surgery and radiotherapy.

CLINICAL CASE EXAMPLE 15.7 – AN INTERSTITIAL CELL TUMOUR IN A RABBIT

By Kevin Eatwell BVSc(Hons) DZooMed(Reptilian) MRCVS, The R(D)SVS, University of Edinburgh.

Signalment

8-year-old entire rabbit.

Presenting signs

Unilateral enlargement of a testicle.

Case history

The relevant history in this case was:
- The rabbit exhibited normal behaviour
- The rabbit was feeding well and passing normal faeces
- The rabbit was presented as the owner noticed a swelling at the rear end
- He was housed alone
- He was vaccinated against myxomatosis virus.

Clinical examination

- The rabbit weighed 2.6 kilos
- The rabbit was bright and alert
- Cardiopulmonary auscultation was unremarkable
- Abdominal palpation was unremarkable
- There was a swelling of the left testicle
- The testicle was non painful and there was no apparent inflammation
- The right testicle was smaller than expected
- There was some mild perineal soiling both with urine and faeces
- No other abnormalities were noted.

Diagnostic evaluation

- The rabbit was admitted for further evaluation
- Haematology demonstrated a mild relative neutrophilia (60%) which was attributed to a stress leucogram. No toxic activity was noted
- Biochemistry was unremarkable
- Plain radiography of the chest and abdomen were unremarkable
- There was some dental pathology but not sufficient to be causing clinical signs.

Presumptive diagnosis

- Testicular neoplasm.

Treatment

Given the clinical history and the physical examination the rabbit was castrated. Both the affected testicle and the smaller right testicle were removed (Figs 15.27, 15.28). The rabbit was anaesthetized using buprenorphine (0.03 mg/kg) pre-operatively and sevoflurane was administered by mask as the rabbit was quite aged. The rabbit was placed in dorsal recumbancy and the pre-scrotal and scrotal areas were carefully shaved. The skin was then prepared aseptically. A scrotal incision on the left side was made using a scalpel and the incision extended using metzenbaum scissors. Blunt dissection separated the tunic from the skin and the testicle was exteriorized. Further blunt dissection freed all attachments allowing a closed castration to be performed. Two artery forceps were placed proximal to the testicle and a crushing ligature of an absorbable suture material (2 metric polydioxone) was applied. The sutured stump was allowed to pass back into the wound and the scrotum was sutured using two single cross mattress sutures. This was repeated for the other testicle, although only a single suture was required. Intraoperatively, meloxicam (0.6 mg/kg), metoclopramide (0.5 mg/kg), trimethoprim/sulfonamide (30 mg/kg) and warmed lactated ringers (10 ml/kg) were given subcutaneously. The animal was discharged home the same day as the procedure.

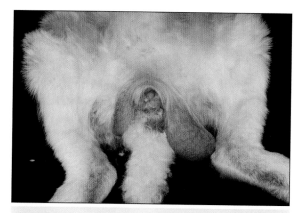

Figure 15.27 *Case 15.7* The appearance of the testicles during the consultation

Diagnosis

- Histopathology confirmed the tumour to be an interstitial cell tumour.

Outcome

- The rabbit made an uneventful recovery and was seen for a post-operative check 72 hours after discharge. Sutures were removed after a further week. The rabbit was reported to be alive and well 6 months later when vaccinated. He was subsequently lost to follow-up.

Theory refresher

Testicular tumours have become increasingly recognized in pet rabbits as owners are increasingly presenting them to veterinarians seeking medical treatment. Four types of neoplasm (seminomas, interstitial cell tumours, sertoli cell tumours and teratomas) have been reported. Other differentials for an enlarged testicle include fight wounds, myxomatosis, *Treponema paraluiscuniculi*, orchitis, epididymitis or a testicular torsion. These can usually be ruled out on clinical history and physical examination of a patient.

Clinical signs are usually limited to a change in the anatomy of the rabbits' genitalia. Occasionally, increased soiling of the area may be evident due to increased difficulty in grooming due to the testicular size. Typically the other testicle is reduced in size. In some rabbits increased libido and aggression may be evident.

The diagnosis is typically based on clinical findings. *Treponema* and myxomatosis can be ruled out by biopsy of the affected scrotal tissues and submitting them for

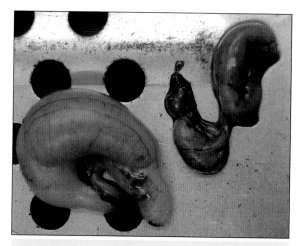

Figure 15.28 *Case 15.7* After removal the difference in testicle size was clearly apparent

histopathology. Medical treatment of these infections is possible, although myxomatosis carries a poor prognosis.

Orchitis and epididymitis usually result in a painful swelling of the testicle within the scrotum. Although medical treatment for these conditions is possible, if the rabbit is not required for breeding then surgical treatment (castration) may be indicated to reduce the risk of ascending infection. In entire males testicular trauma as a result of fight wounds is also possible. In extreme cases involving a breeding male then a fine needle aspirate of the testicle may be required for cytology to try to confirm the diagnosis prior to surgery. Testicular ultrasound may also demonstrate a discrete mass within the testicle.

Treatment is surgical castration using a closed technique to prevent herniation of abdominal contents through the open inguinal canals. This is 100% curative. Metastasis has not been reported. A scrotal ablation may be required to prevent further trauma or abrasion if there has been significant enlargement. Analgesics and gut motility stimulants should be considered routine for all rabbits undergoing anaesthesia.

The definitive diagnosis relies on histopathology of the affected testicle. Typically, a discrete nodule is identified on sectioning of the organ after surgery. Routine castration should be performed to prevent testicular neoplasia in rabbits. Typically this should be performed at 4–5 months of age to control untoward behaviour in male rabbits.

CLINICAL CASE EXAMPLE 15.8 – A SERTOLI CELL TUMOUR IN A DOG

Signalment
13-year-old entire male dog.

Presenting signs
Non-pruritic alopecia affecting his hind legs.

Case history
The relevant history in this case was:
- The dog was fully vaccinated and had no previous medical or surgical history
- The owner had noticed a progressively worsening baldness affecting his hind legs and tail, with his hair coat also thinning on his dorsum and flanks. The owner reported the dog to not appear to be scratching or excessively licking the balding areas

- The dog was otherwise quite well, although the owner described how he had aged recently and that he had become quite slow
- The owner also commented that one testicle was much larger than the other one.

Clinical examination
- The dog was quiet but alert
- Cardiopulmonary auscultation was unremarkable
- Abdominal palpation revealed no abnormalities
- Dermatological examination revealed a bilaterally symmetrical, non-pruritic alopecia with moderate hyperpigmentation of the underlying skin affecting mainly the caudal aspect of his hind legs and all of his tail. His hair coat was generally dry and appeared a little unkempt
- Testicular palpation confirmed significant enlargement of the right testicle (Figs 15.29, 15.30).

Diagnostic evaluation
- Skin scrapes and tape strips were obtained from the alopecic areas but no abnormalities were detected
- In addition to a full serum biochemistry assessment, total T4 and endogenous TSH were measured; these were within normal limits and the dog had no significant biochemical abnormalities
- Digital rectal examination revealed mild-moderate prostatomegaly consistent with an elderly entire male dog but no pain or asymmetry
- His CBC revealed a mild, non-regenerative anaemia (PCV 31%)
- Abdominal ultrasound revealed no enlargement of the abdominal lymph nodes and confirmed the generalized, homogeneous prostatomegaly
- Testicular ultrasound confirmed the presence of a mass within the right testicle.

Diagnosis
- Testicular tumour with paraneoplastic (probably endocrinological) alopecia.

Treatment
The dog was castrated and the testicles submitted for histopathology. The right testicle was confirmed to have contained a Sertoli cell tumour.

Outcome
The hair coat improved and over a period of 6 months the alopecia resolved.

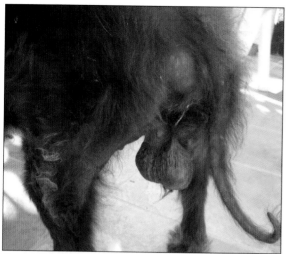

Figure 15.29

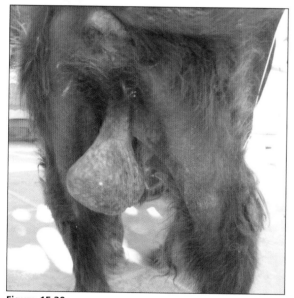

Figure 15.30

Figures 15.29, 15.30 *Case 15.8* The appearance of the dog at presentation

Theory refresher

Tumours of the testicle are statistically the most common form of cancer affecting the male genitalia in dogs and are considered to be rare in cats, but they are uncommonly seen due to the fact that so many dogs are routinely castrated in the UK. It is not known what causes these tumours to develop, but one well-recognized risk factor is cryporchidism, hence the reason that there is a significant health benefit for the dog in finding the

abnormally located testicle and undertaking castration in a cryporchid animal. As cryporchidism is an inherited condition (probably via a sex-limited autosomal recessive trait), cryptorchid animals should undergo bilateral castration and not simply have the abnormally located testicle removed whilst leaving the scrotal testicle in place. Testicular tumours usually only develop in older dogs (mean age of 9.5 years in one study, 10.7 years in another) and in certain breeds such as boxers, cairn terriers, Labrador retrievers, border collies, German shepherds and rough collies. A recent Italian study, which put the incidence of testicular tumours in a post-mortem population as high as 27%, has suggested that the incidence of testicular seminomas in dogs is rising, which interestingly mimics the situation in man in the second half of the 20th century, implying that there may be some causal environmental factors in the development of testicular tumours that are as yet unidentified.

There are three main types of primary testicular tumours in the dog, reflecting three different cells of origin. Interstitial cell tumours (ICT) arise from the interstitial cells of Leydig, Sertoli cell tumours (SCT) arise from the sustentacular cells of Sertoli and seminomas develop from the spermatic germinal epithelium. The recent study from Italy mentioned previously found that 50% of the tumours identified were ICT, 42% seminomas and 8% SCT. Interestingly, this study also found that a significant number of dogs (31%) had more than one tumour type present at the same time.

Testicular tumours usually present simply with testicular enlargement without causing pain. However, as in the case described here, any of the testicular tumours can cause dermatological signs (bilateral, non-pruritic alopecia and hyper pigmentation; Fig. 15.31) and also signs of feminization such as prepucial pendulocity and gynaecomastia. This rather counterintuitive paraneoplastic syndrome appears to be due to the fact that the tumour induces the endogenous production of female reproductive hormones such as oestradiol-17β as well as testosterone and other steroid hormone compounds, so that the relative ratio of sex hormones changes, resulting in the dermatological changes described.

Hyperoestrogenism can also cause much more serious paraneoplastic problems by affecting the bone marrow, resulting in conditions such as aplastic anaemia and pancytopaenia. These problems do not always resolve on removal of the primary tumour, so it is essential to undertake a high quality blood count in the diagnostic evaluation of these patients to ensure that no such

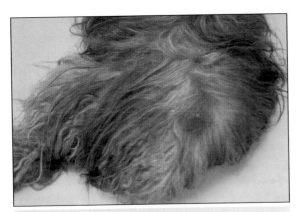

Figure 15.31 An old English sheepdog that presented with alopecia affecting his dorsum. His diagnosis was of a Sertoli cell tumour and the alopecia resolved following castration. Courtesy of Mr Simon Tappin, Dick White Referrals

problems are developing. It also means that a testicular tumour patient could present as a non-regenerative anaemia patient (see Chapter 11). Measuring female hormones such as oestrogen, however, has little role in the diagnostic evaluation of these patients.

The treatment of choice is simple castration in all cases, assuming the patient does not have a potentially life-threatening bone marrow problem. The metastatic rate of testicular tumours is generally quite low (less than 15%), as testicular tumours do not behave in an aggressive manner. Metastatic disease, if it does occur, will be to the local lymph nodes first, then usually the distant lymph nodes secondarily and then to the lungs and other organs. It is to be recommended therefore that cases with a testicular tumour undergo an abdominal ultrasound examination and thoracic radiographs before surgery to ensure that there is no secondary disease present. However, the prognosis for dogs with local disease is generally excellent and surgery is usually curative. The prognosis for dogs with metastatic disease is less clear, mainly because no clearly efficacious chemotherapy for testicular tumours has been described. Cisplatin is commonly used in human medicine and it has been described as being successful in treating canine metastatic testicular tumours but only in a very small number of cases. More work is therefore required to establish the best medical options for dogs with secondary disease.

APPENDICES

Multiple choice questions

1. **Which of the following statements is the most accurate with regard to cytological evaluation of fine needle aspirate biopsy samples?**
   a. Simple, inexpensive but samples usually inadequate to enable tumour grade to be established
   b. Simple, inexpensive and samples very useful for assessing tumour grade
   c. Difficult and expensive and usually not able to establish tumour grade
   d. Requires significant sedation or anaesthesia to be used in order for samples to be of diagnostic quality

2. **The best 'all-purpose' cytological staining solutions that enable clear visualization of cytoplasmic and nuclear detail, consistent mast cell granule staining and bacterial identification are:**
   a. Toludine blue preparations
   b. Diff-Quick and other rapid staining solutions
   c. H&E stains
   d. Romanowski stains, such as Giemsa

3. **Which of the following tumours is classified as a round cell tumour?**
   a. Transitional cell carcinoma
   b. Splenic haemangiosarcoma
   c. Histiocytoma
   d. Peripheral nerve sheath tumour

4. **AgNOR staining (which involves using silver stains to visualize the nucleolar organizing regions within the nucleus of a cell) is potentially useful in both cytology and histopathology to:**
   a. Diagnose the cell of origin of the tumour
   b. Determine whether or not metastatic disease is present
   c. Help establish the grade of the tumour
   d. Help establish the likely response of the tumour to chemotherapy

5. **Which of the following is NOT a feature of a neoplastic cell?**
   a. To have self-sufficient growth ability
   b. To be insensitive to natural anti-growth signals
   c. To be able to promote sustained angiogenesis
   d. To have an increased rate of apoptosis

6. **Chemotherapy should be delayed if the circulating neutrophil count immediately pre-treatment is found to be less than:**
   a. $3.5 \times 10^9/L$
   b. $2.5 \times 10^9/L$
   c. $1.5 \times 10^9/L$
   d. $0.5 \times 10^9/L$

7. **If a dog receiving cyclophosphamide to treat grade III multicentric lymphoma develops signs of haemorrhagic cystitis, which of the following medications could be used in its place?**
   a. Carboplatin
   b. Gemcitabine
   c. Melphalan
   d. Prednisolone

8. **The preparation of cytotoxic medications within a laminar flow fume cupboard is essential to help prevent:**
   a. Direct contact between the drug and the clinician's skin
   b. Inadequate mixing of the drug
   c. Inadvertent splashing of the chemotherapeutic into the clinician's eyes
   d. Inhalation of aerosolized cytotoxic particles

9. **Which is the most appropriate way to initially investigate a suspected mast cell tumour on the pinna of a dog?**
   a. Excisional biopsy
   b. Incisional biopsy
   c. Skin punch biopsy
   d. Fine needle aspirate

10. **For which of these procedures is an excisional biopsy a reasonable choice for initial diagnosis?**
    a. Feline injection site sarcoma
    b. Splenic haemangiosarcoma
    c. Oral melanoma
    d. Cutaneous lymphoma

11. **Which of the following drugs can cause a potentially fatal pulmonary oedema in cats such that its use in this species is contraindicated?**
    a. Cisplatin
    b. Carboplatin
    c. Epirubicin
    d. Vinblastine

12. **Which of the following statements about incisional biopsy is correct?**
    a. It should always be carried out following a fine needle aspirate
    b. The definitive surgery should aim to include the scar from the incisional biopsy
    c. It is not advisable to use this method of biopsy for oral tumours
    d. It is the preferred method of sampling for cutaneous mast cell tumours

13. **What is the main reason for changing gloves when closing an abdominal wound after resection of a colonic adenocarcinoma?**
    a. To avoid contamination of the wound from the environment
    b. To protect the surgeon from contamination from punctured gloves
    c. To avoid seeding of tumour cells from the tumour
    d. To prevent wound breakdown from infection

14. **Which of the following biopsy techniques is most suitable for diagnosing an oral acanthomatous epulis?**

a. Fine needle aspirate
b. Excisional biopsy
c. Incisional biopsy
d. Impression smear

15. **The mechanism of action vincristine is:**
    a. To bind DNA strands together by causing free radicals to be produced
    b. To bind DNA strands together by the insertion of an alkyl group
    c. To inhibit topoisomerase II
    d. To bind to the microtubule assembly, thereby preventing mitosis

16. **Which of the following statements regarding excision of a fibrosarcoma on the elbow of a dog is most correct?**
    a. The tumour should be excised with a 3-cm margin laterally and deeply
    b. The tumour should be excised with a 3-cm margin laterally and one fascial layer deep
    c. Radiotherapy is not useful as an adjunctive treatment for microscopic disease
    d. Chemotherapy is useful as a sole treatment for this tumour type

17. **Which of the following is NOT a diagnostic feature of multiple myeloma in the dog?**
    a. Polyclonal gamma-globulinaemia
    b. Bence-Jones proteinuria
    c. Lytic bone lesions
    d. Plasma cell myelophthisis

18. **Many chemotherapy drugs are metabolized to products that are themselves potentially cytotoxic, which generates important health and safety concerns for the owners. Cisplatin is one such drug and the major route of excretion of its metabolites is:**
    a. Via the liver into bile and therefore into the faeces
    b. Via the liver and then on into saliva
    c. Via the kidneys and therefore into urine
    d. The metabolites are not excreted but accumulate in the fat of the patient

19. **Which of the following describes the relative tissue penetrating power of three different forms of external radiation beam?**
    a. Electron beam < orthovoltage < megavoltage
    b. Orthovoltage < megavoltage < electron beam

c. Megavoltage < orthovoltage < electron beam
d. Electron beam < megavoltage < orthovoltage

20. **Which of these tumours can be effectively treated using a combination of surgery and radiotherapy?**
    a. A rostral maxillary squamous cell carcinoma
    b. A bladder transitional cell carcinoma
    c. A mast cell tumour located on the lateral thoracic wall
    d. A mammary adenocarcinoma

21. **Which of the following suture patterns should be used for an end-to-end anastomosis following resection of a mid-jejunal adenocarcinoma?**
    a. Inverting
    b. Everting
    c. Crushing
    d. Appositional

22. **Which of the following best describes the prevalence of different types of nasal tumour in the dog?**
    a. Lymphoid > epithelial > mesenchymal
    b. Epithelial > mesenchymal > lymphoid
    c. Mesenchymal > lymphoid > epithelial
    d. Epithelial > lymphoid > mesenchymal

23. **Which of the following suture materials is best used for bladder closure following resection of a transitional cell carcinoma?**
    a. Silk
    b. Polypropylene
    c. Catgut
    d. Polydioxanone

24. **Which of the following statements regarding primary lung tumours is correct?**
    a. The preferred surgical approach is via median sternotomy
    b. The prognosis is partly dependent on the size of the local lymph nodes
    c. A needle core biopsy should always be performed preoperatively to determine the tumour grade
    d. Surgical staples are associated with a higher incidence of pneumothorax compared with suture closure methods

25. **Which of these types of surgery is most suitable for removing a mandibular osteosarcoma?**
    a. Compartmental resection
    b. Marginal resection
    c. Intracapsular resection
    d. Wide resection

26. **A ligating dividing stapler is useful for which type of surgery?**
    a. Partial gastrectomy
    b. Hepatectomy
    c. Splenectomy
    d. Lung lobectomy

27. **Which of the following is the most commonly reported malignant oral tumour in the dog?**
    a. Squamous cell carcinoma
    b. Fibrosarcoma
    c. Lymphoma
    d. Melanoma

28. **Which of the following tumour types would be considered least likely to metastasize to the lungs?**
    a. Malignant melanoma
    b. Ulnar osteosarcoma
    c. Mammary adenocarcinoma
    d. Superficial cutaneous haemangiosarcoma

29. **Malignant body cavity effusions can develop for several different reasons, one of which is listed below:**
    a. Reduced vascular permeability
    b. Obstruction of lymphatic vessel flow
    c. Reduced hydrostatic pressure
    d. Increased plasma oncotic pressure

30. **Which one of the following sub-types of ovarian tumour is commonly associated with excessive production of oestrogens, causing signs such as vulval enlargement and alopecia?**
    a. Stromal sex cord tumours
    b. Epithelial cell tumours
    c. Primordial germ cell tumours
    d. Metastatic haemangiosarcoma

31. **The most suitable procedure to remove a mammary mass located in the second cranial mammary gland on the right side in a cat is:**
    a. A local mastectomy involving the second gland only
    b. A regional mastectomy involving the first and second gland
    c. A bilateral chain mastectomy
    d. A unilateral chain mastectomy

32. **Which of the following statements regarding a 2-cm mammary mass in the left inguinal gland of an 8-year-old entire female dog is most correct?**
    a. It is most likely to be malignant
    b. Performing ovariohysterectomy at the time of surgery will prevent recurrence
    c. The prognosis following a unilateral chain mastectomy is better compared with local mastectomy
    d. A fine needle aspirate is not necessary as the results will not influence the extent of the surgery

33. **The best biopsy method for diagnosing a transitional cell carcinoma in a bladder is:**
    a. A catheter suction biopsy
    b. Fine needle aspirate by ultrasound guidance
    c. A tru-cut biopsy by ultrasound guidance
    d. An incisional biopsy

34. **Which of these oral tumours is associated with the most favourable prognosis following aggressive surgery?**
    a. A caudal mandibular osteosarcoma
    b. A caudal maxillary fibrosarcoma
    c. A rostral mandibular squamous cell carcinoma
    d. A rostral maxillary melanoma

35. **If a cancer patient presents with dysphagia as a significant clinical sign, where is the disease unlikely to be?**
    a. Oral cavity
    b. Oesophagus
    c. Stomach
    d. Inner ear

36. **The fine needle aspirate shown below was taken from a soft 2-cm diameter cutaneous mass on a boxer dog. The sample was stained with Giemsa stain. What is the diagnosis?**

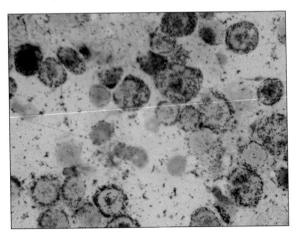

    a. Lymphosarcoma
    b. Histiocytoma
    c. Mast cell tumour
    d. Haemangiosarcoma

37. **Which of the following antibiotic protocols is best practice when used for removal of a large ulcerated infected mast cell tumour on the flank of a dog?**
    a. Subcutaneous administration of amoxicillin clavulanate at the time of the first incision
    b. Intravenous administration of cephazolin 30 minutes prior to the first incision
    c. Intravenous administration of amoxicillin clavulanate at the time of the first incision
    d. Subcutaneous administration of cephazolin at the time of wound closure

38. **Apart from thoracic radiographs, which of the following is a suitable staging procedure for a 3-cm anal sac adenocarcinoma?**
    a. Buffy coat analysis
    b. Fine needle aspirate of contralateral anal sac
    c. Ultrasound examination of medial iliac lymph nodes
    d. Ultrasound examination of descending colon

39. **Which of the following statements regarding mast cell tumours is correct?**
    a. It is recommended to surgically remove intermediate grade tumours with 2-cm lateral margins and include one fascial layer deep

b. Chemotherapy is recommended as adjunctive treatment with all incompletely excised intermediate grade tumours
c. These tumours are normally not radiosensitive
d. Dogs that are prone to multiple mast cell tumours have a poor prognosis

40. Which of the following statements regarding soft-tissue sarcomas is correct?
a. The pseudocapsule is protective and contains tumour cells within the central mass
b. Clinical behaviour and prognosis is dependent on the grade of the tumour
c. Distant metastases are a common finding with these tumours
d. They exfoliate tumour cells readily on fine needle aspirates

41. Which of the following is NOT usually a differential diagnosis for hypercalcaemia in the dog?
a. Hyperparathyroidism
b. Anal sac adenocarcinoma
c. Gastric carcinoma
d. Multicentric lymphoma

42. Which of the following statements regarding colorectal polyps is true?
a. They frequently metastasize and therefore carry a poor prognosis
b. They always require extensive abdominal surgery to remove them
c. Their presence usually causes constipation
d. Although initially benign, if left in situ untreated they can undergo malignant transformation

43. Which of the following treatments is generally considered to be the optimal therapy for nasal tumours in the dog?
a. External beam radiotherapy with a megavoltage linear accelerator
b. Systemic chemotherapy with doxorubicin
c. Surgical excision via a dorsal rhinotomy
d. Endoscopically guided suction debaulking

44. A dog presents with significantly enlarged submandibular and prescapular lymph nodes, from which the following fine needle aspirate was obtained (Giemsa stain, x100 magnification). What is the diagnosis?

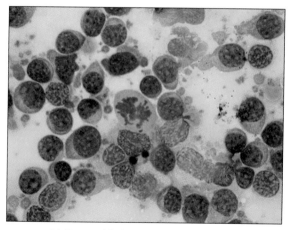

a. Malignant histiocytosis
b. Metastatic oral melanoma
c. Metastatic mast cell tumour
d. Multicentric lymphoma

45. Which of the following chemotherapeutic protocols is generally associated with the longest first remission rates, remission times and lowest relapse rates when used to treat canine lymphoma?
a. CHOP
b. High-dose COP
c. Single-agent doxorubicin
d. Single-agent prednisolone

46. Which of the following statements regarding kidney tumours in dogs is true?
a. Primary renal tumours are most likely to be mesenchymal in nature
b. Renal tumours are more likely to be metastatic lesions rather than primary renal tumours in this species
c. Primary renal tumours are usually associated with marked abdominal discomfort
d. Primary renal carcinoma tumours in the dog are usually bilateral

47. Which of the following statements regarding kidney tumours in cats is true?
a. Renal tumours are more likely to be metastatic lesions rather than primary renal tumours in this species
b. Primary renal tumours are usually associated with marked abdominal discomfort
c. Lymphoma is a more commonly encountered tumour type than carcinoma
d. Renal tumours in cats are usually benign

48. Which of the following treatments offer the highest median survival times for the treatment of a urinary bladder transitional cell carcinoma in the dog?
   a. Surgical resection of the tumour followed by external beam radiotherapy
   b. Surgical resection of the tumour followed by sole agent piroxicam treatment
   c. Surgical resection of the tumour followed by combined piroxicam and mitoxantrone treatment
   d. Piroxicam treatment alone

49. Which of the following are all common clinical signs caused by the presence of a prostatic carcinoma in the dog?
   a. Defaecatory tenesmus, stranguria and lumbar pain
   b. Polyuria, haematuria and vomiting
   c. Urinary incontinence, tail paralysis and abdominal distension
   d. Stanguria, vomiting and pollakiuria

50. Which of the following locations in the gastrointestinal tract is the most common location for an adenocarcinoma in the cat?
   a. Oesophagus
   b. Stomach
   c. Small intestine
   d. Large intestine

51. Which of the following locations in the gastrointestinal tract is the most common location for an adenocarcinoma in the dog?
   a. Oesophagus
   b. Stomach
   c. Small intestine
   d. Large intestine

52. Which of the following tumours is considered the most commonly diagnosed hepatobiliary cancer in the cat?
   a. Bile duct adenoma
   b. Biliary carcinoma
   c. Hepatic carcinoid
   d. Haemangiosarcoma

53. What is a commonly encountered complication associated with splenectomy for removal of a splenic haemangiosarcoma?

   a. Thromboembolic disease
   b. Haemorrhage
   c. Septicaemia
   d. Peritonitis

54. Which of these neoplastic conditions of the oral cavity has the worst reported median survival time in the dog?
   a. Gingival squamous cell carcinoma
   b. Maxillary fibrosarcoma
   c. Tonsillar squamous cell carcinoma
   d. Mandibular acanthomatous epulis

55. Which of the following statements concerning excision of soft-tissue sarcomas is correct?
   a. They should be excised in the reactive zone just outside the pseudocapsule so that any skip metastases are included
   b. They should be excised within their pseudocapsule and then further tissue removed
   c. They should always be excised to include the local lymph nodes
   d. The excision should be wide and the pseudocapsule kept intact

56. Which of the following statements regarding cutaneous histiocytomas in the dog are true?
   a. Their microscopic appearance could be considered consistent with a highly malignant neoplasm to a non-veterinary pathologist but they are actually benign in nature and can sometimes spontaneously resolve
   b. They have a potent malignant potential and need to be treated aggressively with surgery and adjunctive chemotherapy
   c. The prognosis even with surgical treatment is guarded due to their malignant potential
   d. They are also common cutaneous tumours in cats

57. Which of the following axial pattern flaps may be useful in reconstruction of a wound created after removal of a soft-tissue sarcoma on the lateral aspect of the elbow?
   a. Omocervical
   b. Superficial temporal
   c. Cranial superficial epigastric
   d. Thoracodorsal

58. **Which of the following oral tumours is most likely to be associated with local recurrence following aggressive surgical resection?**
    a. Squamous cell carcinoma of the rostral mandible
    b. Malignant melanoma around the upper canine tooth
    c. Fibrosarcoma medial to the caudal upper molar teeth
    d. Acanthomatous epulis of the caudal mandible

59. **What is the approximate median survival time for gastric carcinoma following surgery?**
    a. 6 months
    b. 12 months
    c. 18 months
    d. 24 months

60. **Which is the best way to initially investigate metastasis of an intermediate grade mast cell tumour affecting a digit on a hind limb?**
    a. Thoracic radiographs and ultrasound of liver and spleen
    b. Palpation and aspiration of popliteal lymph node
    c. Bone marrow aspirate from the wing of the ileum
    d. Buffy coat in combination with ultrasound of sublumbar lymph nodes

61. **Bladder tumours are most common in which breed of dog?**
    a. Scottish terriers
    b. Golden retrievers
    c. Boxers
    d. Poodles

62. **Although a number of cases of cutaneous histiocytosis will show spontaneous regression, a significant number require medical treatment. What is the recommended medication type for this condition?**
    a. Systemic chemotherapy with e.g. doxorubicin
    b. COX-2 selective non-steroidal anti-inflammatory drugs e.g. meloxicam
    c. Immunosuppressant with e.g. steroids or cyclosporin
    d. Antibiotics that show good skin penetration e.g. cephalexin

63. **Disseminated histiocytic sarcoma (often termed 'malignant histiocytosis') is more commonly diagnosed in which of the following breeds of dog?**
    a. German shepherd dog
    b. Boxers
    c. Bernese mountain dog
    d. West Highland white terrier

64. **Which of the following forms of feline mast cell tumour is most likely to behave in an aggressive manner?**
    a. Compact cutaneous mastocytic mast cell tumour
    b. Diffuse cutaneous mastocytic mast cell tumour
    c. Cutaneous histiocytic mast cell tumour
    d. Visceral mast cell tumour

65. **Which of the following statements regarding mammary neoplasia in the dog is true?**
    a. Neutering a bitch before her first season offers no protection against the development of malignant mammary tumours in the future
    b. Neutering a bitch after she is allowed to have one litter of puppies offers significant protection against the development of malignant mammary tumours in the future
    c. Neutering a bitch before she has her first season is associated with a significantly lower rate of malignant mammary cancer development
    d. Most mammary tumours in the bitch are benign in nature

66. **Which of the following malignant mammary tumours has the highest malignant potential?**
    a. Non-infiltrating carcinoma
    b. Complex carcinoma
    c. Simple carcinoma
    d. Inflammatory carcinoma

67. **The following picture is of a cluster of neoplastic cells obtained from a canine patient. Which tumour type do the cells represent?**

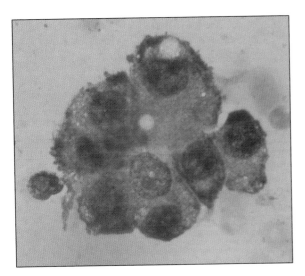

a. A malignant epithelial tumour
b. A benign epithelial tumour
c. A mesenchymal tumour
d. A round cell tumour

68. Which of the following chemotherapeutics is most likely to be associated with causing an anaphylactic reaction following multiple use?
a. Vincristine
b. L-asparaginase
c. Mitoxantrone
d. Prednisolone

69. Canine nasal tumours would be considered more likely to develop in which of the following types of dog?
a. Middle-aged to older dolycephalic dogs
b. Young dolycephalic dogs
c. Young brachycephalic dogs
d. Middle-aged to older brachycephalic dogs

70. The approximate average survival time for dogs following a diagnosis of acute myeloid leukaemia is:
a. 3 days
b. 3 weeks
c. 3 months
d. 3 years

71. Which of the following would be an unusual presenting sign for a rabbit with a uterine adenocarcinoma?
a. Haematuria
b. Weight loss

c. Decreased faecal output
d. Coughing

72. Which breed of dog appears to have a higher than normal incidence of prostatic carcinoma?
a. German shepherd dog
b. Boxer
c. Bouvier de Flandres
d. Irish wolfhound

73. Which of the following statements relating to osteosarcoma is most true?
a. Osteosarcoma of the appendicular limb is most commonly seen in middle-aged to older large-breed dogs
b. Osteosarcoma of the appendicular limb is most commonly seen in young large-breed dogs
c. Osteosarcoma of the rib is most commonly seen in older large-breed dogs
d. Osteosarcoma of the rib is not a malignant tumour

74. Which of the following treatments relating to osteosarcoma in the cat are most true?
a. Feline osteosarcoma is generally a benign disease
b. Feline osteosarcoma is a malignant disease but with a much slower metastatic potential than in dogs
c. Feline osteosarcoma is a common problem in cats
d. Feline osteosarcoma requires aggressive management with amputation and then postsurgical radiation therapy and chemotherapy to generate any hope of a long-term survival

75. The diagnosis of a tumour on a digit of a cat is most likely to be:
a. A benign primary tumour of little concern
b. A malignant primary digit tumour with a low metastatic potential
c. A malignant primary digit tumour with a high metastatic potential
d. A metastatic lesion with the primary in a distant location

76. Which of the following tumours could a xenogenic DNA vaccine be useful in the management of?

a. Injection site sarcoma
b. Mammary adenocarcinoma
c. Oral melanoma
d. Multicentric lymphoma

77. Which of the following malignant digital tumours occur most frequently in the dog?
a. Osteosarcoma, mast cell tumour, cutaneous lymphoma
b. Squamous cell carcinoma, malignant melanoma, soft-tissue sarcoma
c. Osteosarcoma, squamous cell carcinoma, malignant melanoma
d. Cutaneous lymphoma, mast cell tumour, soft-tissue sarcoma

78. Which of the following suture materials is recommended for closure of an end-to-end anastomosis following resection of a colonic adenocarcinoma?
a. Polypropylene
b. Monofilament nylon
c. Polyglecaprone
d. Polydioxanone

79. Which of the following statements regarding injection-site sarcomas in the cat is correct?
a. Their behaviour is similar to a low grade soft-tissue sarcoma and should be excised with 2-cm margins
b. They should be removed with a minimum of 2-cm margins following diagnosis by needle core or incisional biopsy
c. Their behaviour is similar to a high-grade soft-tissue sarcoma and diagnosis should be made by excisional biopsy
d. Prognosis is usually good following marginal excision

80. The most effective method to treat nasal adenocarcinoma in the dog is?
a. Chemotherapy
b. Cryosurgery
c. Radiotherapy
d. Surgery

81. Which of the following possible side effects is particularly associated with doxorubicin use in the dog?

a. Hepatotoxicity
b. Nephrotoxicity
c. Cardiotoxicity
d. Neurotoxicity

82. Which of the following possible side effects is particularly associated with lomustine (CCNU) use on the dog?
a. Hepatotoxicity
b. Nephrotoxicity
c. Cardiotoxicity
d. Neurotoxicity

83. Flow cytometry is a technique that can be extremely useful in the diagnosis of:
a. Lymphoid neoplasia
b. Epithelial neoplasia
c. Mesenchymal neoplasia
d. Meylofibrosis

84. Which of the following statements regarding the general presenting signs of diarrhoea originating in the large bowel (colon) is most true?
a. Reduced defecatory frequency, haematochezia and mucus are usually reported
b. Increased defecatory frequency, haematochezia and mucus are usually reported
c. Normal defecatory frequency, but no haematochezia or mucus are usually reported
d. Weight loss and hypoalbuminaemia are common

85. Which of the following features of a small intestinal adenocarcinoma has the most important prognostic significance in the dog?
a. The size of the primary tumour
b. The location within the small intestine
c. The presence or absence of lymphatic metastasis
d. Whether or not the tumour is causing the dog to vomit

86. Which of the following assessments is the most important to make in order to establish whether or not anaemia is regenerative or non-regenerative?

a. The reticulocyte percentage
b. The absolute reticulocyte count
c. The degree of polychromasia
d. The degree of erythroid anisocytosis

87. **Which of the following mesenchymal tumours is most frequently associated with metastatic disease to the brain in the dog?**
    a. Oral fibrosarcoma
    b. Cutaneous haemangiosarcoma
    c. Splenic haemangiosarcoma
    d. Liposarcoma

88. **Which of the following type of testicular tumour is considered to be the most prevalent in the dog?**
    a. Seminoma
    b. Sertoli cell tumour
    c. Interstitial cell tumour
    d. Teratoma

89. **The biggest clinical concern regarding injection site sarcomas in the cat is:**
    a. The extensive local invasion that develops making complete excision of the primary tumour difficult
    b. The tough fibrous capsule that makes complete excision difficult
    c. The reduced immune response of the cat making them more prone to post-operative infection
    d. The postoperative analgesia requirement for these patients considering the proximity of the tumour to the spinal cord

90. **Cisplatin is an extremely useful chemotherapeutic used in a variety of different diseases. Which of the following points regarding its use is NOT true?**
    a. Its metabolites are excreted renally and reach high concentrations in the urine, meaning that urine should be collected and handled as cytotoxic waste for the first 24 hours after administration
    b. It is highly emetogenic, necessitating the use of anti-emetics in all cases
    c. It is not particularly nephrotoxic in comparison to carboplatin and therefore intravenous fluids are not required when it is given to patients

d. Its use cannot be recommended in the cat due to the development of acute pulmonary oedema in this species in response to cisplatin

91. **The approximate average disease-free period for a dog with a transitional cell carcinoma of the bladder treated with piroxicam and mitoxantrone is:**
    a. 19 days
    b. 190 days
    c. 290 days
    d. 390 days

92. **The approximate average increase in survival time in dogs with an appendicular limb osteosarcoma treated with amputation plus adjunctive chemotherapy as opposed to amputation alone is:**
    a. A four-fold increase
    b. A three-fold increase
    c. A two-fold increase
    d. No increase in survival time is seen

93. **Which of the following statements regarding appendicular limb osteosarcoma in the cat is most true?**
    a. Osteosarcoma in the cat is an aggressive malignant neoplasm with poor survival times regardless of the treatment undertaken and as such is considered a more aggressive cancer than it is in dogs
    b. Osteosarcoma in the cat is an aggressive malignant neoplasm that frequently metastasizes despite amputation and adjunctive chemotherapy, leading to similar survival times to that reported in dogs
    c. Osteosarcoma in the cat is a potentially malignant tumour but post-amputation survival times are frequently considerably longer than those reported in the dog, so treatment should always be considered unless gross secondary disease is identified
    d. Appendicular limb osteosarcoma has not been reported in the cat

94. **The biggest problem causing poor survival times in cases of canine malignant oral melanoma is:**

a. The rapid recurrence of the primary tumour resulting in inappetance and cachexia
b. The very poor sensitivity of the tumour to radiotherapy
c. The high rate of metastatic disease that is seen with this tumour
d. The toxicity side effects seen with the chemotherapeutics available for treatment

95. **Which of the following pulmonary neoplastic diseases frequently responds well to chemotherapy?**
a. Primary bronchial carcinoma
b. Pulmonary lymphoma
c. Mesothelioma
d. Pulmonary lymphomatoid granulomatosis

96. **Intraplueral chemotherapy has been described as a useful and efficacious treatment for which of the following conditions?**
a. Primary bronchial carcinoma
b. Malignant pleural effusions
c. Thymic lymphoma
d. Unresectable lung tumours

97. **Which of the following colorectal tumour types would usually be associated with the longest survival times following surgical excision?**
a. Canine colonic gastrointestinal stromal tumour (GIST)
b. Canine colonic adenocarcinoma
c. Feline colonic adenocarcinoma
d. Feline colonic mast cell tumour

98. **Approximately what percentage of splenic masses in the dog have been found *not* to be malignant when assessed histopathologically?**
a. 25%
b. 45%

c. 65%
d. 85%

99. **Which hormone is primarily responsible for causing hypercalcaemia of malignancy in cases such as lymphoma or an anal sac adenocarcinoma?**
a. Parathyroid hormone (PTH)
b. Calcitonin
c. 1,25 dihydroxy vitamin D
d. Parathyroid hormone related peptide (PTHrP)

100. **A mass has been found by the owner on the right foreleg of a 6-year-old male Labrador dog. The mass measures approximately 2 cm in diameter, feels fixed to the deep tissues and is only a little movable. Fine needle aspirates of the mass are obtained. The sample was poorly cellular but a small number of cells with the appearance shown below were identified. What is the most likely diagnosis from the list below?**

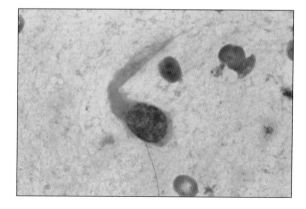

a. Mast cell tumour
b. Histiocytoma
c. Soft-tissue sarcoma
d. Cutaneous lymphoma

MCQs – Answers

1. A
2. D
3. C
4. C
5. D
6. B
7. C
8. D
9. D
10. B
11. A
12. B
13. C
14. C
15. D
16. B
17. A
18. C
19. A
20. A
21. D
22. B
23. A
24. B
25. A
26. C
27. D
28. D
29. B
30. A
31. D

32. D
33. A
34. C
35. C
36. C
37. B
38. C
39. A
40. B
41. C
42. D
43. A
44. D
45. A
46. B
47. C
48. C
49. A
50. C
51. D
52. B
53. B
54. C
55. D
56. A
57. D
58. C
59. A
60. B
61. A
62. C

63. C		82. A	
64. D		83. A	
65. C		84. B	
66. D		85. C	
67. A		86. B	
68. B		87. C	
69. A		88. C	
70. B		89. A	
71. D		90. C	
72. C		91. C	
73. A		92. B	
74. B		93. C	
75. D		94. C	
76. C		95. D	
77. B		96. B	
78. D		97. A	
79. B		98. B	
80. C		99. D	
81. C		100. C	

APPENDIX 1
World Health Organization clinical staging scheme for lymphoma in domestic animals

This classification system divides lymphoma firstly according to the anatomical location of the disease and then secondly by the extent of the disease, as shown below:

A Generalized
B Alimentary
C Thymic
D Skin
E True leukaemia
F Other sites

Stage I   Disease confined to a single node or to just a single organ (excluding the CNS and bone marrow)

Stage II   Disease affecting a regional group of lymph nodes, usually only on one side of the diaphragm

Stage III Generalized lymph node involvement

Stage IV   Disease affecting the liver and/or spleen with or without stage III disease

Stage V   Disease affecting the bone marrow and/or other organs not listed above

In addition to the I–V staging system, the stage can be subclassified as either 'a' or 'b', in which animals with no clinical signs of illness are subclassified as being in group 'a' and those animals who have systemic signs of illness are in sub-group 'b'.

2 APPENDIX
Chemotherapy protocols

MODIFIED MADISON-WISCONSIN CHEMOTHERAPY PROTOCOL

Week 1:	Vincristine 0.7 mg/m² i.v. L-asparaginase 400 iu/kg i.m. Prednisolone 2 mg/kg SID p.o.
Week 2:	Cyclophosphamide 250 mg/m² i.v. or p.o. Prednisolone 1.5 mg/kg SID p.o.
Week 3:	Vincristine 0.7 mg/m² i.v. Prednisolone 1.0 mg/kg SID p.o.
Week 4:	Doxorubicin 30 mg/m² i.v. Prednisolone 0.5 mg/kg SID p.o.
Week 5:	No treatment and wean off prednisolone
Week 6:	Vincristine 0.7 mg/m² i.v.
Week 7:	Cyclophosphamide 250 mg/m² i.v. or p.o.
Week 8:	Vincristine 0.7 mg/m² i.v.
Week 9:	Doxorubicin 30 mg/m² i.v.

For weeks 10–25, the above protocol is repeated (without the l-asparaginase or prednisolone) with a 14-day gap between each treatment. Total treatment time 25 weeks.

It has been reported that effective treatment can be achieved by just the first 9-week induction protocol, which is then used again should a relapse occur.

HIGH-DOSE COP PROTOCOL

Week 1:	Vincristine 0.7 mg/m² i.v. Cyclophosphamide 300 mg/m² Prednisolone 2 mg/kg SID
Week 2:	Vincristine 0.7 mg/m² i.v. Prednisolone 2mg/kg SID

Week 3:	Vincristine 0.7 mg/m² i.v. Prednisolone 1 mg/kg SID
Week 4:	Vincristine 0.7 mg/m² i.v. Cyclophosphamide 300 mg/m² Prednisolone 0.5 mg/kg EOD
Week 7:	Vincristine 0.7 mg/m² i.v. Cyclophosphamide 300 mg/m² Prednisolone 0.5 mg/kg EOD

This is continued for 6 months, after which time the treatment interval moves from 3 weeks to 4 weeks.

MOPP CHEMOTHERAPY PROTOCOL

- Mechlorethamine 3 mg/m² by i.v. injection on days 1 and 7
- Vincristine 0.7 mg/m² by i.v. injection on days 1 and 7
- Procarbazine 50 mg/m² by mouth once a day on days 1–14
- Prednisolone 30 mg/m² by mouth once a day on days 1–14
- No treatment is then given between days 15 and 28 and the protocol is repeated at week 4

D-MAC CHEMOTHERAPY PROTOCOL

Day 1:	Dexamethasone 1 mg/kg p.o., s.c. or i.v. Actinomycin D 0.75 mg/m² i.v. Cytosine arabinoside 300 mg/m² as a slow 4-hour intravenous infusion or s.c.
Day 8:	Dexamethasone 1 mg/kg p.o., s.c. or i.v. Melphalan 20 mg/m² p.o.

This cycle is then repeated continuously every 2 weeks until either a remission or stable disease is achieved. If there is evidence of bone marrow suppression, especially in the form of thrombocytopaenia, then chlorambucil can be used instead of the melphalan at a dose of 20 mg/m².

If the dog does achieve a complete remission, then it is recommended after 5–8 cycles to swap onto a maintenance 'LMP' protocol, which is:

- Chlorambucil 20 mg/m² p.o. once every other week
- Methotrexate 2.5–5.0 mg/m² p.o. twice a week
- Prednisolone 20 mg/m² every other day

VINBLASTINE AND PREDNISOLONE CHEMOTHERAPY FOR MAST CELL TUMOURS

Week 1:	Vinblastine 2 mg/m² i.v. Prednisolone 40 mg/m² once daily by mouth
Week 2:	Continue prednisolone 40 mg/m² once daily by mouth
Week 3:	Vinblastine 2 mg/m² i.v. Reduce prednisolone to 20 mg/m² once daily by mouth
Week 4:	Continue prednisolone at 20 mg/m² once daily by mouth
Week 5:	Vinblastine 2 mg/m² i.v. Reduce prednisolone to 20 mg/m² every other day
Week 6:	Continue prednisolone at 20 mg/m² every other day
Week 7:	Vinblastine 2 mg/m² i.v. Continue prednislone at 20 mg/m² every other day
Week 8:	Continue prednisolone at 20 mg/m² every other day
Week 9:	Vinblastine 2 mg/m² i.v. Wean off prednisolone altogether
Week 11:	Vinblastine 2 mg/m² i.v.
Week 13:	Vinblastine 2 mg/m² i.v.
Week 15:	Vinblastine 2 mg/m² i.v.

An alternative approach is to give the vinblastine at weekly intervals for the first four injections.

CHLORAMBUCIL AND PREDNISOLONE CHEMOTHERAPY FOR MAST CELL TUMOURS

Week 1 & 2:	Chlorambucil 4–5 mg/m² every other day by mouth Prednisolone 40 mg/m² once daily by mouth
Week 3 & 4:	Chlorambucil 4–5 mg/m² every other day by mouth Prednisolone 20 mg/m² once daily by mouth
Week 5 onwards:	Chlorambucil 4–5 mg/m² every other day by mouth Prednisolone 20 mg/m² every other day by mouth

Treat for 6 months and then wean off the prednisolone and stop the chlorambucil.

DOXORUBICIN AND CARBOPLATIN CHEMOTHERAPY FOR OSTEOSARCOMA

Week 1:	Carboplatin 300 mg/m² by intravenous infusion over 20 minutes
Week 4:	Doxorubicin 30 mg/m² by intravenous infusion over 20 minutes
Week 7:	Carboplatin 300 mg/m² by intravenous infusion over 20 minutes
Week 10:	Doxorubicin 30 mg/m² by intravenous infusion over 20 minutes
Week 13:	Carboplatin 300 mg/m² by intravenous infusion over 20 minutes
Week 16:	Doxorubicin 30 mg/m² by intravenous infusion over 20 minutes

The authors recommend chlorpheniramine is administered intravenously prior to any administration of doxorubicin to reduce the possible risk of acute anaphylaxis caused by mast cell degranulation.

CYCLOPHOSPHAMIDE AND PIROXICAM CHEMOTHERAPY FOR INCOMPLETELY EXCISED SOFT-TISSUE SARCOMAS

- Cyclophosphamide 10 mg/m² given either once a day or once every other day by mouth
- Piroxicam 0.3 mg/kg given once a day by mouth

Continue treatment for at least 6 months, aiming for the treatment to be continuous for the duration of the remission achieved.

5-FLUOROURACIL AND CYCLOPHOSPHAMIDE CHEMOTHERAPY FOR MAMMARY CARCINOMA

Week 1:	5-Fluorouracil 150 mg/m^2 Cyclophosphamide 100 mg/m^2 Given one after the other by intravenous injection
Week 2:	5-Fluorouracil 150 mg/m^2 Cyclophosphamide 100 mg/m^2 Given one after the other by intravenous injection
Week 3:	5-Fluorouracil 150 mg/m^2 Cyclophosphamide 100 mg/m^2 Given one after the other by intravenous injection
Week 4:	5-Fluorouracil 150 mg/m^2 Cyclophosphamide 100 mg/m^2 Given one after the other by intravenous injection

This protocol should be commenced 1 week after the surgery to remove the primary tumour.

MITOXANTRONE AND PIROXICAM CHEMOTHERAPY FOR TRANSITIONAL CELL CARCINOMAS OF THE URINARY BLADDER

Week 1:	Mitoxantrone 5 mg/m^2 by intravenous infusion over 20 minutes Start piroxicam at 0.3 mg/kg once a day by mouth
Week 4:	Mitoxantrone 5 mg/m^2 by intravenous infusion over 20 minutes Continue piroxicam at 0.3 mg/kg once a day by mouth
Week 7:	Mitoxantrone 5 mg/m^2 by intravenous infusion over 20 minutes Continue piroxicam at 0.3 mg/kg once a day by mouth
Week 10:	Mitoxantrone 5 mg/m^2 by intravenous infusion over 20 minutes Continue piroxicam at 0.3 mg/kg once a day by mouth
Week 13:	Mitoxantrone 5 mg/m^2 by intravenous infusion over 20 minutes Continue piroxicam at 0.3 mg/kg once a day by mouth for as long as the dog remains in remission

3 APPENDIX
Protocol for a water deprivation test

1. Fast the patient for 12 hours and then place an intravenous catheter
2. Completely empty the urinary bladder (ideally by means of an indwelling catheter), measure the specific gravity (USG) of the urine and weigh the patient
   a. If the facilities are available to measure osmolality, then urine osmolality and plasma osmolality should be measured now and at all points in the remainder of the protocol where USG measurement is referred to
3. Calculate what 5% of the patient's pre-test weight would be
4. Completely withdraw water availability from the patient
5. Empty the urinary bladder every 1–2 hours, measure the USG and then weigh the patient after the bladder has been emptied
6. Continue the test until either:
   a. The USG measurement rises to within the normal range
   If the USG rises to 1.015 or greater, then a diagnosis of diabetes insipidus is highly unlikely
   b. The patient loses 5% of their bodyweight
7. If a 5% bodyweight loss is realized with little or no elevation in the USG, then the patient has diabetes insipidus (DI). To differentiate between central and nephrogenic diabetes insipidus, the injectable form of the vasopressin analogue, DDAVP is administered by intramuscular injection. In cases of nephrogenic DI, there will be little or no response to this treatment and the USG will remain extremely low and the patient is at great risk of losing more body weight and becoming severely dehydrated. In most cases of central diabetes insipidus, however, the USG/urine osmolality should rise significantly within 2–4 hours of the DDAVP injection

4 APPENDIX
Daily calorie calculations for dogs and cats

In a normal animal, there are energy stores within the body in three main forms:

- Hepatic glycogen
- Triglycerides within adipocytes
- Amino acids.

If an animal begins to starve then the hepatic glycogen is used first, the triglycerides second and then the proteins used thirdly and the metabolism is reduced to preserve energy. In a sick animal, instead of conservation of energy, an accelerated form of catabolism develops in which there is:

- Early use of the hepatic glycogen
- A higher requirement for amino acids
- It becomes impossible for fat breakdown to meet energy needs, so the protein demand increases. This causes an elevation in the concentrations of stress hormones such as cortisol and catecholamines, which result in an increased metabolic rate.

Sick animals therefore need special attention to their diet and this is especially the case for cancer patients. All hospitalized patients should have their daily calorie requirements calculated and this can be done as follows:

- Dog
  - [(30 × body weight in kg) + 70] × illness factor

The illness factor varies between 1.2 and 1.7, but for most hospitalized patients, the illness factor can be taken as being a factor of 1.4

- Cat
  - 50 × body weight in kg

These calculations give the number of kilocalories a patient requires a day and from this, as all reputable food manufacturers publish the calorie content per gram of their foods, a very accurate feeding plan can be established.

For human cancer patients there is much spoken and published regarding the potential health benefits of different food types. In veterinary nutrition, it also makes sense for foods fed to cancer patients to be of the highest quality and biological value. However, there are few good veterinary scientific publications to show the health benefits of one particular diet type against another, or comparing home cooked food, or raw diets with commercially available diets. Studies have certainly supported a beneficial effect of omega-3 fatty acid supplementation in canine lymphoma patients. Furthermore, there is evidence to show that feeding a canine lymphoma patient a high fat, high protein, low carbohydrate diet can increase the chances of a patient going into remission and also help to increase the length of that remission. This is thought to be because lymphoma cells preferentially utilize glucose and then produce lactate which is re-cycled, meaning that the surrounding healthy cells actually expend ATP in order to metabolize the lactate which is then potentially re-used by the lymphoma cells, leading ultimately to cancer cachexia. Feeding a high fat diet may help to reduce the metabolic rate of the cancer cells by 'starving' the cancer cells of their prime energy substrate. Ensuring that veterinary cancer patients eat properly whilst hospitalized is one of the most important jobs of the attending veterinary nurse/animal technician and this can help significantly in both the degree of response and length of response that a patient may have to his or her treatment.

5 APPENDIX
Protocol for performing a prostatic wash

Under acepromazine and butorphanol sedation or a brief general anaesthetic, a lubricated, sterile dog urinary catheter should be placed into the urethra and advanced slowly in a retrograde fashion. The clinician then performs a digital rectal examination and feels for the catheter advancing underneath his fingertip, placed over the mid-line of the prostate (i.e. along the line of the urethra). When the tip of the catheter is at the tip of his/her finger, the advancement is stopped. 10 ml of saline is introduced into the catheter and the tip of the catheter pushed a little ventrally. The prostate is massaged before the saline is withdrawn back into a syringe and the sample submitted for cytology.

6 APPENDIX
Suppliers list

CHEMOTHERAPY

Hospira, Queensway, Leamington Spa, Warwickshire, CV31 3RW

Unidrug Distribution Group, Amber Park, Berristow Lane, South Normanton, Derbyshire, DE55 2FH

FLOW CYTOMETRY

Central Diagnostic Services, The Queen's Veterinary School Hospital, The University of Cambridge, Madingley Road, Cambridge, CB3 OE5
Tel: 01223 337625

SURGICAL STAPLING DEVICES

Direct Medical Services, Suite 19, Newal's Corner, 2 Bath Road, Hounslow, Middlesex, TW3 3HJ

Index